Animal Models of Retrovirus Infection and Their Relationship to AIDS

Academic Press Rapid Manuscript Reproduction

Animal Models of Retrovirus Infection and Their Relationship to AIDS

Edited by

Lois Ann Salzman

Office of the Scientific Director
National Institute of Allergy and Infectious Diseases
National Institutes of Health
Bethesda, Maryland

1986

ACADEMIC PRESS, INC.

Harcourt Brace Jovanovich, Publishers

Orlando   San Diego   New York   Austin
London   Montreal   Sydney   Tokyo   Toronto

ACADEMIC PRESS, INC.
Orlando, Florida 32887

United Kingdom Edition published by
ACADEMIC PRESS INC. (LONDON) LTD.
24–28 Oval Road, London NW1 7DX

Library of Congress Cataloging in Publication Data

Animal models of retrovirus infection and their
   relationship to AIDS.

   Includes bibliographies and index.
   1. AIDS (Disease)—Animal models.   2. Retroviruses.
3. Virus diseases—Animal models.   I. Salzman, Lois
Ann.   [DNLM: 1. Acquired Immunodeficiency Syndrome.
2. Disease Models, Animal.   3. Retrovirus Infections—
veterinary.   WD 308 A598]
RC607.A26A5   1986   616.97'92   86-70473
ISBN 0–12–617330–3 (alk. paper)

PRINTED IN THE UNITED STATES OF AMERICA

86 87 88 89   9 8 7 6 5 4 3 2 1

Contents

Introduction

Virology of Retrovirus Model Systems

Pathogenesis of Retrovirus Infection

Host Immunity and Retrovirus Disease

Vaccines and Immunotherapy

Human AIDS in the Chimpanzee

Contributors

Numbers in parentheses indicate the pages on which the authors' contributions begin.

Harvey J. Alter (443), Department of Transfusion Medicine, Clinical Center, National Institutes of Health, Bethesda, Maryland 20892.

David M. Asher (457), Laboratory of Central Nervous System Studies, National Institute of Neurological and Communicative Disorders and Stroke, National Institutes of Health, Bethesda, Maryland 20892

I. M. Bause (301), Department of Pathobiological Sciences, School of Veterinary Medicine, University of Wisconsin, Madison, Wisconsin 53706

P. Bentvelzen (233), Radiobiological Institute TNO, Rijswijk, The Netherlands

Raoul E. Benveniste (335), Laboratory of Viral Carcinogenesis, National Cancer Institute, Frederick Cancer Research Facility, Frederick, Maryland 21701

David Boettiger (17), Department of Microbiology, University of Pennsylvania, Philadelphia, Pennsylvania 19104

C. Bruck (107), Department of Molecular Biology, University of Brussels, Brussels, Belgium

Delia Budzko (325), National Institute of Neurological and Communicative Disorders and Stroke, National Institutes of Health, Bethesda, Maryland 20892

A. Burny (107), Department of Molecular Biology, University of Brussels, Brussels, Belgium

B. A. Buxton (301), School of Veterinary Medicine, Auburn, Alabama 36849

Bruce Chesebro (279), Laboratory of Persistent Viral Diseases, Rocky Mountain Laboratories, National Institute of Allergy and Infectious Diseases, National Institutes of Health, Hamilton, Montana 59840

Y. Cleuter (107), Department of Molecular Biology, University of Brussels, Brussels, Belgium

Leroy Coggins (203), North Carolina State University, School of Veterinary Medicine, Raleigh, North Carolina 27605

Susan M. Cotter (403), Department of Veterinary Medicine, Tufts University School of Veterinary Medicine, Boston, Massachusetts 02155

D. Couez (107), Department of Molecular Biology, University of Brussels, Brussels, Belgium

Ronald Desrosiers (145), New England Regional Primate Research Center, Southborough, Massachusetts 01772

Gordon R. Dressman (443), Virology and Immunology Department, Southwest Foundation for Biomedical Research, San Antonio, Texas 78284

Jorg W. Eichberg (443), Virology and Immunology Department, Southwest Foundation for Biomedical Research, San Antonio, Texas 78284

Leon G. Epstein (457), Laboratory of Central Nervous System Studies, National Institute of Neurological and Communicative Disorders and Stroke, National Institutes of Health, Bethesda, Maryland 20892

Nancy R. Ernst (403), Immune Response Program, Pacific Northwest Research Foundation, Seattle, Washington 98104

M. E. Essex (223), Department of Cancer Biology, Harvard School of Public Health, Boston, Massachusetts 02115

L. D. Foil (95), Department of Entomology, Louisiana State University, Baton Rouge, Louisana 70803

Donald Francis (161), Center for Infectious Diseases, Centers for Disease Control, Atlanta, Georgia 30333

Torgny N. Fredrickson (193), Laboratory of Immunopathology, National Institute of Allergy and Infectious Diseases, National Institutes of Health, Bethesda, Maryland 20892

D. Carleton Gajdusek (457), Laboratory of Central Nervous System Studies, National Institute of Neurological and Communicative Disorders and Stroke, National Institutes of Health, Bethesda, Maryland 20892

Murray Gardner (325, 431), Department of Pathology, School of Medicine, University of California, Davis, California 95616

Peter W. Gasper (59), Department of Pathology, Colorado State University, Fort Collins, Colorado 80523

Clarence J. Gibbs, Jr. (457), Laboratory of Central Nervous System Studies, National Institute of Neurological and Communicative Disorders and Stroke, National Institutes of Health, Bethesda, Maryland 20892

W. Ellis Giddens, Jr. (335), Division of Animal Medicine and Department of Pathology, School of Medicine, University of Washington, Seattle, Washington 98195

Jaap Goudsmit (457), Laboratory of Central Nervous System Studies, National Institute of Neurological and Communicative Disorders and Stroke, National Institutes of Health, Bethesda, Maryland 20892

Chris K. Grant (403), Immune Response Program, Pacific Northwest Research Foundation, Seattle, Washington 98104

Maneth Gravell (325), National Institute of Neurological and Communicative Disorders and Stroke, National Institutes of Health, Bethesda, Maryland 20892

D. Gregoire (107), Department of Molecular Biology, University of Brussels, Brussels, Belgium

Ashley T. Haase (121), Department of Microbiology, University of Minnesota, Minneapolis, Minnesota 55455

William D. Hardy, Jr. (75), Laboratory of Veterinary Onocology, Memorial Sloan-Kettering Cancer Center, New York, New York 10021

Janet W. Hartley (41, 193), Laboratory of Immunopathology, National Institute of Allergy and Infectious Diseases, National Institutes of Health, Bethesda, Maryland 20892

Roy V. Henrickson (325), California Regional Primate Center, Davis, California 95616

Edward A. Hoover (59), Department of Pathology, Colorado State University, Fort Collins, Colorado 80523

R. D. Hunt (223), New England Regional Primate Research Center, Southborough, Massachusetts 01772

James N. Ihle (369), National Cancer Institute, Frederick Cancer Research Facility, Frederick, Maryland 21701

C. J. Issel (95), Department of Veterinary Science, Louisiana State University, Baton Rouge, Louisiana 70803

Frank R. Jones (403), Immune Response Program, Pacific Northwest Research Foundation, Seattle, Washington 98104

P. J. Kanki (223), Department of Cancer Biology, Harvard School of Public Health, Boston, Massachusetts 02115

Ronald C. Kennedy (443), Virology and Immunology Department, Southwest Foundation for Biomedical Research, San Antonio, Texas 78284

R. Kettmann (107), Department of Molecular Biology, University of Brussels, Brussels, Belgium

David A. Lawlor (443), Virology and Immunology Department, Southwest Foundation for Biomedical Research, San Antonio, Texas 78284

William T. London (325), National Institute of Neurological and Communicative Disorders and Stroke, National Institutes of Health, Bethesda, Maryland 20892

L. J. Lowenstine (233), California Primate Research Center, Davis, California 95616

David L. Madden (325), National Institute of Neurological and Communicative Disorders and Stroke, National Institutes of Health, Bethesda, Maryland 20892

M. Mammerickx (107), Faculty of Agronomy, Gembloux, Brussels, Belgium

T. O. Manning (301), James A. Baker Institute for Animal Health, Cornell University, Ithaca, New York 14853

G. Marbaix (107), Department of Molecular Biology, University of Brussels, Brussels, Belgium

Preston A. Marx (131, 325), California Primate Research Center, University of California Davis, Davis, California 95616

Donald Maul (325), California Regional Primate Center, Davis, California 95616

Travis C. McGuire (295), Department of Veterinary Microbiology and Pathology, Washington State University, Pullman, Washington 99164

B. D. Miles (169), Worcester Foundation for Experimental Biology, Shrewsbury, Massachusetts 01545

Janice Miller (421), National Animal Disease Center, Ames, Iowa 50010

Luc Montagnier (265), Viral Oncology Unit, Institut Pasteur, Paris, France

R. C. Montelaro (95), Department of Biochemistry, Louisiana State University, Baton Rouge, Louisiana 70803

Richard P. Morrison (279), Laboratory of Persistent Viral Diseases, Rocky Mountain Laboratories, National Institute of Allergy and Infectious Diseases, National Institutes of Health, Hamilton, Montana 59840

Herbert C. Morse III (41, 193, 285), Laboratory of Immunopathology, National Institutes of Allergy and Infectious Diseases, National Institutes of Health, Bethesda, Maryland 20892

William R. Morton (335), Regional Primate Research Center, University of Washington, Seattle, Washington 98195

Donald E. Mosier (285), Institute for Cancer Research, Philadelphia, Pennsylvania 19111

James I. Mullins (59), Department of Cancer Biology, Harvard School of Public Health, Boston, Massachusetts 02115

Opendra Narayan (355), Departments of Neurology and Comparative Medicine, Johns Hopkins University School of Medicine, Baltimore, Maryland 21205

Jane Nishio (279), Laboratory of Persistent Viral Diseases, Rocky Mountain Laboratories, National Institute of Allergy and Infectious Diseases, National Institutes of Health, Hamilton, Montana 59840

Richard Olsen (393), The Ohio State University, Department of Veterinary Pathobiology, Columbus, Ohio 43210

V. S. Panangala (301), School of Veterinary Medicine, Auburn, Alabama 36849

D. Portetelle (107), Department of Molecular Biology, University of Brussels, Brussels, Belgium

Sandra L. Quackenbush (59), Department of Pathology, Colorado State University, Fort Collins, Colorado 80523

J. C. Rhyan (301), School of Veterinary Medicine, Auburn, Alabama 36849

H. L. Robinson (169), Worcester Foundation for Experimental Biology, Shrewsbury, Massachusetts 01545

Lois Ann Salzman (3), Office of the Scientific Director, National Institute of Allergy and Infectious Diseases, National Institutes of Health, Bethesda, Maryland 20892

W. Carl Saxinger (443), Laboratory of Tumor Cell Biology, National Cancer Institute, National Institutes of Health, Bethesda, Maryland 20892

R. D. Schultz (301), James A. Baker Institute for Animal Health, Cornell University, Ithaca, New York 14853

Kenneth W. Sell[1] (3), Office of the Scientific Director, National Institute of Allergy and Infectious Diseases, National Institutes of Health, Bethesda, Maryland 20892

---

[1]Present address: Emory University School of Medicine, Department of Pathology, Atlanta, Georgia 30322.

John Sever (155, 325), National Institute of Neurological and Communicative Disorders and Stroke, National Institutes of Health, Bethesda, Maryland 20892
William M. Shannon (241), Kettering-Meyer Laboratory, Southern Research Institute, Birmingham, Alabama 35255
David T. Shen (387), Veterinary Micropathology, Washington State University, Pullman, Washington 99163
Mitra C. Singhal (403), Immune Response Program, Pacific Northwest Research Foundation, Seattle, Washington 98104
Harry W. Snyder, Jr. (403), Immune Response Program, Pacific Northwest Research Foundation, Seattle, Washington 98104
Kurt Stromberg (335), Laboratory of Viral Carcinogenesis, National Cancer Institute, Frederick Cancer Research Facility, Frederick, Maryland 21701
S. E. Tracy (169), Worcester Foundation for Experimental Biology, Shrewsbury, Massachusetts 01545
Che-Chung Tsai (335), Regional Primate Research Center, University of Washington, Seattle, Washington 98195
Martin J. Van Der Maaten (213), National Animal Disease Center, U.S. Department of Agriculture, Ames, Iowa 50010
A. A. van Es (233), Primate Center TNO, Rijswijk, The Netherlands
W. van Vreeswijk (233), Primate Center TNO, Rijswijk, The Netherlands
L. Willems (107), Department of Molecular Biology, University of Brussels, Brussels, Belgium
W. C. Yang (301), Department of Pathobiological Sciences, School of Veterinary Medicine, University of Wisconsin, Madison, Wisconsin 53706
Robert A. Yetter (193, 285), Laboratory of Immunopathology, National Institutes of Allergy and Infectious Diseases, National Institutes of Health, Bethesda, Maryland 20892
Lois H. Yoshida (403), Immune Response Program, Pacific Northwest Research Foundation, Seattle, Washington 98104

Preface

The acquired immune deficiency syndrome (AIDS) has reached epidemic proportions since it was first recognized in 1981. The number of patients diagnosed as suffering from AIDS doubles every 15 months. It is a fatal syndrome that may become apparent months to years after infection with the underlying causative retrovirus, HTLV-III/LAV (human T cell lymphotropic virus type III/lymphadenopathy-associated virus), and leaves its victims to die from opportunistic diseases, months to years after diagnosis. No patient diagnosed as having AIDS has regained his lost immunity.

In an attempt to understand, control, treat, and prevent this human syndrome, we have compiled this book comparing AIDS to related retrovirus diseases in selected animals. The chapters are a comprehensive source of up-to-date information written by scientists who have made major contributions in their fields. The book is divided into five sections: Virology of Retrovirus Model Systems, Pathogenesis of Retrovirus Infection, Host Immunity and Retrovirus Disease, Vaccines and Immunotherapy, and Human AIDS in the Chimpanzee. The animal model systems reviewed include the feline, simian, sheep, murine, equine, and bovine systems. The authors compare the similarities and differences between the human and animal retroviruses, the opportunistic diseases related to virus infection, and their treatment. The problems associated with development of a vaccine for AIDS are also discussed, using as a model the only marketed retrovirus vaccine, one developed for feline leukemia virus in cats.

Much progress has been made in understanding the syndrome known as AIDS. Use of the knowledge that we have gained and will gain from related animal retrovirus infections can make this progress even more rapid.

Lois Ann Salzman

Acknowledgments

The preparation of *Animal Models of Retrovirus Infection and Their Relationship to AIDS* required the work of a number of people. I wish to acknowledge specifically the editorial assistance of Ms. Betty J. Sylvester, whose good judgment and advice were essential to the book, and to Dr. Ruth Guyer, who coordinated the initial preparation of the manuscript. The volume would not have been possible without the efforts of Dr. Kenneth W. Sell, who initiated and sponsored the meeting that was the basis for the contents of the book, as well as Dr. Gordon Wallace, who was Acting Scientific Director of the National Institute of Allergy and Infectious Diseases (NIAID), and Dr. Anthony S. Fauci, who was Director of NIAID during the preparation of this manuscript and supported its publication.

Lois Ann Salzman

INTRODUCTION

THE ACQUIRED IMMUNE DEFICIENCY SYNDROME
PAST, PRESENT AND FUTURE

Lois Ann Salzman[1]
Kenneth W. Sell[2]

Office of the Scientific Director
National Institute of Allergy
and Infectious Diseases
Bethesda, Maryland

The acquired immune deficiency syndrome (AIDS) first reported about 5 years ago remains as one of the most devastating and challenging human acquired diseases. It is also one of the diseases best known to the entire general public. Taxicab drivers will tell you most of the details of the disease, who gets it, how it is transmitted, that it is caused by a virus, the rapid advances in understanding it and that there is a recent test to detect it. AIDS has become a prime focus of study, classified by the Public Health Service as the number one infectious disease target because it is a disease of enormous, increasing proportions. It has threatened our blood and blood product supply, although that threat is now under increasing control with the use of commercial detection kits. It affects homosexual and and bisexual males, female contacts, hemophiliacs, intravenous drug users and pediatric cases usually born of infected parents.

---

[1]Present address: National Institute of Dental Research, National Institutes of Health, Bethesda, Maryland.
[2]Present address: Emory University School of Medicine, Department of Pathology, Atlanta, Georgia.

ANIMAL MODELS OF RETROVIRUS INFECTION
AND THEIR RELATIONSHIP TO AIDS

3

The original surveillance definition of AIDS by the Communicable Disease Centers was the occurrence of a disease predictive of a defect in cell-mediated immunity and occurring in a person with no known cause for diminished resistance to that disease (1). These diseases include opportunistic infections causing fatal illnesses from pneumonia to cancer and caused often by unusual human pathogens including protozoa, fungi, mycobacteria and severe virus infections of long duration (2,3). AIDS as described here is the end stage of the disease.

In order to improve diagnostic specificity for a less severe disease state, the term AIDS-related complex (ARC) is used. The diagnosis of ARC requires the presence of two clinical conditions such as fever greater than 100°F for at least 3 months, weight loss, lymphadenopathy for at least 3 months, diarrhea, fatigue or night sweats as well as two laboratory abnormalities such as decreased helper T cell number, altered helper T cell-suppressor T cell ratio, anergy to skin tests, elevated serum globulins, leukothrombocytopenia anemia or depressed blastogenesis. The designation ARC does not necessarily imply that the patient will progress to AIDS.

As released by the Centers for Disease Control (CDC), on August 5, 1985, there were 12,256 reported cases of AIDS in the United States. Of the 12,107 adult patients, 21% were in the 20 to 39 year age group, 47% were in the 30 to 39 year age group and 21% were 40 to 49 years of age at the time of diagnosis. As seen in Table I, 149 (1%) of the cases were in children under 13 years of age where epidemiological data suggests transmission from infected mother to child before, at or shortly after the time of birth. The CDC report given in Table I uses a hierarchical classification system for patient assignment with cases belonging to multiple risk groups being tabulated arbitrarily to the group that appears first on the list. Thus the cases of intravenous drug users excludes those who are also homosexual or bisexual and so forth. The groups at risk have remained stable since AIDS was

TABLE I.   Cases of U.S. AIDS Listed by Risk Group,
Age Group and Sex Reported to the CDC
as of August 5, 1985

Patient group	Male		Female		Total	
	No.	%	No.	%	No.	%
Adult and Adolescent AIDS						
Homosexual or bisexual men	8861	78	–	–	8861	73
Intravenous (IV) drug users	1661	15	421	53	2082	17
Hemophilia/coagulation disorder	71	1	4	1	75	1
Heterosexual contact	14	0	106	13	120	1
Blood transfusion/blood product recipient	107	1	77	10	184	2
None of the above/other	598	5	187	24	785	6
Total	11312	100	795	100	12107	100
Pediatric AIDS (under 13 years of age at diagnosis)						
Hemophilia/coagulation disorder	8	9	–	–	8	5
Parent with AIDS or at increased risk for AIDS	53	60	51	84	104	70
Blood transfusion/blood product recipient	18	20	5	8	23	15
None of the above/other	9	10	5	8	14	9
Total	88	100	61	100	149	100

recognized. Homosexual or bisexual males comprise 78% of the
total cases of AIDS, nonhomosexual IV drug users account for 15%
of male and 53% of female AIDS patients. Patients with hemophilia
and coagulation disorders and AIDS are 1 to 2% of the total number. Thirteen percent of women with AIDS have had heterosexual
contact with a person with AIDS or at risk of AIDS. Five percent
of males and 24% of female patients with AIDS have had transfusions with blood or blood products containing the AIDS virus
HTLV-III/LAV (human T cell lymphotropic virus type III/lymph-
adenopathy-associated virus). The "None of the Above" catagory
includes 334 persons born in countries in which most AIDS cases
have not been associated with known risk factors.

Table II reminds us of the increase in the case rate and the
case-fatality ratio since 1979. The rapid increase in cases during 1981 to 1983 has been followed in 1984 and 1985 by a less
steep increase although the lag time between diagnosis and the
report of cases to CDC may account for some of the decrease. The
doubling time for new cases may be up from 6 months to 13 months;
however, a more accurate estimate would include the increase for
the individual at risk groups of patients and their location in
the United States. As noted in the case-fatality ratio column,
50% of the diagnosed cases have died. Unless there is some break-
through in treatment of AIDS and the associated fatal opportunistic infections, 50% of AIDS patients can be expected to die
within 18 months of diagnosis and some 80% will die within 36
months of diagnosis. As of August 5, 1985, 57% of the AIDS
patients died from Pneumocystis carinii pneumonia (PCP), a pro-
tozoan pneumonia, 20% with Kaposi's sarcoma (KS), a cancer, 6%
with both PCP and KS and the remaining 17% with other opportunistic infections.

Thirty-nine states have reported nine or more cases of AIDS.
The largest number of cases are in five states: New York, 36%;
California, 23%; Florida, 7%; New Jersey, 6% and Texas, 5%.
Together they account for 77% of the total number of cases

TABLE II. Number of Reported Cases of AIDS
and Case-Fatality Ratio[a]

Year	No. of cases	No. of known deaths	Case-Fatality ratio %
1979	12	9	75
1980	47	42	89
1981	260	218	84
1982	989	728	74
1983	2692	1866	69
1984	5132	2529	49
1985[b]	3124	775	25
Totals[c]	12256	6167	50

[a]Data supplied by the Centers for Disease Control.

[b]As of August 5, 1985.

[c]Includes eight cases diagnosed prior to 1979. Of these
eight cases, four are known to have died.

reported. Within these states the largest proportion of AIDS
cases are in five cities. As seen in Table III, the largest number of cases are reported in New York city followed by San Francisco, Los Angeles, Miami and Newark. Men in New York city and
San Francisco clearly have higher incidence rates (number of
cases/million population) than those in other areas of the
United States.

As shown in the information given above, AIDS is recognized
as a severe public health problem. It has been addressed with an
enormous infusion of interest and concern on the part of scientists and a spontaneous development of funding for support of
research. In fiscal year 1982, which started in October of 1981,
there was a total in the Public Health Service of about 5.5

TABLE III.   Comparison of the Incidence Rate
in the U.S. Cities with the Most Cases of AIDS

City	No. of cases	Percent of total	Cases per million population[a]
New York, NY	4045	33	443.5
San Francisco, CA	1383	11	425.5
Miami, FL	425	3	261.4
Newark, NJ	310	3	157.7
Los Angeles, CA	1045	9	139.8
Elsewhere	5048	41	24.7
Total	12256	100	53.8

[a]Based on the 1980 census by standard Metropolitan statistical area of residence from June 1, 1981, to August 5, 1985.

million dollars distributed as shown in Table IV. The largest
amount of money came from the CDC, which was responsible for
first identifying and making the scientific community aware of
this disease, and the National Cancer Institute (NCI). By fiscal
year 1983, money was appropriated for AIDS research and increased
to 28 million dollars. In 1984 $61,460,000 was spent of directly
identifiable funds not including indirect funds spent in related
fields. In 1985, it is estimated that over 108 million dollars
will be spent and in 1986 $126,000,000 is obligated to AIDS
research. What has this money been spent for? What have we
learned about AIDS since 1981? This is a short period of time
in the field of medical research.

The National Heart, Lung and Blood Institute has been very
interested in a diagnostic test to remove the threat of AIDS
virus transmission through transfusion and blood products. Within
the last 6 months, a screening test called ELISA (for enzyme-

linked immunosorbent assay) has been made widely available by
three commercial companies. The test detects antibodies to the
virus believed to cause AIDS in the blood of exposed persons. It
identifies those at risk for the disease and prevents this contaminated blood from being used for transfusions and the blood
coagulation products needed principally by hemophiliacs. Improve-
ments on this initial test and other tests with greater specificity for both the AIDS virus and the antibodies synthesized to
the virus are being investigated.

Much of the initial funds were spent looking for the etiological (causative) agent of AIDS. We are indebted to the
researchers in the Pasteur Institute in France (4) and the NCI
in the United States (5,6) who described the retroviruses LAV
and HTLV-III and provided the evidence relating these viruses
to the disease AIDS. Since these two retroviruses are so closely
related (7), we will designate them here as one virus, HTLV-III/
LAV. The CDC, the National Institute of Allergy and Infectious
Diseases (NIAID) and the NCI have conducted epidemiological
studies to understand the natural history of the disease, how it
spreads, how it develops and what a positive test for HTLV-III/
LAV antibody in the blood means.

Many research scientists, including those in NIAID and NCI,
have struggled to define the mechanism used by retrovirus HTLV-
III/LAV, to produce its profound effect. The virus has a selective affinity for the helper/inducer subset of T lymphocytes
defined by the T4 or Leu3 cell surface marker. Destruction or
latent infection of these T4 cells has a profound effect since
they play a role in the induction and orchestration of the entire
immune system (8). AIDS also induces a hyperactivity of the B
lymphocytes (antibody producers) and reduces their ability to
respond to new stimulation. There is much more to learn in trying
to understand this disease. Some researchers feel that in order
for AIDS to occur, HTLV-III/LAV may need a co-factor to permit
it to be active. Two herpes viruses--cytomegalovirus, which has

TABLE IV. AIDS Obligations (in Thousands of Dollars)[a]

	1982 Actual	1983 Actual	1984 Actual	1985 Estimate	1986 Estimate
Public Health Service:					
National Institutes of Health:					
National Cancer Institute	2,400	9,790	16,627	26,951	28,441
National Heath, Lung, and Blood Institute	5	1,202	4,871	10,153	11,200
National Institute of Dental Research	25	25	81	54	684
National Institute of Neurological and Communicative Disorders and Stroke	31	684	1,510	1,150	1,500
National Institute of Allergy and Infectious Diseases	297	9,223	19,616	23,262	27,067
National Eye Institute	33	45	60	200	100
Division of Research Resources	564	699	1,356	1,731	1,731
Total, NIH	3,355	21,668	44,121	63,501	70,723

(continued)

TABLE IV (continued)

	1982 Actual	1983 Actual	1984 Actual	1985 Estimate	1986 Estimate
Food and Drug Administration	150	350	798	9,005	6,630
Centers for Disease Control	2,050	6,202	13,750	33,231	45,645
Alcohol, Drug Abuse, and Mental Health Administration	—	516	2,791	3,242	3,459
Total, PHS	5,555	28,736	61,460	108,979	126,457

[a] Money obligated supplied by the National Institutes of Health, Division of Financial Management, Budget Formulation and Presentation Branch as of August 13, 1985.

11

a high incidence among male homosexuals, and the Epstein-Barr
virus--are being studied in this regard. The co-factor could
also be some other susceptibility factor that relates to the
infection and results in some populations being more at risk
than others. Multiple infections, antigen overload and the allo-
genic effects of sperm may also affect the disease progress.

Treatment of this devastating disease is being intensively
studied in many places, including NCI and NIAID. Antiviral agents
being tested at the NIH or at AIDS clinics nationwide include
alpha-interferon, suramin, ribavirin and a Swedish drug called
forcarnet. These antiviral drugs act on different stages of virus
replication. Once the virus is contained, different experimental
therapies can be used designed to restore the damaged immune system, including interleukin-2, manufactured in the bone marrow,
and bone marrow transplantation. Other agents used to control the
opportunistic infections include DHTG used in cytomegalovirus
infections. Researchers are also working on a vaccine which may
still be several years away. In spite of all our efforts, however, AIDS is still a terminal illness.

Traditionally, many of our questions about the stages in
viral diseases, its treatment and protection offered by vaccination have been answered by the use of animal models. Animals
with their own specific, closely related retrovirus diseases and
those infected with the human virus HTLV-III/LAV would be of tre-
mendous help in the understanding and treatment of AIDS. They can
also tell us about the role and treatment of opportunistic infections since that is what the AIDS patients die from. Information
about vaccines and which viral protein would be the best to use
in vaccine studies can be gained from animal studies.

We have tried to cover some of the knowledge that we have
gained about AIDS, the research data, the problems and the gaps
in our knowledge. We feel that the retrovirus diseases that
occur in animals may well provide some of the most important
clues as to what is going on in the human AIDS patients. Many of

the things that represent problems in humans can, in one form or another, be seen in animal retrovirus infections. The only effective retrovirus vaccine has been developed for cats for protection against the feline leukemia virus. This vaccine will be discussed in another chapter in this book.

We hope that two things happen as a result of the discussions in this book. We hope that the development of the AIDS problem stimulates our support of, and interest in, working on the animal models. They deserve work in their own right. We also hope that the study of these models will provide important information for those who are interested in trying to deal with the devastating lethal and difficult problem in humans--the problem of AIDS.

REFERENCES

1. Centers for Disease Control. (1982). MMWR 507, 513.
2. Masur, H., Michelis, M.A., Green, J.B. et al. (1981). N. Engl. J. Med. 305, 1431.
3. Mildvan, D., Mathur, U., Endlow, R.W. et al. (1982). Ann. Intern. Med. 96, 700.
4. Barré-Sinoussi, I.F., Chermann, J.C., Rey, F. et al. (1983). Science 220, 868.
5. Popovic, M., Sarngadharan, M.G., Read, E. et al. (1984). Science 224, 497.
6. Gallo, R.C., Salahuddin, S.Z., Popovic, M. et al. (1984). Science, 224, 500.
7. Rabson, A.B. and Martin, M.A. (1985). Cell 40, 477.
8. Bowen, D.L., Lane, H.C. and Fauci, A.S. (1985). In "AIDS" (V.T. DeVita, S. Hellman and S.A. Rosenberg, eds.). Lippincott Publishing Co., Philadelphia, Pennsylvania.

VIROLOGY OF
RETROVIRUS MODEL SYSTEMS

AVIAN RETROVIRUS MODEL SYSTEMS:
VIRUSES AND HOST CELL TYPES

David Boettiger

Department of Microbiology
University of Pennsylvania
Philadelphia, Pennsylvania

These discussions focus on animal model systems for the elucidation of the mechanisms which may be involved in the genesis of diseases induced by retroviruses. Beginning this volume with the avian retrovirus systems seems appropriate since this group of viruses was first identified in chickens. These chicken-derived viruses have remained the major model system for the development of the now familiar genetics and molecular biology of retroviruses.

The discovery of this group of agents by the Danish scientists Ellermann and Bang (1) resulted in the description of an avian leukosis which could be transmitted by a filterable agent. Rous and his associates (2) soon thereafter isolated and characterized a filterable agent which induced sarcomas. The modern development of the Rous sarcoma virus as the prototype model system for retroviruses (then called RNA tumor viruses) was initiated by Temin and Rubin (3) with the development of a quantitative focus assay using cultured chick embryo. This assay provided a means for titrating the virus, a system for investigating the biology of the virus replication process and a means for cloning the virus, thus giving rise to the beginnings of retroviral genetics.

The avian system flourished as a model because of three inherent advantages: The avian viruses are easier to propagate than many other retroviruses, and the avian virus particles are more stable than many other retroviruses. Most important was the existence of nondefective transforming strains of Rous sarcoma virus. The same viral genome coded for the essential replication functions and the transformation function and thus enabled a direct approach to both the assay and the viral genetics studies.

The following sections provide an abbreviated summary of the genetics and fundamental biology of the avian retroviruses. For additional information about these systems, the reader is referred to "RNA Tumor Viruses: The Molecular Biology of Tumor Viruses," 2nd ed. (4). The majority of this chapter focuses on the development of avian retrovirus model systems for the analysis of the virology and biology of these viruses in the context of hematopoietic cell differentiation. The significance of this model is that retroviruses are generally transmitted by blood and generally have their primary effects on the hematopoietic cells. The development of sarcomas and solid tissue tumors would usually be a dead end for these viruses were it not for the intervention of the curious scientist.

CLASSES OF AVIAN RETROVIRUSES

Retroviruses appear to be widespread at least among vertebrate groups. They have been isolated from the fishes (5) and reptiles (6). The avian retroviruses isolates have come either from the domestic chicken and related galliformes or from ducks. Two major groups of avian retroviruses are distinguished on the basis of RNA genome homology, the avian leukosis-sarcoma virus complex and the avian reticuloendotheliosis viruses. An additional unrelated retrovirus which causes a lymphoproliferative disease in turkeys has been reported and may represent a third

group (7). The basic classification of the avian retroviruses is
given in Table I.

In the avian leukosis-sarcoma virus complex, the common field
isolates are the leukosis viruses from domestic chickens (ALV).
These viruses induce avian leukosis which is a B cell neoplasm
limited often to the lymph nodes. The Rous-associated viruses
(RAV) are very similar to the ALVs but have been isolated from
stocks of sarcoma viruses in the laboratory and have rather different passage histories, although many are able to induce the
typical leukosis. The viral subgroups are based on different
envelope glycoproteins and utilize different receptors on the
host cells, at least for the A, B, C and E subgroups. The ALVs
are primarily of the A subgroup although some B subgroup viruses
have been isolated; the RAV's inclusion of C and D subgroups
probably reflects their different laboratory passage history
either on cells resistant to A and B subgroups or through mammalian hosts. The endogenous viruses are also similar but have been
induced from uninfected cells; their ability to replicate and to
induce disease in the species of origin is generally low. The
different subgroups reflect different species of origin within
the galliformes. The sarcoma viruses and the acute leukemia
viruses have arisen originally from the ALVs by the introduction
of oncogenes from the chicken host. Those found in the sarcoma
viruses include: src, fps, yes and ros; and the acute leukemia
viruses include: erb A, erb B, ets, mil, myb and myc. The rapid
onset of disease induced by the sarcoma viruses and the acute
leukemia viruses is dependent on the expression of these host-
derived oncogenes. During the course of the recombination events
involved in the capture of these host oncogenes there is generally a deletion of viral genes resulting in viral genomes which
are defective or no longer capable of independent replication
and which therefore require a helper virus. The helper function
is usually supplied by the ALV involved in the generation of the

TABLE I. Classification of Avian Retroviruses

Virus	Subgroups	Pathogenesis
Avian Leukosis-Sarcoma Virus Complex		
Avian leukosis viruses (ALV)	A (few B)	Leukosis
Rous-associated viruses (RAV)	A, B, C, D	Leukosis (most)
Avian endogenous viruses	E, F, G, H	None (in species of origin)
Avian sarcoma viruses (ASV, or Rous sarcoma virus [RSV])	A, B, C, D	Sarcomas (primarily)
Acute leukemia viruses (AEV)	A, B (primarily)	Erythroblastosis
(MC29)		Monocytic leukemia
(AMV)		Monoblastic leukemia
Reticuloendotheliosis Viruses		
Spleen necrosis group (SNV, DIAV, REV-A, CSV)	(1)[a]	Anemia, visceral lesions, leukosis, nerve lesions, immunosuppression
REV-T	(1)	Reticuloendotheliosis rapid pre-B cell tumors
Lymphoproliferative Disease Virus		
LPDV	?	Lympholiferative disease distinct from those above

[a]Common subgroup for REV.

sarcoma or acute leukemia virus. The only exception to the
defective nature of these viruses are certain src containing
strains of Rous sarcoma virus from European laboratories. These
nondefective strains have been particularly useful in the
development of retroviral genetics.

The range of pathology induced by the reticuloendotheliosis
virus group is a little different than that of the leukosis-
sarcoma virus complex. The nondefective SNV group tend to produce
some cell killing effects particularly in culture, and the pathology of the diseases appears to reflect this tendency. However,
they also can induce a leukosis similar to that induced by the
ALVs. The defective REV-T strain carries the rel oncogene which
appears to have originated in turkeys. The rapidly fatal disease
induced by this strain appears to involve early B cells and may
require the immunosuppressive effect of the REV-A helper virus
contained in these virus stocks.

MOLECULAR GENETICS OF ROUS SARCOMA VIRUS

Because of the early development of the viral assay system
for Rous sarcoma virus and to the relative ease of handling of
this virus, it has become the prototype for investigation of the
replication scheme of this virus class and for the development
of viral genetics. From this model system, the familiar prototype
for the retroviral genome has been developed. Figure 1 shows the
genetic structure of the prototype Rous sarcoma virus as it
exists in the integrated proviral state. In this DNA form the
viral genome is linked at either end to the host cell DNA producing a small direct repeat at either end of the viral genome
suggestive of integration occurring via a staggered cut in the
host cell DNA. At either end of the genome is the long terminal
repeat (LTR) consisting of 330 nucleotides and containing the
major regulatory elements for viral RNA transcription including

GENETIC STRUCTURE OF RETROVIRUSES

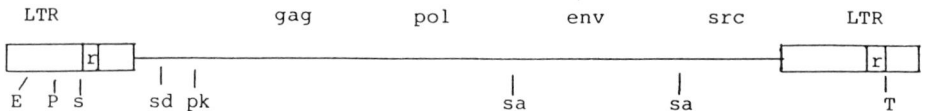

Fig. 1. E = enhancer; P = promoter; S = mRNA start; sd = splice donor; pk = viral RNA packaging signal; sa = splice acceptor; T = mRNA termination; r = terminal redundance of viral RNA.

enhancer (E), promoter (P), poly-A addition site which results in mRNA termination (T) and the initiation site for mRNA synthesis (s). The genome consists of four genes gag, pol, env and src. The first three are common to all replication competent retroviruses and encode respectively for the internal viral structural proteins, the reverse transcriptase and the viral envelope glycoprotein. Several retroviruses carry a fourth gene, in this case represented by src which may be important for the pathogenesis of these viruses either by producing an oncogenic product as in the case of src or in regulation of viral replication as in the bovine and human retroviruses. The gag and pol genes are translated from a genome length unspliced mRNA, whereas the env and src genes are translated from subgenomic spliced mRNAs. A splice donor site (sd) exists just downstream of the LTR region and splice acceptor sites (sa) exist at the beginning of the env and src genes. The location of the packaging site (pk) for the viral RNA downstream of the splice donor site ensures that it is not included in the spliced RNAs and that they are not incorporated into the maturing virions.

MODEL FOR AVIAN EMBRYONIC HEMATOPOIESIS

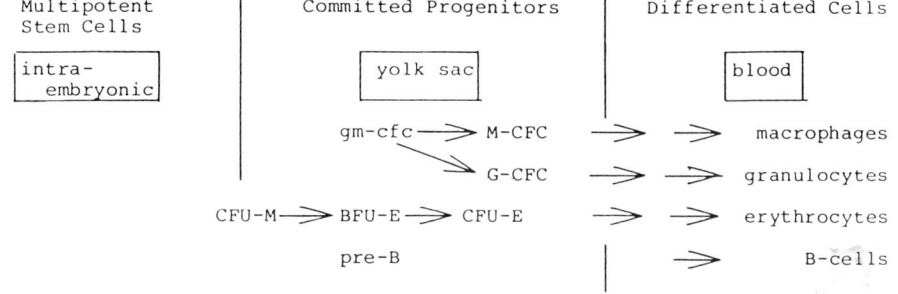

Fig. 2. Proposed models for the association of pathogenic effects with particular viral genes.

RELATIONSHIP OF VIRAL GENES TO PATHOGENESIS

Most of the focus on the pathogenic effects of avian retroviruses has been on their ability to induce tumors. This is particularly dramatic in the cases of the acute leukemia viruses and the REV-T strain in which the neoplastic process can kill the host in 7 to 10 days with massive tumor cell invasion of the hematopoietic tissue. In addition to the oncogenic potential there are reports of cell toxic and immunosuppressive effects associated with certain virus strains, although the mechanism of these effects has received little attention. The proposed models for the association of pathogenic effects with particular viral genes are summarized in Figure 2.

The oncogene-mediated pathogenesis is determined by viral oncogenes, such as src, which are relatively recently acquired from the host genome and participate in transformation of host cells but are dispensable for viral replication (Table II). This is a collection of 20, or so, distinct genes each of which is capable of inducing a characteristic range of tumor types. Three basic types of mechanism have been proposed to explain the

TABLE II. Models for Pathogenesis by Retroviruses

Oncogene-mediated	Expression of virus transduced cell gene	1. Mutated cell gene 2. Inappropriate level 3. Inappropriate context (cell type)
LTR-mediated	Enhancer activation of cell genes	
	Viral RNA synthesis	1. Quantity 2. Cell type
Glycoprotein-mediated		1. Toxic 2. Cell signals 3. Cell proliferation (chronic antigenic stimulation)

difference between the action of these viral oncogenes and of the
resident cellular homologues from which they are derived. First,
all viral oncogenes for which we have sufficient information
differ from the host cellular homologue and hence represent
mutant "alleles." The differences include: point mutations,
truncation (usually missing certain exons) and fusion with viral
genes to produce hybrid genes. Second, the oncogene product may
be expressed at inappropriately high levels. Generally the level
of expression of the viral oncogenes has been found to be dramatically elevated in comparison to expression of their cellular
homologues, although there are some exceptions (8; Duprey, S.P.
and D. Boettiger, manuscript submitted) and it is likely that
more will be elucidated as more different cell types are analyzed
for expression of the cellular homologues to the viral oncogenes.
Third, expression of the viral oncogene may occur in a cell type

in which the cellular homologue is never expressed. Both these
latter mechanisms can occur due to the loss of normal regulatory
signals and the acquisition of the viral regulatory signals in
the transition from host to viral gene.

The LTR-mediated models for pathogenesis focus on the role of
sequences in the LTR region as regulators of gene expression. The
enhancer region of the viral LTR can serve to inappropriately
activate cellular genes (the "promoter insertion" model) as has
been demonstrated for the myc oncogene in many B cell tumors (9).
Also the LTR regulates viral synthesis both in terms of the level
of viral transcription and the cell types in which transcription
occurs. For example the level of transcription in the nononcogenic avian retrovirus RAV-0 is significantly lower than its
oncogenic relative RAV-1 (10). Also some recent evidence from
the murine system has demonstrated that the LTR is an important
determinant of the type of tumor produced in retroviruses which
do not carry specific oncogenes, presumably as a result of tissue
specific replication (11).

Of the genes involved in viral replication, only the env
gene encoding the viral glycoprotein has been proposed to have
a direct role in the development of pathogenesis. Viruses of the
avian leukosis-sarcoma virus complex which fall into the B subgroup serotype and viruses of reticuloendotheliosis virus group
often exert cytotoxic effects on the infected cells. This cytotoxicity has been employed in the development of plaque assays
for several of these viruses (12,13). Perhaps more interesting
for the pathogenesis of disease is that these same viruses are
immunosuppressive in chickens. Birds infected with these viruses
exhibit a reduced blastogenic response to phytohemagglutinin,
concanavalin A and pokeweed mitogen (14). Additional experiments
with the reticuloendotheliosis virus system have implicated
direct contact, presumably of the lymphocytes with virus-infected
cells or surface proteins from the infected cells, as essential

for the inhibition of the blastogenic response (15). The immunosuppression parallels immunosuppression found in other retroviral
systems but the availability of different serotypes in the avian
sarcoma-leukosis viruses and the correlation of viral subgroup
with cytotoxic and immunosuppressive effects implicates the gene
in the process. However, the essential recombination studies to
map this viral function remain to be done in the avian system.
The association of immunosuppression with the viral glycoprotein
is consistent with data from other model systems. The mechanism
by which the viral glycoprotein exerts this "toxic" effect is not
understood and has not been extensively investigated. In addition
to this suppressive effect of the viral glycoprotein, other
models have proposed that the expression of particular viral
glycoproteins on the cell surface may mimic signals for cell
proliferation (16).

PATHOGENESIS IN THE CONTEXT OF (HEMATOPOIETIC) CELL DIFFERENTIATION

The process of cell differentiation produces a diversity of
cell types which are distinguished on the basis of differential
gene expression. The generation of a pathogenic state either by
the introduction of a virus into the cell or other by means is
dependent on the particular constellation of genes products found
in that cell. These host gene products form the substrate for
pathologic alteration and the presence or absence of certain substrates can profoundly affect both the ability of the agent to
induce the disease and the course of the disease. This caveat is
particularly important in the case of the retroviruses since
their mode of replication and generation of pathogenic effect is
intimately tied to the biology of the host cell. The retrovirus
replication cycle is dependent on cell division; this restricts
potential host target cells. Both the synthesis of viral-coded
gene products and their effect on host cells is dependent on the

particular molecules present in the host cell. There is increasing evidence that these elements are often developmentally regulated gene products. Hence understanding the interaction of the
virus with its significant target cells is important to understanding the genesis of the pathology. The approach to investigating this interaction is hampered by the complexity and limited
manipulability of the in vivo situation, so such studies need to
be supplemented with studies on differentiated cells in culture.
Here again certain caution needs to be maintained to assure that
the in vitro studies are an accurate reflection of the in vivo
situation.

The mechanism of retroviral replication involves production
of a DNA provirus which is integrated into the host cell genome.
This stable association of the viral genome and the host cell
means that the fate of the virus depends to some extent on the
fate of the host cell. During the course of hematopoietic cell
differentiation, which takes place throughout the life of the
animal, cells differentiate into terminal cell phenotypes which
are often short lived. In these cell populations, continual rein-
fection would be required to maintain the virus. On the other
hand, infection of the stem cell populations which is a self-
renewing population would provide for indefinite maintenance of
the virus in the absence of continual replication cycles. Furthermore, the differentiation of this cell population into the
various hematopoietic cell types provides a changing set cellular
substrates which may affect both the expression of the viral
genes and their ability to induce the pathogenic state. In the
following sections, I shall use the avian retrovirus system to
illustrate the importance of the differentiated phenotype of
potential target cells of the hematopoietic system and how different stages of differentiation in the same lineage may influence the development of the pathology.

Hematopoietic Development in the Chicken Embryo

While considerable work has focused on the particular cell
types involved in the production of tumors by these viruses,
these have generally been viewed as static states of development.
I wish to widen the issue to consider the dynamic process of
differentiation and examine how the virus and the pathogenesis
develop at successive stages of differentiation. In order to take
such an approach it is necessary to be able to examine not only
the functionally defined mature cell types, but also the earlier
stages of progenitors to these more mature cell types. For many
of these studies the chicken embryo is the experimental system of
choice, since large numbers of embryos may be obtained at a pre-
defined stage of differentiation; and, hence, sufficient numbers
of the relatively rare progenitor cell populations may be
obtained. The hematopoietic system is particularly convenient
because several stages of maturation are separated anatomically
as shown in Figure 3. The stem cell for the hematopoietic lineages (the cell which is multipotential and produces daughters for
several lineages) is resident at some as yet to be determined
embryonic site, the committed progenitors to several hematopoietic lineages are in the yolk sac in the process of active population expansion and the more mature cells are released into the
embryonic circulation (17,18). This has allowed us to examine
separately the effects on at least the committed progenitor and
the mature cell populations for several related cell lineages.

Differentiation Affects the Susceptibility of Cells to Infection

The susceptibility of cell populations to infection by particular retroviruses has usually been restricted to examination
of fibroblasts, or mixed populations of cells in tissue culture.
In the case of the avian sarcoma-leukosis virus complex about
which most is known, it appears that most cell types from susceptible birds are infectable by the viruses as long as they retain

their proliferative potential. There are some large differences
in the degree of susceptibility to the virus (19) and the total
range of cell types which have been examined carefully is small.
Since the more mature stages of differentiation usually predomi-
nate in these systems, there is very little information on the
susceptibility of the progenitor cell populations. The potential
significance for the infection of the progenitor cell populations
by retroviruses is that the retroviral provirus remains in the
infected cell and proliferates with the infected cell. These progenitor cell populations undergo extensive expansion, and hence
the provirus would multiply passively; differentiation alters the
cellular environment and presents a new series of substrates to
the viral gene products. These elements can affect the course of
pathogenesis.

In the course of the infection of yolk sac cells with high
multiplicities of avian myeloblastosis virus (AMV) (>20 IU/cell)
it became apparent that the majority of the cell population
failed to express viral antigens. This appeared to provide an
explanation for the failure of the granulocyte lineage cells to
fail to transform in response to infection by AMV. To investigate the problem further, one group of chicken embryos was inoculated with AMV intravenously into a chorioallantoic membrane vein
at 11 days of incubation. A parallel set of embryos was used at
11 days as a source of yolk sac cells, which were infected with
AMV. Two days later both the in vitro and the in vivo infected
cells were analyzed for expression of viral antigens, FACS analysis using a rabbit anti-envelope glycoprotein and immunofluorescence using a monoclonal anti-p19 gag. Table III demonstrates
that infection in vivo was quite efficient, whereas infection
in vitro led to minimal levels of viral antigen expression.
Further examination of the cells during in vitro differentiation
demonstrated that the mature granulocytes were able to express
the viral antigens when the progenitors were infected in vivo.

TABLE III.   In Ovo and In Vitro Infection
by Avian Myeloblastosis Virus

	Total cells by FACS	Nonerythroid cells by immunofluorescence[a]
IV inoculation of day 11 embryos	70%	95%
In vitro infection of day 13 yolk sac cells	>4%	Not detected

[a]Includes granulocyte progenitors which continue to express viral antigens during in vitro differentiation, and transformed cells.

The committed granulocyte progenitors in 11 to 13 day chicken embryo yolk sac will survive for 3 to 5 days under our culture conditions during which they both divide (preliminary evidence suggests at least one obligatory cell division for full maturation) and mature into fully developed granulocytes. The simplest interpretation of the results is that either the granulocyte progenitors present in the yolk sac are resistant to infection, but that an earlier progenitor is susceptible, or that additional factors not available in the tissue culture system are required. In spite of this infection of the granulocytes, inoculated embryos which were allowed to develop to day 19, at which time they die of myeloblastosis, showed no pathological evidence for transformation of granulocyte lineage cells. Thus the pathological effect of the virus was absolutely dependent on the differentiation of the infected cells into the target lineage. As long as some of its progenitor cells are susceptible to infection, it is not necessary that the ultimate target cell be susceptible; the pathology can be induced by specific differentiation. Because of the absence of erythropoietin in the in vitro culture system, the data on the erythroid cells are open to

broader interpretation, but it is likely that the more mature
cells are also resistant to infection by retroviruses.

The Differentiation Process Affects Pathogenic Expression

Previous experiments had demonstrated that functionally
mature macrophages could serve as target cells both for infection
and transformation by AMV (20,21). This did not mean that this is
the only stage in the lineage which can serve as target cells. To
more fully examine this question, we took advantage of the
compartmentalization of hematopoiesis in the chicken embryo and
utilized the macrophage progenitors in the yolk sac as target
cell for the virus. These cells were efficiently infected by the
virus and produced transformed cells of indistinguishable phenotype from those in which mature macrophages were used as the
target cell population. There was however one difference in the
transformation process. The transformation of yolk sac cells by
the virus was more sensitive to the level of chicken serum than
for target cells derived from bone marrow or from mature macrophages. Figure 3 shows the dose response curve for yolk sac cells
and for bone marrow cells. The fundamental difference between
these two starting populations is in maturity. In bone marrow
there is a high proportion of myelocytes and promonocytes which
are absent from yolk sac. The function of the chicken serum is
to supply the specific factors required for hematopoietic cell
proliferation and differentiation since it cannot be replaced by
serum of other species and these factors tend to be species
specific. The result suggests that the cells from yolk sac have
a different factor requirement for transformation and that this
difference is not related to survival or growth of the transformed cells. The simplest interpretation is that the factor is
required for a differentiation step which must precede the transformation process. Or phrased in another manner, the macrophage
progenitors in the yolk sac can be infected by AMV but only their

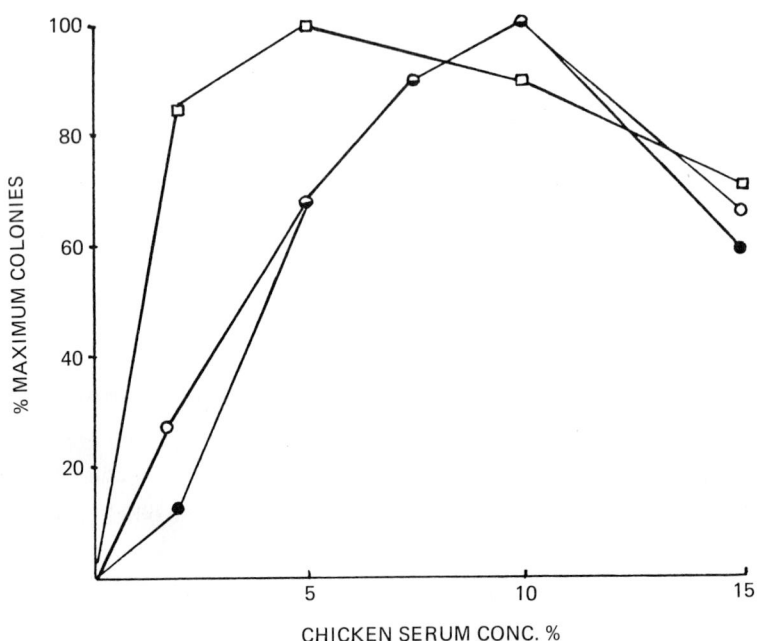

Fig. 3. Serum dependence for normal macrophage colony formation and for transformation by AMV. ●——● = normal macrophage
colonies from yolk sac cells; o——o = AMV-transformed colonies
from yolk sac cells; □——□ = AMV-transformed colonies from bone
marrow cells.

progeny which differentiate along the macrophage lineage can

undergo transformation.

The failure to transform the committed progenitor to the

macrophage present in the yolk sac may be viewed in the larger

developmental context. At this stage of differentiation the

cell population is undergoing rapid expansion. Expression of

the mature macrophage markers at this time could impede the

proliferation process and would, at the least, divert energy and

raw materials from the proliferation process. The expression of

the myb oncogene carried by AMV has precisely this effect, the

suppression of the synthesis of the majority of the mature macro-

phage differentiation products (22). If the cellular homologue

TABLE IV. Number of Copies of myb RNA
           Transcripts per Cell

v-myb	
AMV-transformed cells	1000
E26-transformed cells	50-100
c-myb	
Enriched yolk sac	200-400
cell fraction	

of the viral myb had an analogous function, it might be expressed
at high levels in this cell population. Table IV shows that elevated levels of myb expression are found in the yolk sac and
that when the macrophage progenitors are purified from this population, the myb expression appears to be confined to this subpopulation. When the actual level is calculated from dot blot
hybridizations, the level of myb expression in the macrophage
progenitor cell is as high or higher than in the virally transformed macrophages (Duprey, S.P. and D. Boettiger, manuscript
submitted). The prediction was validated both that the level of
myb expression in the macrophage progenitors was elevated, and
that expression was restricted to the macrophage progenitors.

Specificity of Cell Response to Particular Retroviruses

Pure cultures of functionally mature macrophages were prepared by the in vitro differentiation of the macrophage progenitors from chicken embryo under conditions which select for
macrophages. Using phagocytosis and cytoplasmic lipids as markers
more than 5000 cells were scored and no immature macrophages or
other cell types could be detected. This cell population was then
infected with four different avian retroviruses, Rous sarcoma
virus (Prague B [PR-B] strain), avian myelocytomatosis virus
(MC29), AMV (BAI strain) and myeloblastosis-associated virus
(MAV-2 strain). Parallel cultures were used for the determination

TABLE V. Response of Macrophages to Avian Retroviruses

Virus	IC[a]	Growth[b]	Morphology	Differentiation		
				Im. phag.	Acid Phos.	Lipid
None	0	1.00	Large macrophage	+++	+++	+++
MAV-2	82	0.99	Large macrophage	+++	+++	+++
PR-B	70	1.28	Large macrophage	+++	+++	+++
MC29	80	5.90	Small macrophage	+++	+++	+++
AMV	Trans-formed	9.14	Promyelocyte (transformed)	-	+	+

Mature macrophages were infected with the various viruses and tested.

[a] IC (%), infectious center assay to determine infected, virus-producing cells; the AMV cells were selected for morphological transformation.

[b] Relative growth rates were determined by [³H]TdR incorporation in a 4 hour labeling period.

of infectious centers as a measure of the proportion of infected,
virus-producing cells, pulse labeled with [^{3}H]TdR to measure
relative rates of DNA synthesis, examined for cell morphology and
analyzed for the expression of several macrophage differentiation
markers. Table V demonstrates that the majority of the cell population in each case was infected and producing progeny virus.
Cell phenotype based on the differentiation and proliferation
measurements showed specific differences in the effects of these
viruses on the cells. Rous sarcoma virus and myeloblastosis-
associated virus produced no phenotypic changes and the infected
cells were essentially indistinguishable from the control cells.
AMV altered both the cell proliferation and the expression of the
macrophage markers, while MC29 affected primarily the proliferation of the cells with no major effects on the expression of the
differentiation markers (22).

The failure of Rous sarcoma virus to alter the morphology or
proliferation of the macrophages was surprising in the light of
its dramatic effects on cell phenotype for most other cell types
which have been tested. One possible reason for the failure to
transform the macrophages could have been the failure to produce
the src oncogene product in the infected cells. When this was
examined in more detail, it was found that pp60^{src}, the product
of the viral oncogene, was produced, showed both a similar
pattern of phosphorylation and intracellular distribution as in
transformed fibroblasts, and the p36 putative target of the
pp60^{src} kinase activity also exhibited increased phosphorylation
(23). An unusual feature of the system was that the level of
pp60^{src} and gp85^{env} expression in the macrophages were reduced
in comparison to the level of pr76^{gag}. This suggests the possibility of reduced splicing efficiency for the viral RNA in the
macrophage.

The effect of AMV on the macrophage population demonstrated
that the functionally mature macrophage could be transformed by

the virus and that the phenotype of the transformed cells was indistinguishable from that found in the in vivo tumor or cells from other sources transformed in vitro by the virus (21). This also demonstrates that the transformed phenotype does not occur due to a block in the total maturation pathway as had been proposed. We will return to the mechanism of this transformation event below.

The MC29 virus is known to alter a variety of cell types and to cause a variety of tumor phenotypes. This virus carries the prototype myc oncogene, which is thought to play a role in cell proliferation. The result with the macrophage system supports this view. The morphology of the infected cells differs somewhat from the control cultures, but on closer examination they resemble the smaller faster proliferating macrophages with no change in the expression of the differentiation markers. This effect of MC29 to alter the proliferation potential of cells with little or no effect on the expression of the differentiated cell markers has also been demonstrated in the chondroblast differentiation system (24). It is interesting to note that in the chondroblast system the effect of the src gene is primarily to suppress the expression of differentiated cell markers much the same as the effect of the myb gene of AMV in the macrophage system. Thus there may be a class of oncogenes represented by myb and src which display a cell type specificity and have their primary effect on the expression of differentiated cell products, and another class represented by myc which have their primary effect on cell differentiation.

CONCLUSIONS AND DISCUSSION

The biology of the retroviruses is quite distinct from other groups of viruses. The fundamental basis of this difference is the obligatory (generally) integration into the host cell DNA.

Since it is an obligatory step, retroviruses have evolved efficient means to effect this specific integration. Such integration
events can disrupt genes and create mutations (25), disrupt gene
regulation by separating genes from their normal regulatory
sequences (26) or introduce viral regulatory elements into host
cell genes (9). The high efficiency of retrovirus integration
means that these disruptions may play major roles in the pathogenesis induced by these viruses. The second aspect of the integration process is that, unlike other virus groups, transcription
of viral RNA is completely dependent on the host cell enzymes and
factors. Since transcription is a primary level for regulation
of expression of cell differentiation, expression of viral genes
may be developmentally regulated. This mode of viral replication
is particularly adapted for the induction of chronic disease
states either of a neoplastic, hyperplastic or degenerative type.
It also means that the tracing of the etiology of diseases to
retroviruses will be more difficult than for other virus groups.

In the examples above, taken from the interaction of several
avian retroviruses with the developing hematopoietic systems,
there are several elements which may apply to other retroviral
systems.

1. Susceptibility of cells to infection by retroviruses
    can be regulated as a function of the maturity of
    the cell along a particular developmental pathway.
    This dependence can be separated from the require-
    ment for proliferating cells.
2. Infection of a progenitor cell can lead to virus
    gene expression in the differentiated progeny, even
    when the differentiated progeny are themselves
    resistant to infection.
3. The expression of a pathologic phenotype can be
    dependent on the differentiation of the initially
    infected cell to a more mature phenotype.

4. The specific pathology induced can depend both on
    the cell type and on the particular retrovirus.

The avian retrovirus model system has provided much of the
pivotal information on the biology of retroviruses and on their
potential for pathogenesis. While much of the lead in the characterization of retroviral genetics followed the lead of the
avian viruses, many of the other families of retroviruses have
reached a similar level of sophistication. However, the particular biology of the chicken and of the avian retroviruses still
provide certain advantages for the unraveling of the more complex factors that contribute to the pathogenesis which may be
peculiar to the retrovirus group.

REFERENCES

1. Ellermann, V. and Bang, O. (1908). Zentralbl. Bakteriol. 46,
    595.
2. Rous, P. (1911). J. Exp. Med. 13, 397.
3. Temin, H.M. and Rubin, H. (1958). Virology 6, 669.
4. Weiss, R.A., Teich, N., Varmus, H. et al. (1982). In "RNA
    Tumor Viruses: The Molecular Biology of Tumor Viruses," 2nd
    ed. Cold Spring Harbor, New York.
5. Mulcahey, M.F. and Leary, A.O. (1970). Experientia 26, 891.
6. Clark, H.F., Anderson, P.R. and Lunger, P.D. (1979). J. Gen.
    Virol. 43, 673.
7. Gazit, A., Yaniv, A., Ianconescu, M. et al. (1979). J. Virol.
    31, 639.
8. Muller, R., Verma, I.M. and Adamson, E.D. (1983). EMBO J. 2,
    679.
9. Hayward, W.S., Neel, B.G. and Astrin, S.M. (1981). Nature
    290, 475.
10. Tsichlis, P.N. and Coffin, J.M. (1980). J. Virol. 33, 238.
11. Lenz, J., Celender, D., Crowther, R.L. et al. (1984). Nature
    308, 467.
12. Graf, T. (1972). Virology 50, 567.
13. Temin, H.M. and Kassner, V. (1974). J. Virol. 13, 291.
14. Rup, B.J., Hoelzer, J.D. and Bose, H.R., Jr. (1982). Virology
    116, 61.
15. Carpenter, C.R., Rubin, A.S. and Bose, H.R., Jr. (1978).
    J. Immunol. 120, 1313.
16. McGrath, M.S. and Weissman I.L. (1979). Cell 17, 65.

17. LeDouarin, N., Joterau, F., Houssaint, E. et al. (1983). In
    "The Reticuloendothelial System " (N. Cohen and M.M. Sigel,
    eds.), vol. 3. Plenum, New York.
18. Boettiger, D. and Durban, E.M. (1984). J. Virol. 49, 841.
19. Boettiger, D., Roby, K., Brumbaugh, J. et al. (1977). Cell
    11, 881.
20. Moscovici, C., Gazzolo, L. and Moscovici, M.G. (1975).
    Virology 68, 173.
21. Durban, E.M. and Boettiger, D. (1981). J. Virol. 37, 488.
22. Durban, E.M. and Boettiger, D. (1981). Proc. Natl. Acad. Sci.
    78, 3600.
23. Lipsich, L., Brugge, J. and Boettiger, D. (1984). Mol. Cell.
    Biol. 4, 1420.
24. Alema, S., Tato, F. and Boettiger, D. (1985). Mol. Cell.
    Biol. 5, 538.
25. Copeland N.G., Hutchinson, K.W. and Jenkins, N.A. (1983).
    Cell 33, 379.
26. Mitchell, K.F., Battey, J., Hollis, G.F. et al. (1984).
    J. Cell. Physiol. (Suppl.) 3, 171.

BIOLOGY OF MURINE LEUKEMIA VIRUSES

Herbert C. Morse III
Janet W. Hartley

Laboratory of Immunopathology
National Institute of Allergy and Infectious Diseases
National Institutes of Health
Bethesda, Maryland

Murine leukemia viruses (MuLV), like other retroviruses, are usually thought of in terms of their role in induction of leukemias and lymphomas. The mouse shown in Figure 1 has the typical appearance of an animal dying with a retrovirus-induced nonthymic lymphoma in exhibiting splenomegaly, lymphadenopathy of both peripheral and mesenteric nodes and slight hepatomegaly. However, this particular animal does not have a true lymphoma; it is suffering from a massive, non-neoplastic proliferation of B cells associated with severe immunosuppression. Although we have a remarkably thorough understanding of these infectious agents and their interactions with the host species, we still have much to learn about the mechanisms that result in neoplastic and non-neoplastic diseases as a consequence of their expression.

The transmission of retroviruses in different species has been found to occur as a result of vertical transmission of proviruses integrated in germ cells and, less often, horizontally by exogenous routes of infection. In the mouse, the only documented modes of transmission are vertical--either through the germ line or by maternal transmission from transplacental infections or passage through the milk.

ANIMAL MODELS OF RETROVIRUS INFECTION
AND THEIR RELATIONSHIP TO AIDS

41

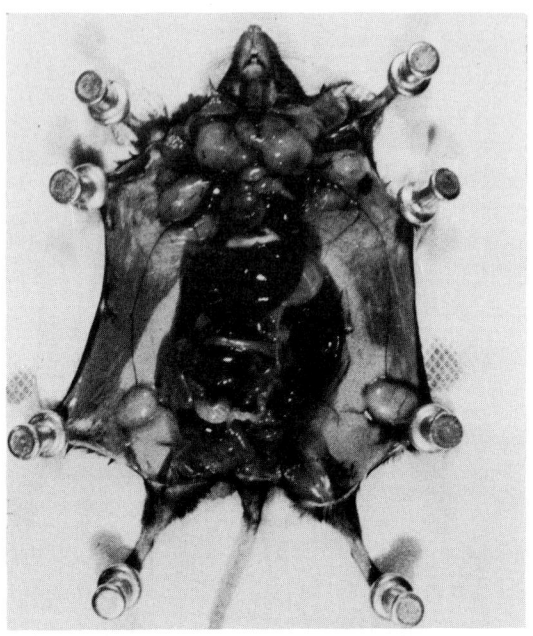

Fig. 1. A C57BL/6 mouse infected with LP-BM5 MuLV exhibiting
nonmalignant lymph adenopathy and splenomegaly.

The characteristics of MuLV are shown in Table I.

These viruses mature by budding through the host cell membrane, leading to their acquisition of a lipid envelope containing host gene products as well as the virus-coded gp70 and p15E
antigens which form characteristic knobs on the surface of the
virion (Fig. 2). The envelope surrounds an icosahedral core
structure which contains the viral RNA genome, the polymerase
enzyme and the virus-coded proteins p15, p30, p12 and p10.

The RNA genome of MuLV contains three coding regions flanked
by short repeats unique to the 5' and 3' ends of the genome. The
repeats contain within U5, the signal of reverse transcription
and in U3 region, sequences important for the initiation and
termination of RNA transcription. The internal regions termed
gag, pol and env code respectively for core proteins, polymerase
and the envelope proteins.

TABLE I. Properties of MuLV

Morphology

Spherical enveloped virions (80-120 nm); variable surface projects (8-12 nm); icosahedral capsid composed of a core shell and a ribonucleic acid complex; buds from cell surface

Nucleic acid

Two identical subunits (30-353; ∿8.8 kb) of positive-sense, single-stranded RNA, coding for repeated sequences at the 3' and 5' ends and three genes (gag, pol, env)

Protein

∿60% by weight; gag, internal protein structures p15, p12, p30, p10; pol, reverse transcriptase; env, envelope proteins gp70, p15(E)

Lipid

∿35% by weight; derived from cell membrane

Carbohydrate

∿4% by weight; associated with env gene products

Physicochemical properties

Density 1.16 to 1.18 g/ml in sucrose, 1.16-1.21 g/ml in cesium chloride; sensitive to lipid solvents, detergents, heat inactivation (56°C, 30 min); highly resistant to UV- and X-irradiation

Antigenic characteristics

Antibodies to all proteins, glycoproteins have been produced in mice, rats, rabbits or goats; "autoantibodies" to gp70, p15E and p30

Modes of transmission

Vertical as chromosomally integrated proviruses or by maternal passage

---

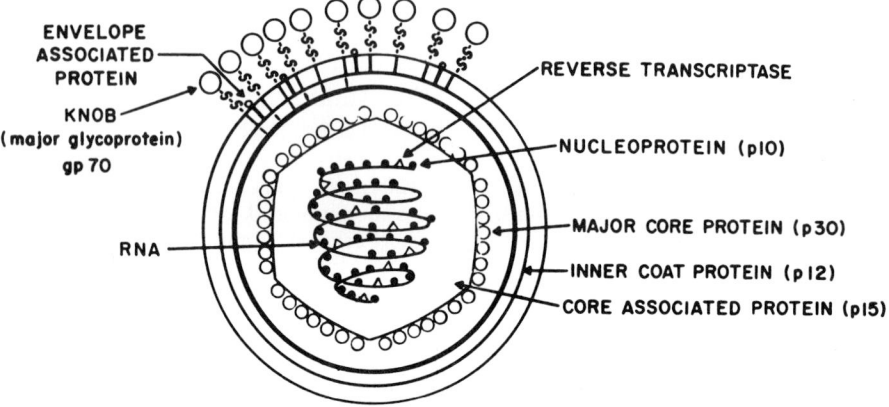

Fig. 2.   Morphologic features and structural components of
mature, enveloped type C MuLV.

The life cycle of these viruses is understood in reasonably
great detail (Fig. 3). After the virions bond to virus-specific
receptors on the cell surface, the RNA genome is introduced into
the cytoplasm. There, by the action of reverse transcriptase, a
double-stranded DNA copy of the virus is made which is colinear
with the viral RNA with the exception that both ends of the coding region are now flanked by long terminal repeats (LTRs) with
the U5 and U3 regions being represented at both ends of the
genome. After circularization of the proviral DNA, it is
inserted, apparently randomly, in cellular DNA. Expression of the
integrated provirus involves the utilization of normal cellular
mechanisms for the translation of the two viral mRNA species and
their translation to produce the proteins required for the
production of the virion.

MuLV are traditionally classified on the basis of their
host-range characteristics, or said another way, their ability
to infect cells of mice or cells from xenogeneic species (Table
II). Another important determinant in classification is the ability of the different viruses to produce foci of transformation in

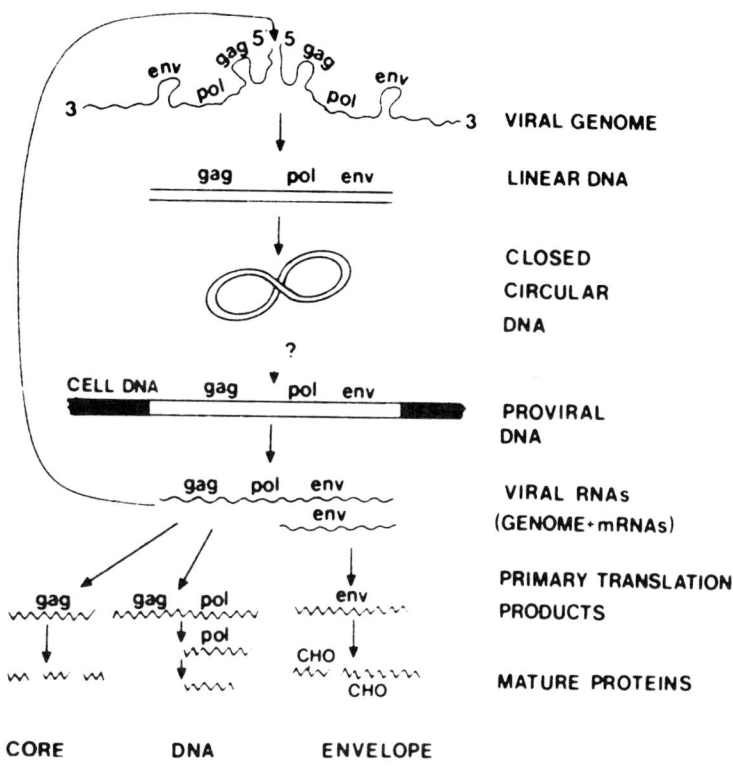

Fig. 3.   Generation of a DNA copy of the MuLV genome, insertion of the viral DNA into cellular DNA and expression of the
integrated provirus.

XC cells. Ecotropic MuLV are infectious for mouse cells but not
xenogeneic cells and induce XC plaques. The prototype ecotropic
viruses are the AKR viruses first detected by Ludwig Gross. By
comparision, xenotropic MuLV, first described in NZB mice, cannot
infect mouse cells but do infect xenogeneic cells and do not
induce XC plaques. The third class of viruses are amphotropic
viruses. These agents infect both murine and xenogeneic cells and
do not induce XC foci. Viruses belonging to this class have only
been recovered from some California wild mice and will not be
considered further. The fourth class of MuLV is also infectious
for mouse and xenogeneic cells and does not give XC foci.

TABLE II. Classification of Type C Viruses of Mice

Class	Host range	Assays			Prototype
		XC	Mink S^+L^-	Mink CPE	
Ecotropic	M$\underline{^a}$	+	-	-	AKV-1
Xenotropic	X$\underline{^b}$	-	+	-	NZB-1
Amphotropic	M and X	-	+	-	Wild mouse
MCF	M and X	-	(+)	+	AKR lymphomas

$\underline{^a}$Mouse cells.

$\underline{^b}$Xenogeneic cells.

However, it does induce characteristic foci in mink lung cells leading to their designation as mink cell focus (MCF)-inducing viruses. Another name for this class is polytropic viruses.

Among inbred strains, only ecotropic and xenotropic viruses are transmitted in the germ line as complete proviruses. Amphotropic viruses are passaged vertically in feral mice and MCF viruses are formed by recombination events involving infectious ecotropic virus and endogenous nonecotropic viral sequences.

Early studies of Wally Rowe, Janet Hartley and others showed that expression of infectious ecotropic viruses varied greatly among strains of inbred mice. Strains such as AKR and C58 produced high levels of infectious virus from early in life, whereas strains such as C57BL/6 or BALB/c produced only intermediate or low levels of virus late in life. Finally, no virus was recovered from other strains such as C57L, 129 or NFS. Studies of genetic crosses between high virus strains like AKR and virus-negative mice, like NFS, showed that the high virus phenotype was determined by two or more independently assorting dominant loci that behaved like classic cellular genes. The genes controlling

TABLE III.   Characteristics of Ecotropic Virus Induction Loci

---

1. Induction rate can be high or low
    - A function of the locus itself
    - IUDR induction rate parallels the spontaneous rate

2. Locus contains viral genomic DNA

3. Normally carries N-tropic virus, but a few B-tropic loci found in $\underline{Fv-1}^b$ strains

4. Not at allelic sites in various strains

5. Multiple loci (2 to >4) in many high virus strains, one in low virus strains

6. Viral genome can excise

7. Viral genome can insert back into germ line DNA

---

expression of infectious ecotropic virus were termed induction loci. The characteristics of induction loci are given in Table III. Studies of the induction loci in different strains of mice showed that the rate of virus induction from a locus could be high or low and that this induction characteristic was a function of the locus itself. It was also found that treatment of cells with agents such as IUDR could lead to virus production and that the rate of induction following treatment paralleled the spontaneous induction rate.

Classic studies by Wally Rowe and his collaborators showed that the loci contained viral genomic DNA and was thus coded for the virus itself. Most of the proviral loci were found to carry N-tropic virus, but a few B-tropic loci have been identified in C57BL mice.

Subsequent investigations showed that among different strains, the induction loci were not at allelic sites and could be mapped to a variety of chromosomal locations, including loci on chromosomes 5, 7, 8, 9, 11 and 16 (Fig. 4).

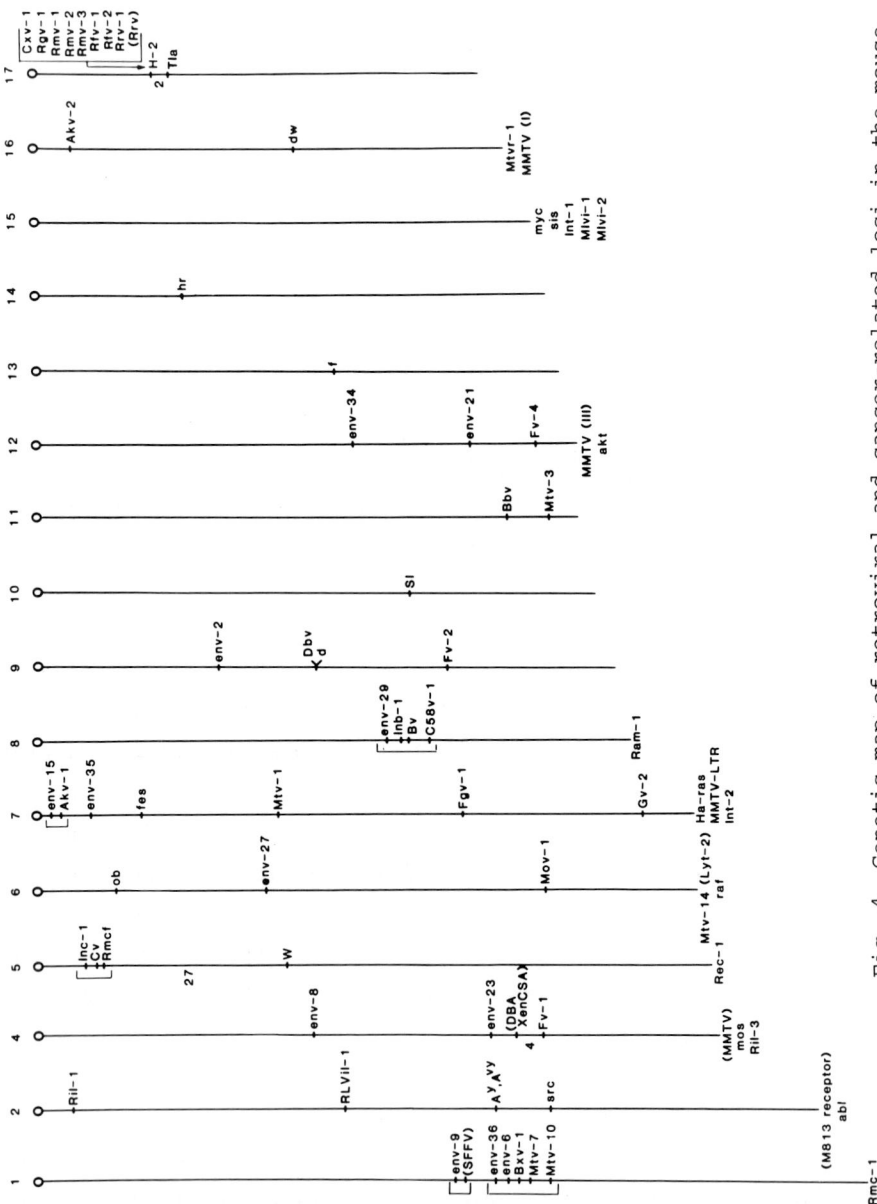

Fig. 4. Genetic map of retroviral and cancer-related loci in the mouse.

Studies of xenotropic MuLV have closely paralleled those of ecotropic MuLV. Various inbred strains have been shown to differ in their spontaneous production of infectious xenotropic MuLV. Rare strains such as NZB or F/St produce high levels of virus, whereas others produced intermediate or low levels of virus and others, including NFS, were virus-negative. Analyses of crosses between high-virus and virus-negative mice showed that virus expression was controlled by induction loci that assorted in Mendelian fashion and that the loci had high and low induction phenotypes either spontaneously or after treatment of cells with IUDR. However, the xenotropic induction loci differ from the ecotropic induction loci in several important respects.

First, even though ecotropic induction loci are scattered throughout the genome, the xenotropic induction locus for at least four unrelated strains was found to be at single site on chromosome 1, termed Bxv-1 (Fig. 4).

Second, virus-coded gp70 antigens can sometimes be expressed at high levels on cells of mice that produce little infectious virus (Fig. 5). Figure 5 shows fluorescence profiles of cells from different mouse strains stained with antibodies specific for the gp70 of xenotropic and MCF viruses. Although DBA/2 mice produce little infectious virus, they express high levels of gp70 on their spleen cells and thymocytes in comparison to NFS mice.

Third, genes that are not linked to xenotropic virus induction loci can have a profound effect on virus expression. F/St mice are one of the few inbred strains that spontaneously produce high levels of infectious xenotropic virus. This strain was found to have a single induction locus on chromosome 1, apparently allelic with that of the low xenotropic virus strains AKR, BALB and others. In contrast to the dominant phenotype for virus expression for ecotropic induction loci, high expression of xenotropic virus was found to be a recessive trait in F_1 mice. When F_1 mice were backcrossed to F/St, thymocytes from 50% of the mice produced high levels of virus; whereas the other half produced

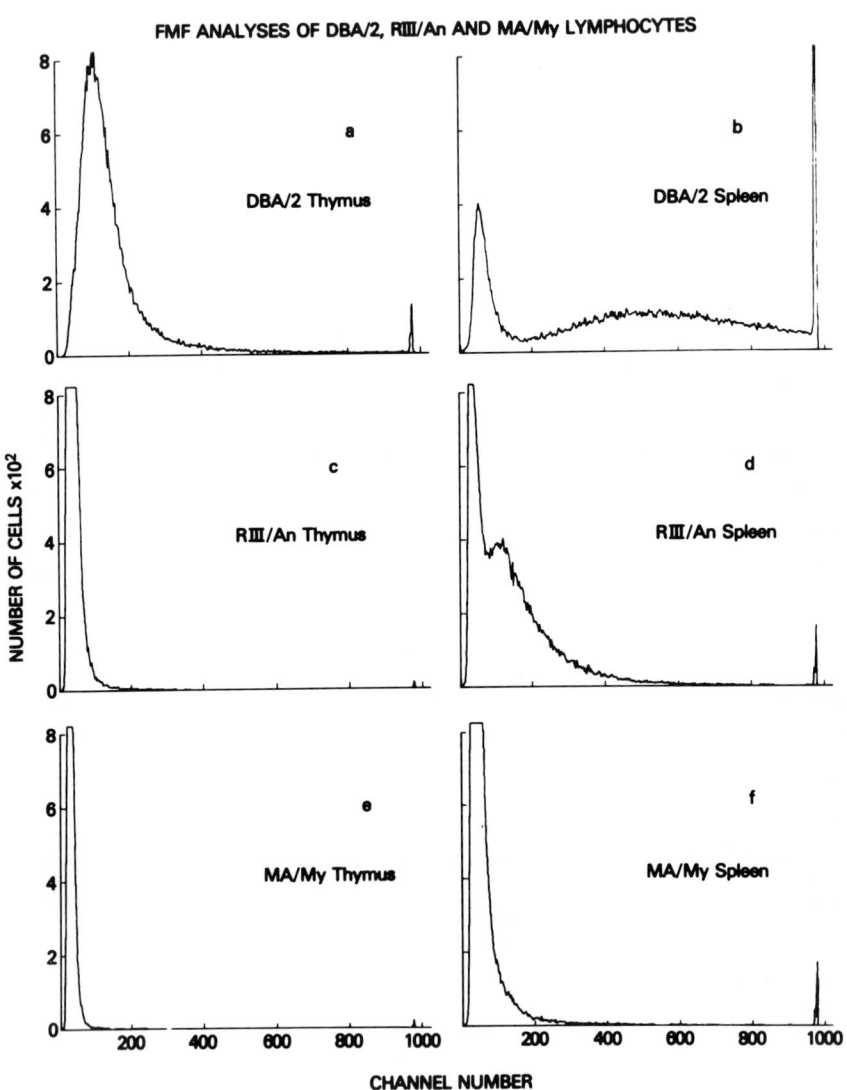

Fig. 5. Fluorescence profiles of thymocytes and spleen cells from DBA/2, RIII and MA mice stained with fluorescein-labeled antibodies to XenCSA.

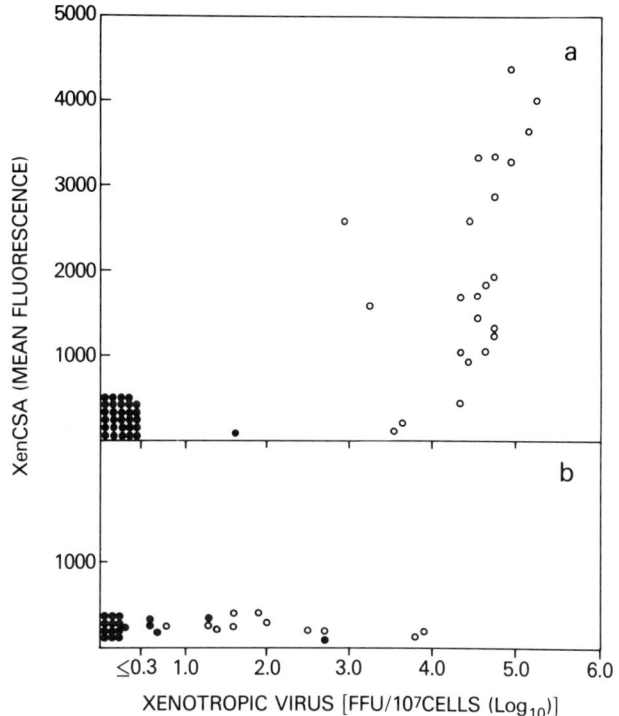

Fig. 6. Relation of infectious xenotropic MuLV expression and XenCSA expression by thymocytes (a) and spleen cells (b) of (AKR × F/St)F_1 × F/St mice to alleles of H-2. Values for H-2^p homozygotes are given as open circles and values for H-2$^{k/p}$ heterozygotes as closed circles.

essentially none, as shown in Figure 6. Also indicated in this figure is the typing of backcross mice for alleles at H-2K. All the high virus mice were homozygous for the H-2K^p of F/St or all the low virus mice were heterozygous H-2^p/H-2^k. These results showed that a gene on chromosome 17 that we have called Cxv-1 controls the expression of infectious xenotropic virus from a chromosome 1 induction locus.

The characteristics of the Cxv-1 locus are presented in Table IV.

Finally, molecular studies of these viruses have shown that multiple copies of sequences related to xenotropic env genes are

TABLE IV.   Characteristics of Cxv-1

---

1. Resistance allele is present in non-H-2^P mice

2. Cxv-1^r mice are resistant to expression of X-MuLV from
    a chromosome 1 induction locus possibly allelic with
    Bxv-1

3. Cxv-1^s mice are permissive for expression of X-MuLV from
    Fxv-1 but not Bxv-1

4. Resistance is dominant

5. Cxv-1 maps to chromosome 17 in linkage to H-2

---

present in all strains of mice, whereas ecotropic proviral loci
are present in some strains but not others. Figure 7 shows
HindIII digests of cellular DNA from three strains of mice,
Molossiniss, F/St and NFS, hybridized with three different
probes. On the left a generalized MuLV probe that will react with
all proviral sequences, one specific for ecotropic env sequences
and one specific for xenotropic env sequences. Multiple copies of
MuLV-related DNA were found in all strains. However, the ecotropic virus specific probe showed that NFS mice differed from
Molossiniss and F/St in lacking totally ecotropic virus information. By comparison, all three strains had multiple copies of
xenotropic virus-related DNA.

Other studies have shown that very few of these xenotropic-
like proviral loci can be expressed as infectious virus but
importantly that they can participate in recombination events
with infectious ecotropic viruses to produce MCF viruses.

In comparison to ecotropic MuLV isolates some MCF viruses
were shown to be highly leukemogenic when reinoculated into
newborn mice.

Molecular studies of the genomes of these viruses showed
that complete proviral copies that corresponded to the viral RNA
genome could not be found in cellular DNA. Rather it was apparent

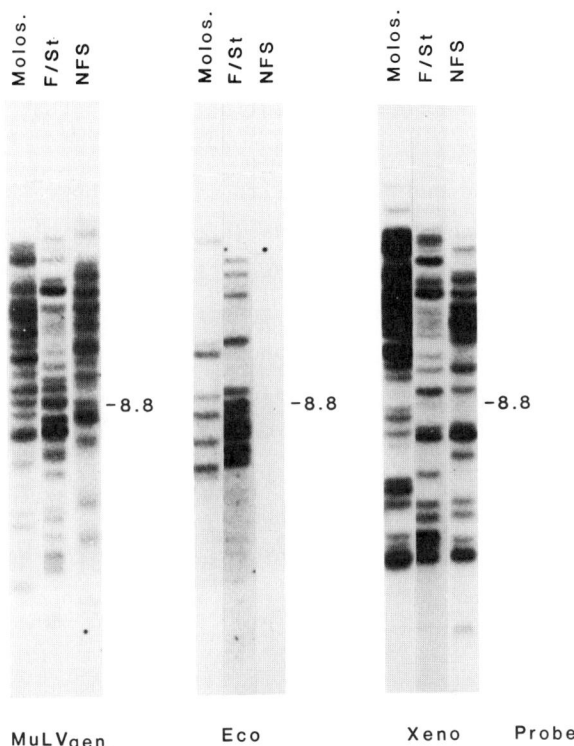

Hind III Digests

Fig. 7. HindIII digests of liver DNA from M. molossinus,
F/St and NFS mice hybridized with probes reactive with all
endogenous proviral sequences (MuLVgen), ecotropic MuLV only
(eco) or xenotropic/MCF MuLV (xeno).

that portions of their genome derived from ecotropic viruses
while other parts came from endogenous nonecotropic viral
sequences. These nonecotropic sequences could be localized to
three regions of the genome: the 5' end of the gp70 region, the
3' end of p15E and the LTRs. Changes in the gp70 region were
found to be responsible for the altered host range characteristics of the MCFs in comparison to ecotropic viruses while changes

in the p15E-LTR region were found to control the leukemogenic
potential of this virus class.

The LTR substitutions have been localized primarily to the
U3 region which contains the 70 bp direct repeats that function
as enhancer sequences as well as the viral promoters.

Studies of Friend and Moloney viruses have shown that repli-
cation-competent Friend helper virus induces erythroleukemias in
NFS mice, whereas Moloney virus induces lymphomas. Recombinants
between these viruses were made to generate a Friend virus that
was substituted with the Moloney genome in the p15 and LTR
regions only. The importance of these regions in leukemogenesis
was shown by the observations that while Friend virus alone produces erythroleukemias, the Friend virus with these small substituted areas gave Moloney-like lymphomas.

In addition to our detailed knowledge of the characteristics
of MuLV structure and function, we have also developed considerable knowledge about how these viruses are controlled in their
expression by host genes (Fig. 8). This scheme broadly outlines
the role of viruses in induction of neoplasia and indicates the
sites at which particular host genes can influence the development of leukemia. The three that I will mention include Fv-1
which restricts the intracellular growth of both ecotropic and
MCF viruses, Fv-4 that completely restricts spread of ecotropic
viruses and Rmcf which controls spread of MCF viruses.

The characteristics of Fv-1 locus are given in Table V.

The classic studies of Lilly, Pincus, Rowe and Hartley showed
that the Fv-1 locus controls the replication of the two forms of
ecotropic virus termed N-tropic and B-tropic. Studies of these
viruses showed that cells from some strains of mice were sensitive to replication of N-tropic virus but not B-tropic virus,
whereas cells from other mice had the opposite sensitivity
pattern. This effect was found to be due to a single codominant
gene on chromosome 4 called Fv-1. The effects of this locus can
be observed both in vivo and in vitro and affect both ecotropic

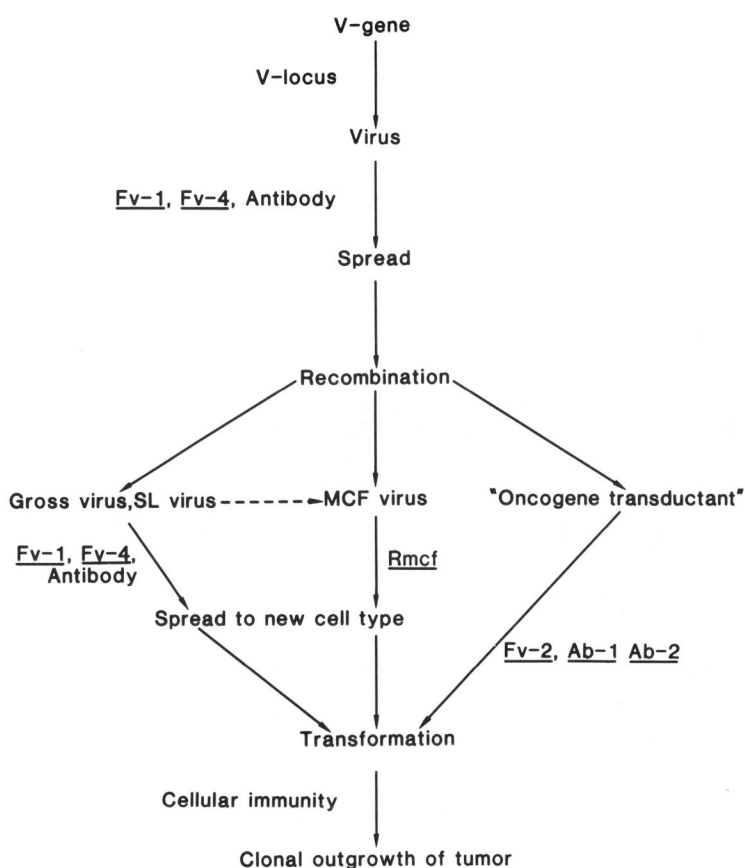

Fig. 8.   Pathogenesis of MuLV infections resulting in
neoplasia.

and MCF viruses. Production of these viruses in mice with the
nonpermissive alleles greatly affects their ability to spread
and thus to participate in the development of neoplasms. The
nature of this effect in cellular terms is incompletely understood but clearly alters the ability of viruses to reinsert in
the genome after they enter the cell.

The Fv-4 locus (Table VI) restricts spread of ecotropic
viruses in an entirely different manner. The dominant

TABLE V.   Characteristics of Fv-1

1. Two types of MuLV: N-tropic and B-tropic

2. $Fv-1^n$ mouse cells are sensitive to N-tropic and rela-
    tively resistant to B-tropic MuLV

3. $Fv-1^b$ mouse cells show the opposite pattern

4. Alleles are codominant for resistant: $Fv-1^{n/b}$ mice are
    resistant to N-tropic and B-tropic MuLV

5. Effects are observed in vitro and in vivo

TABLE VI.   Characteristics of Fv-4 (Akrv-1)

1. Resistance is present in Asian and California wild mice

2. In vivo

    • Restricts spread of endogenous and exogenous ectropic
      virus

    • Resistance is dominant

    • Maps to chromosome 12

3. In vitro

    • Fv-4 mouse cells are relatively resistant (1-2 logs)
      to ecotropic MuLV

    • Sensitivity is dominant

TABLE VII.   Characteristics of Rmcf

---

1. Resistant allele (r) is present in DBA and some CBA
    sublines

2. Rmcf^r cells are relatively resistant (2 logs) to MCF
    virus

3. Resistance is dominant

4. Maps to chromosome 5

5. Rmcf^r strains are relatively resistant to MCF-mediated
    leukemogenesis

---

restrictive allele at this locus leads to receptor blockade such
that ecotropic viruses are unable to enter cells.

This effect was shown to be due to a partial viral genome
that contains an env sequence like that of ecotropic gp70.
Genetic studies showed that mice carrying this new sequence were
completely resistant to infection with ecotropic virus, whereas
those mice that resembled BALB/c were sensitive.

More recently Drs. Hartley and Yetter defined a third
extremely important locus involved in leukemogenesis, the Rmcf
locus. This locus acts to limit the spread of recombinant MCF
viruses.

The characteristics of the Rmcf locus are given in Table
VII.

A large number of other host genes have also been shown to
influence the development of disease caused by MuLV. A partial
list of these genes and their effects are presented in Table
VIII.

In summary our knowledge of MuLV and their biology is possibly better understood than for any other infectious agent. The
genomes of these viruses and the functions of the various portions are known in great detail. In addition, a large variety of
host genes have been described that are permissive or restrictive

TABLE VIII.   Classes of Genes Involved
in the Biology of MuLV

---

1. Loci for induction of virus (Akv-1, Bxv-1) or of viral
    components (Akvp, Gv-1)

2. Loci controlling expression of induction loci (Cxv-1)

3. Genes controlling cell-surface receptors for virus
    (Rec-1, Ram-1, Rmc-1)

4. Genes affecting growth of virus (Fv-1, Rmcf, Fhe)

5. Genes affecting immune responses to virus or virus-
    transformed cells (H-2-linked Ir genes, Rgv-1, Rfv-1)

6. Genes for resistance of cells to transforming defective
    variants (Fv-2, Av-2)

7. Genes modifying the physiology of target cells (Sl, W,
    f)

---

for the production and spread of virus in vivo and which determine if the end result of virus expression will be disease or
lack thereof. Nonetheless, considerable work remains to be done
before we have a comprehensive understanding of how these agents
can contribute to pathology in their host species.

SELECTED REFERENCES

1. "RNA Tumor Viruses. Molecular Biology of Tumor Viruses"
    (R. Weiss, N. Teich, H. Varnus et al., eds.), 1st ed. (1982),
    2nd ed. (1985). Cold Spring Harbor Laboratory, Cold Spring
    Harbor, New York.
2. Morse, H.C., III and Hartley, J.W. (1986). In "Viral and
    Mycoplasmal Infection of Laboratory Rodents: Effects on
    Biomedical Research (P. Bhatt, R. Jacoby, H.C. Morse, III
    et al., eds.). Academic Press, New York.

PATHOGENESIS OF FELINE RETROVIRUS-INDUCED CYTOPATHIC DISEASES: ACQUIRED IMMUNE DEFICIENCY SYNDROME AND APLASTIC ANEMIA

Edward A. Hoover,[1] James I. Mullins,[2]
Sandra L. Quackenbush[1] and Peter W. Gasper[1]

[1]Department of Pathology
Colorado State University
Fort Collins, Colorado

[2]Department of Cancer Biology
Harvard School of Public Health
Boston, Massachusetts

Although less infamous than leukemia, cytosuppressive diseases constitute the major pathologic manifestation of feline leukemia virus (FeLV) infection in cats. The most significant cytopathic diseases caused by FeLV are acquired immune deficiency syndrome (AIDS) and aplastic anemia (AA), diseases which have been recognized in cats for over 15 years (1-6) and which now can be rapidly and consistently reproduced by experimental inoculation of outbred specific pathogen-free (SPF) cats with FeLV (7,8). Prototype pathogenic FeLV strains that induce either feline AIDS (FAIDS) or AA have been identified by serial in vivo passage in SPF cats and recently have been molecularly cloned and shown to possess disease-specific pathogenicity in inoculated SPF cats (9-13; Hoover, E.A., J.I. Mullins, S.L. Quackenbush et al., manuscript submitted). The early pathogenesis of experimental FeLV infection and the specific induction of immunodeficiency syndrome and AA will be discussed in this chapter.

59

FeLV is an exogenous, contagiously transmitted, retrovirus
of domestic cats (14,15). An estimated one million (2%) of the
52 million pet cats in the United States are actively infected
(persistently viremic) with FeLV; over 80% of these cats will
die of FeLV-related disease within 3 years (15). FeLV is a typical replication competent type C retrovirus comprised of gag,
pol and env genes and long terminal repeat regions containing
unique and common regions (10). Three FeLV subgroups (A,B,C)
have been identified by viral interference assays and subgroup-
specific neutralizing antibody and reflect polymorphism in the
gp70 envelope glycoprotein (16,17). Studies of the occurrence of
subgroup viruses in naturally and experimentally infected cats
by Sarma (18) and Jarrett (19,20) have contributed much to our
understanding of the pathobiology of feline retroviruses. FeLV-A,
the most common virus type, replicates only in feline cells and
may occur in combination with subgroup B or C viruses (16,19).
FeLV-A isolates are associated with long periods of relatively
asymptomatic viremia and eventual lymphosarcoma. FeLV-B viruses
always are associated with FeLV-A in nature, have the widest host
range in vitro and are associated with lymphosarcoma, immunodeficiency syndrome and myeloproliferative diseases (18-20).
FeLV-C are least common, always are associated with FeLV-A or A
and B subgroup viruses in nature, replicate in guinea pig as well
as cat cells and induce AA in experimentally infected cats (18,
20-22). Current information suggests that FeLV-C viruses, and
probably other FeLV variants less clearly defined at present, are
generated via recombinational events between FeLV-A and endogenous DNA sequences in feline cells (22).

All naturally occurring pathologic manifestations associated
with FeLV infection can be reproduced experimentally and studied
prospectively in outbred cats. Experimental studies have shown
that the pathogenicity of feline retroviruses is determined by
interplay between virus genotype and host resistance in which
the early containment vs. amplification of viral replication in

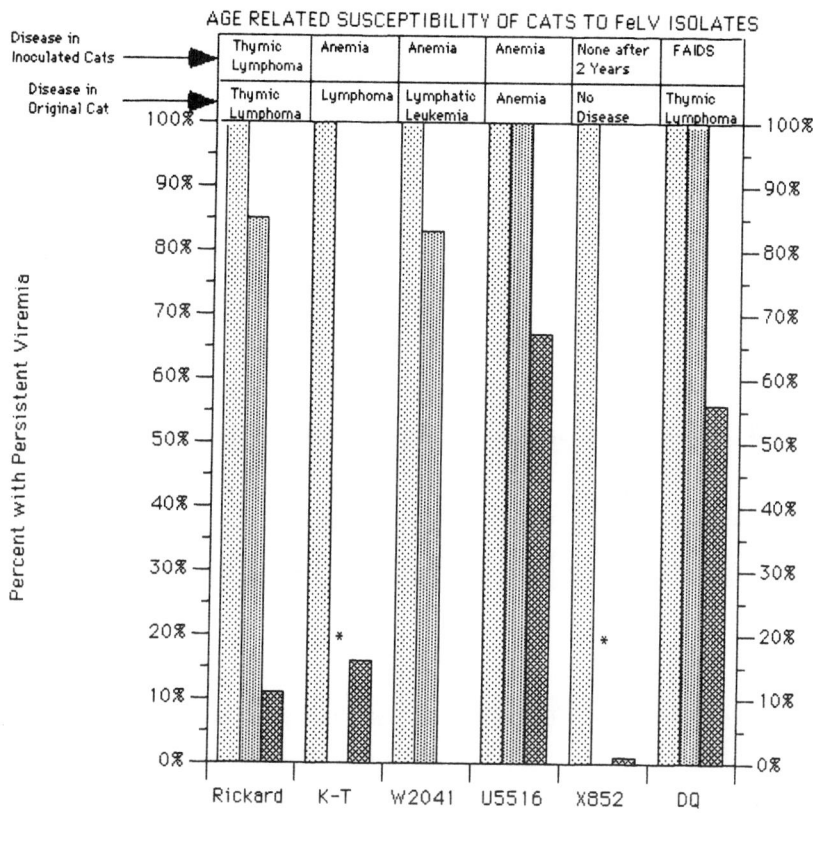

Fig. 1. Age-related susceptibility of cats to FeLV isolates. Schematic summary of experimental studies defining the sequential pathogenesis of progressive FeLV Rickard infection in SPF cats with immunofluorescence for FeLV p27 antigen in paraffin-embedded tissue sections (23). From Hoover et al. In "Feline Leukemia." CRC Press, Boca Raton, Florida, 1980 (8). Age of inoculated cats: ▦ = newborn; ▦ = 8 weeks; ▦ = >4 months. * = not tested.

target hemolymphatic cells is central and pivotal (23,24). The resistance of cats to FeLV is virus strain- and cat age-related (3) (Fig. 1), macrophage-dependent, corticosteroid-sensitive (25,26) and can be modulated experimentally by introducing various cofacts during the early period after virus exposure (8,27).

Within 2 to 6 weeks after virus exposure, either of two major
host/virus relationships evolve in cats infected with FeLV (3,4,
24): 1) progressive infection characterized by persistent viral
replication in lymphoid, hemopoietic and certain mucosal and
glandular epithelial cells, persistent viremia, ineffectual
antiviral immune response and a high incidence of FeLV-related
disease or 2) regressive infection characterized by early cur-
tailment of viral replication in local or systemic hemolymphatic
tissues, abrogation of viremia due to effective antiviral immune
responses, subsequent viral latency of variable duration in bone
marrow cells and a minimal incidence of disease.

The early pathogenesis of progressive feline retrovirus
infection in cats (23) involves sequential virus replication in
1) macrophages in local lymphoid tissues, 2) small numbers of
circulating mononuclear leukocytes, 3) B and T lymphocytes in
systemic lymphoid tissues, 4) bone marrow myeloid, megakaryocytic
and erythroid progenitor cells, 5) circulating leukocytes and
platelets and, finally, 6) mucosal and glandular epithelial cells
with subsequent viral excretion and horizontal transmission
(Fig. 2). Cats which manifest regressive infection curtail viral
replication in the phase of lymphoid or early hemopoietic cell
replication (23,24).

In regressively infected cats in which FeLV replication has
reached the bone marrow prior to containment, FeLV may persist in
a latent state in the marrow. Latent FeLV is controlled by host
immunologic mechanisms in vivo but can be reactivated by in vitro
culture of marrow cells or, less readily, by in vivo treatment of
cats with large doses of corticosteroids over a period of several
weeks (28). The pathologic significance of latent FeLV infection
and the viral subgroups involved remain to be fully elucidated.

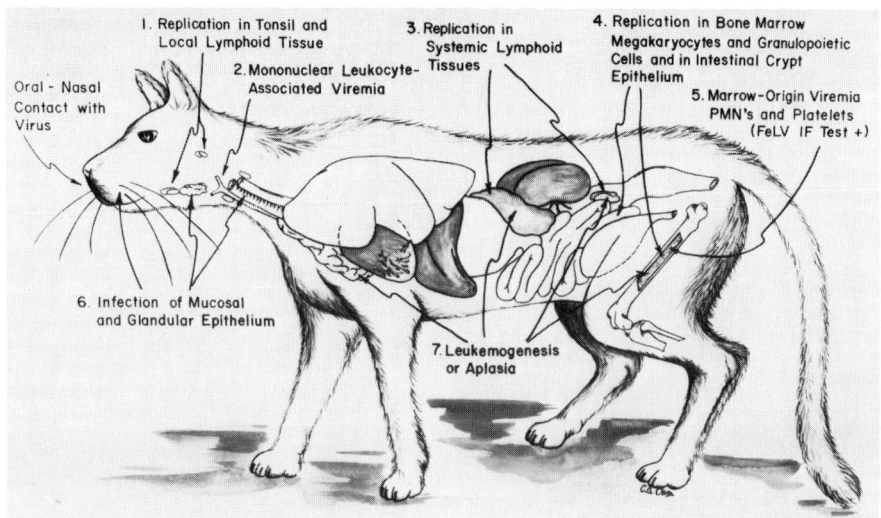

Fig. 2. Pathogenesis of feline leukemia virus infection. Relationship between FeLV isolate and cat age in determining the susceptibility of age-matched SPF cats to induction of persistent viremia (progressive infection) after intraperitoneal inoculation of 5×10^4 to 1×10^5 focus-forming units of each FeLV isolate.

FELINE ACQUIRED IMMUNE DEFICIENCY SYNDROME

Recent studies indicate that FAIDS is induced preferentially by certain variants of FeLV which are associated with and may be related to leukemogenic FeLVs. We have identified a powerfully immunosuppressive isolate of FeLV (FeLV-FAIDS) which induces a lethal AIDS in 100% of viremic cats after intervals of <2 months to >12 months after inoculation (Hoover, E.A., J.I. Mullins, S.L. Quackenbush et al., manuscript submitted) (Table I).

Experimentally induced FAIDS, like the naturally occurring disease, is characterized by persistent viremia, progressive weight loss leading to emaciation, intractable diarrhea, lymphocytosis and elevated lymphocyte blastogenic responses to mitogens followed by lymphopenia and suppressed lymphocyte mitogenic responses, systemic lymphoid hyperplasia followed by severe

TABLE I. Experimental Transmission of Feline Acquired Immune Deficiency Syndrome (FAIDS) in SPF Cats of FeLV

Age of cat when inoculated	Route of inoculation	Virus passage number	Total no. of cats inoculated	No. of cats with persistent viremia	No. with FAIDS	Survival time for viremic cats (days)	Absolute lympho-cytopenia	Suppressed mitogen-induced lymphocyte blastogenesis	Prolonged skin allograft rejection	Lesions induced
Newborn	Intrathymic	I	6	5	5	59 (55-62)[a]	3/3	ND[b]	ND	Thymic-lymphoid depletion, necrotizing enterocolitis
8 weeks	Intraperi-toneal	I, III	10	9	9	81 (25-159)	5/5	5/5[c]	2/2[d]	Thymic-lymphoid depletion or oral-nasal or lymphoid hyperplasia, necrotizing or granulomatous stomatitis, hepatitis, enterocolitis
14 weeks	Oral-nasal	I, II	10	6	6	191 (96-319)	4/4	2/2	ND	Enterocolitis, severe thymic-lymphoid depletion or lymphoid hyperplasia, severe weight loss
23 weeks	Oral-nasal	I	6	3	3	380 (351->425)	3/3	3/3	2/3	Severe weight loss, diarrhea, lymphoid depletion, anemia
1 year	Intraperi-toneal	I	6	0	1[e]	292[e]	1/1	ND	ND	Severe weight loss, lymphoid depletion, thrombocytopenia, petechial hemorrhage

[a]Mean (range).

[b]None done.

[c]Number with significantly decreased responses/total number test (decreased response both total dpm and stimulation index of >2 standard deviations less than control mean).

[d]Number with significantly prolonged graft rejection/total number tested (significantly delayed rejection = 15 days or longer (mean rejection time in central CPF cats = 13.1 ± 1.5 days).

[e]One cat developed FeLV-negative FAIDS, the remaining five cats remained asymptomatic and were not followed beyond 365 days.

lymphoid depletion (Figs. 3 and 4), chronic enteritis and opportunistic infections including oral mycotic infections (thrush).
Prodromal lymphoid hyperplasia in cats inoculated with FeLV-FAIDS
appears to be correlated with intense viral replication in follicular lymphocytes, whereas subsequent lymphoid depletion is
correlated with extinction of viral replication in affected lymphoid tissues (Figs. 5 and 6). FeLV-FAIDS, like other feline
retrovirus strains, replicates extensively in salivary gland,
pharyngeal and esophogeal epithelium and is shed in saliva (Fig.
7). The pathogenesis of experimental FAIDS model is summarized
in Figure 8.

Our current studies of the molecular pathogenic mechanisms
of experimentally induced FAIDS have revealed that after the
onset of persistent FeLV-FAIDS viremia but prior to the onset of
clinical FAIDS, a common form of proviral DNA present as 1 to 2
copies per cell was discernible in bone marrow cells of all
viremic cats (12; Mullins, J.I., C.S.Chen, and E.A. Hoover,
manuscript submitted). Coincident with the onset of the acute
clinical syndrome of FAIDS, both the production of large quantities (>15 copies per cell) and of predominantly unintegrated
viral DNA and the appearance or selective amplification of characteristic FeLV variants, recognizable by acquisition of a new
internal Kpn 1 restriction site generating viral DNA fragments
of 2.1 kb vs. the 3.65 kb fragment common to FeLV isolates, in
bone marrow from five of five cats tested thus far but not in
cats with either thymic lymphosarcoma, AA or myeloproliferative
syndrome induced by experimental infection of SPF cats with three
other characterized strains of FeLV (13). The occurrence of the
unintegrated FeLV-FAIDS variant in bone marrow, therefore,
appears to be both a disease- and tissue-specific marker of
incipient FAIDS and may be an important mechanism of the lympho-
cytopathic activity of feline and human retroviruses (Mullins,
J.I., C.S. Chen, and E.A. Hoover, manuscript submitted).

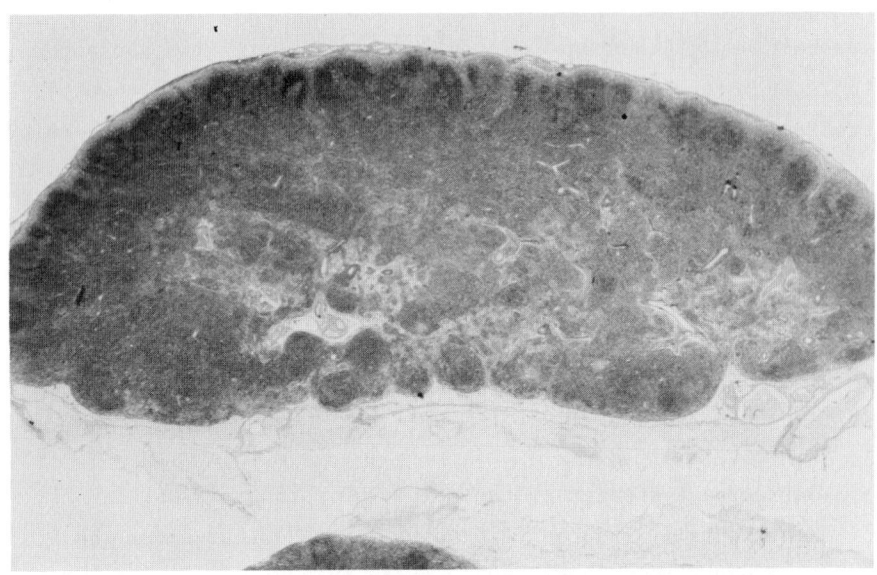

Fig. 3. Normal lymph node from a control SPF cat. Dense cortical and paracortical lymphocyte populations are present (H & E stained histologic section).

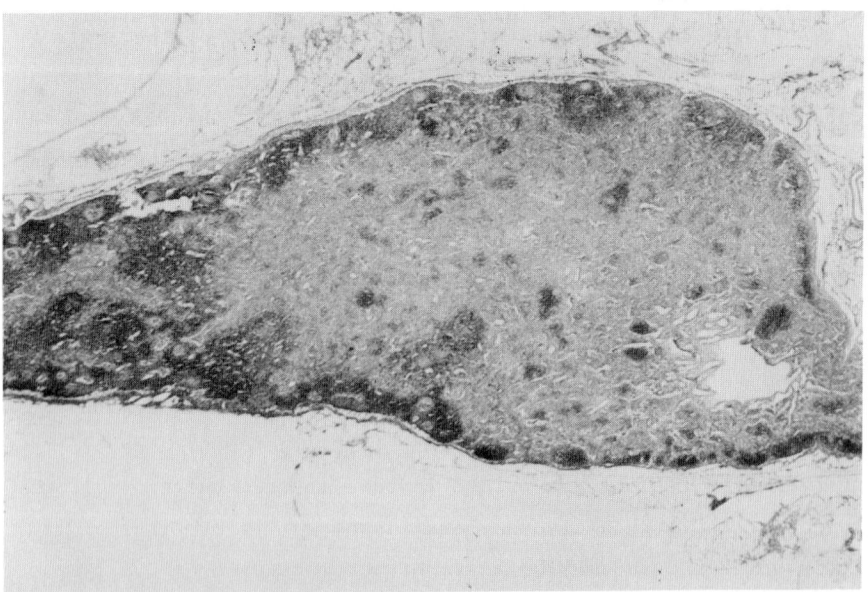

Fig. 4. Lymph node from a cat with advanced experimentally induced FAIDS. Extensive depletion of cortical follicular and paracortical, and medullary lymphocytes.

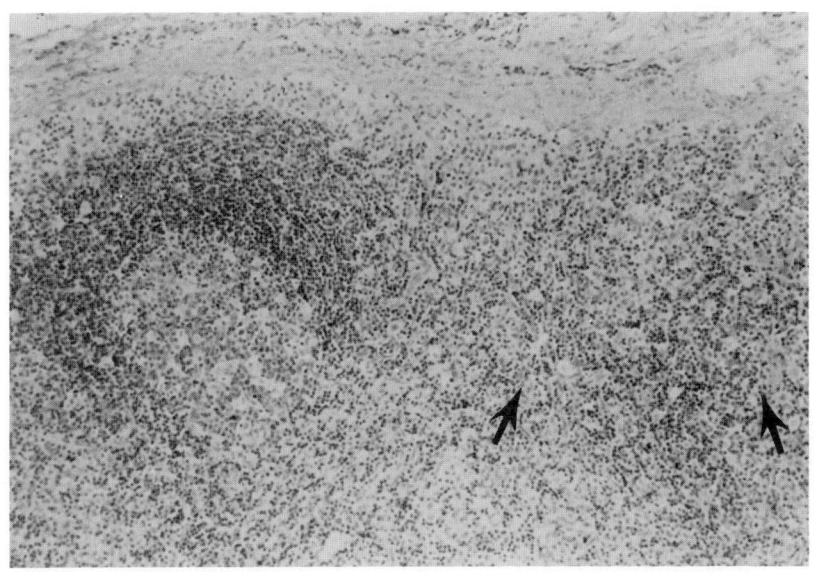

Fig. 5. Development of cortical and paracortical lymphoid depletion in a lymph node from a cat inoculated with FeLV-FAIDS. Region of ablation of one cortical follicle (arrows) is contrasted with adjacent less severely affected follicle zone at left. (Lymph node, H & E stained section).

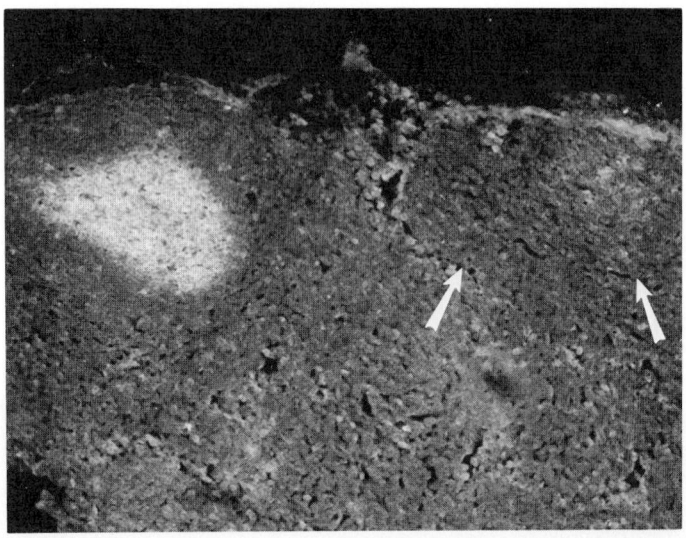

Fig. 6. FeLV-FAIDS replication demonstrated by immunofluorescence (23) in the lymph node from the same cat depicted
in Figure 5. Regional ablation of cortical follicular lymphocytes
correlates with extinction of viral replication in such areas
(arrows), whereas intense viral replication is evident in replete
follicles (at left).

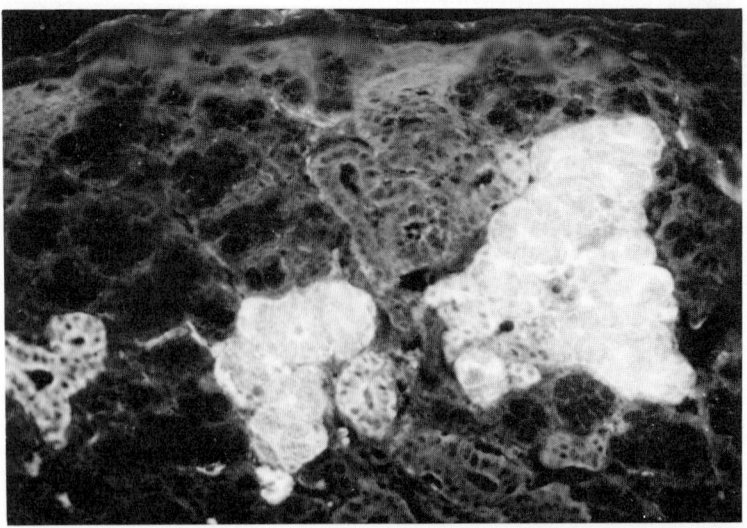

Fig. 7. FAIDS retrovirus replication in the salivary gland
of an experimentally infected cat (immunofluorescence for FeLV
p27 antigen).

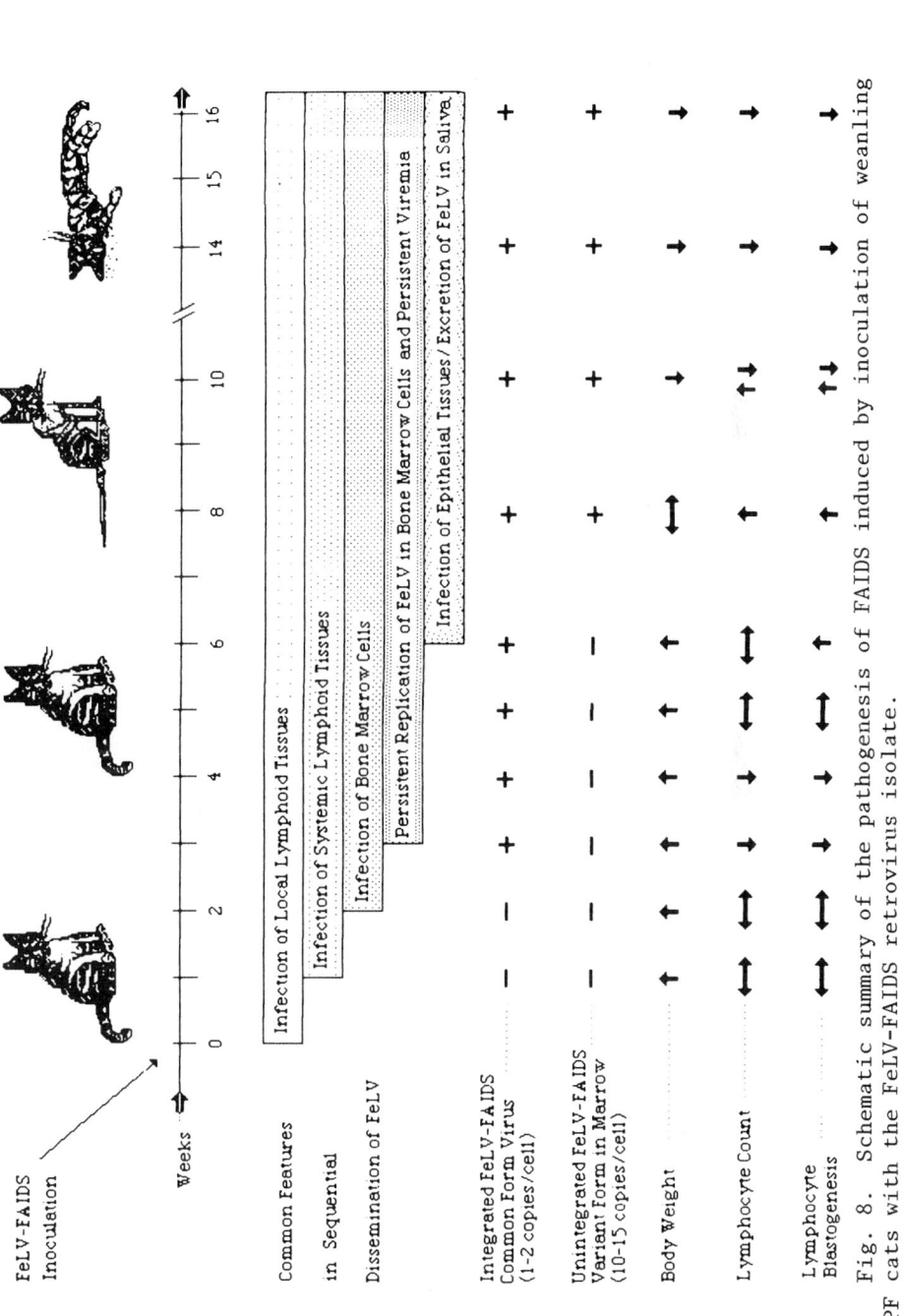

Fig. 8. Schematic summary of the pathogenesis of FAIDS induced by inoculation of weanling SPF cats with the FeLV-FAIDS retrovirus isolate.

Our present work with the experimental FAIDS system is
directed toward identification of the viral genetic elements
responsible for and the pathogenetic mechanisms of retrovirus-
induced immunodeficiency syndrome in cats.

FeLV-INDUCED APLASTIC ANEMIA

AA has been recognized as a major fatal cytosuppressive
disease caused by FeLV for over a decade (5,6). FeLV-induced AA
was transmitted initially by serial passage of FeLV-KT and other
field isolates in newborn cats (3,5,29) and subsequently in cor-
ticosteroid treating weanling and adult cats (30,31). Incubation
period for induction of viremia and progressive marrow aplasia is
4 weeks or less and survival 9 weeks or less in weanling cats
infected with biologically passaged anemogenic isolates such as
FeLV-KT. The studies of Jarrett and colleagues (21,22) have
established that feline AA is induced preferentially by subgroup
C FeLV and suggest that FeLV-C virions represent recombinants,
perhaps generated in bone marrow cells infected with FeLV-A.
Serial analyses of bone marrow cell colony-forming progenitor
cells from cats infected with FeLV-C containing isolates have
demonstrated the most sensitive hemopoietic cell to the erythrosuppressive effect of anemogenic FeLV-C is the burst-forming unit
(BFU-e), the most primitive feline erythroid progenitor cell
detectable by clonigenic assay in semisolid medium cultures (21,
32,33) (Fig. 9). Moreover, the FeLV-C has been molecularly cloned
by Mullins and shown to retain its striking erythrosuppressive
capacity in experimentally infected cats (13; Hoover, E.A., J.I.
Mullins, S.L. Quackenbush et al., manuscript submitted). Marrow
myeloid (granulocyte-macrophage) progenitor cells are depleted in
cats infected with anemogenic FeLV-C; however, this decline lags

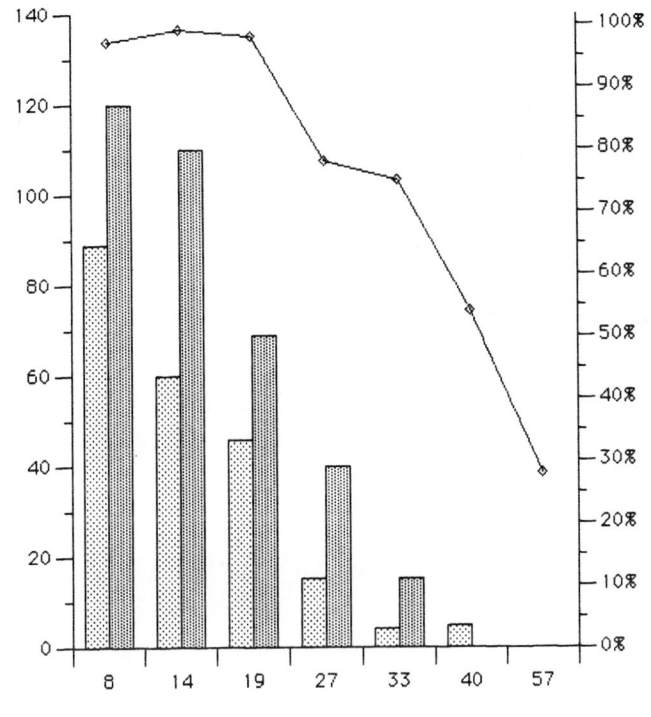

Days Post Inoculation

Fig. 9. Erythroid aplasia induced by experimental FeLV-infection in SPF cats (seven FeLV-KT infected and seven age-matched control cats). Sequential analysis of clonigenic colony-forming hemopoietic progenitor cells in weanling SPF cats inoculated with FeLV-KT demonstrating that early impairment in the burst-forming erythroprogenitor cell population is the primary cytopathic effect produced by anemogenic FeLV-C (32). ▦= BFU-e; ▦ = colony-forming units-erythroid; ◇ = percent cell volume.

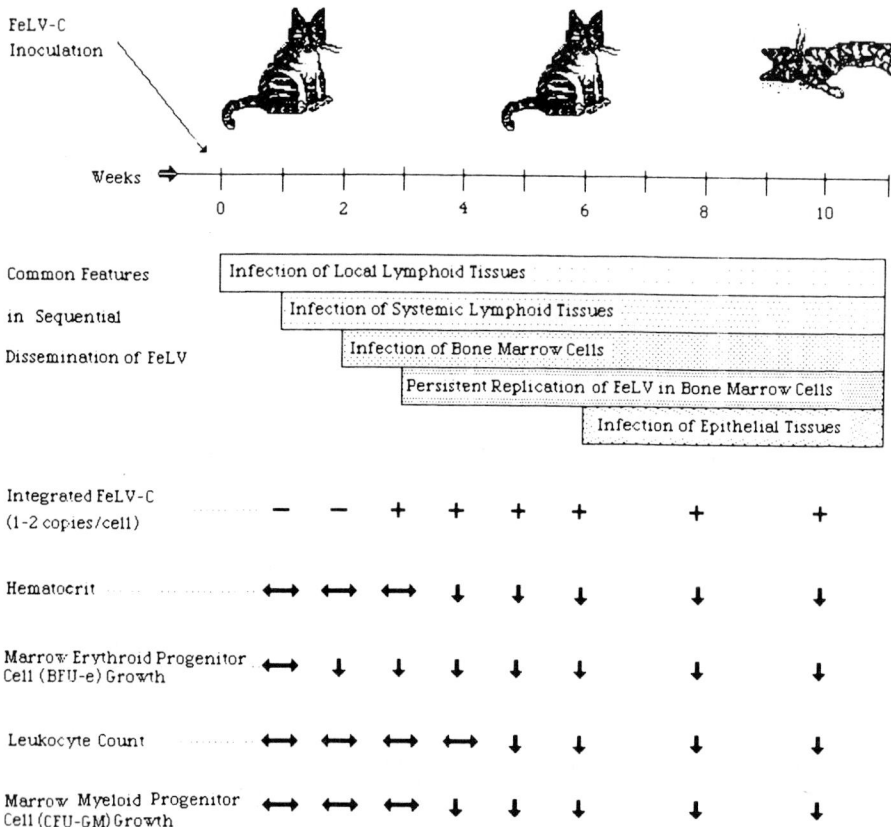

Fig. 10. Schematic summary of the pathogenesis of AA induced by inoculation of weanling SPF cats with anemogenic FeLV-C containing retrovirus isolates.

substantially behind the paralysis of erythrogenesis. The pathogenesis of experimental FeLV-C induced AA is summarized in
Figure 10.

Thus, experimental FeLV-induced AA and AIDS in cats represent
rapid and consistent models of irreversibly fatal cytopathic
retrovirus diseases in which the causative viral genotypes and
the principal cytopathic target cells can be identified and the
molecular pathogenetic mechanisms of selective cytopathicity and
disease can be approached prespectively and intimately.

REFERENCES

1. Anderson, L.J., Jarrett, W.F. and Jarrett, O. (1971).
   J. Natl. Cancer Inst. 47, 817.
2. Mackey, L.J., Jarrett, W.F.H., Jarrett, O. et al. (1972).
   J. Natl. Cancer Inst. 48, 1663.
3. Hoover, E.A., McCullough, B. and Griesemer, R.A. (1972).
   J. Natl. Cancer Inst. 9, 973.
4. Hardy, W.D., Jr., Hess, P.W., MacEwen, E.G. et al. (1976).
   Cancer Res. 36, 582.
5. Hoover, E.A., Kociba, G.J., Hardy, W.D. Jr. et al. (1974).
   J. Natl. Cancer Inst. 53, 1271.
6. Mackey, L., Jarrett, W., Jarrett, O. et al. (1975). J. Natl.
   Cancer Inst. 54, 209.
7. Hoover, E.A., Olsen, R.G., Hardy, W.D., Jr. et al. (1976).
   J. Natl. Cancer Inst. 5, 365.
8. Hoover, E.A., Jojko, J.L. and Olsen, R.G. (1980). In "Feline
   Leukemia" (R.G. Olsen, ed.), p. 32. CRC Press, Boca Raton,
   Florida.
9. Mullins, J.I., Casey, J., Nicolson, M.O. et al. (1980).
   Nucleic Acids Res. 8, 3287.
10. Mullins, J.I., Casey, J.W., Nicolson, M.O. et al. (1981).
    J. Virol. 38, 688.
11. Hoover, E.A. and Mullins, J.I. (1985). In "RNA Tumor Viruses,
    1985." Cold Spring Harbor Laboratory, New York.
12. Mullins, J.I., Hoover, E.A., Overbaugh, J. et al. (1985). In
    "RNA Tumor Viruses, 1985." Cold Spring Harbor Labortory, New
    York.
13. Hoover, E.A., Mullins, J.I. and Gasper, P.W. (1985). In "RNA
    Tumor Viruses, 1985." Cold Spring Harbor Labortory, New York.
14. Jarrett, W.F., Martin, W.B., Crighton, G.W. et al. (1965).
    Nature 202, 566.
15. Hardy, W.D., Jr., Old, L.J., Hess, P.W. et al. (1973).
    Nature, 244, 266.

16. Sarma, P.S. and Log, T. (1973). Virology 54, 160.
17. Jarrett, O., Laird, H.M. and Hay, D. (1973). J. Gen. Virol. 20, 169.
18. Sarma, P.S., Log, T., Skuntz, S. et al. (1978). J. Natl. Cancer Inst. 60, 871.
19. Jarrett, O., Hardy, W.D., Jr., Golder, M.C. et al. (1978). Int. J. Cancer 21, 334.
20. Jarrett, O. and Russel, P.H. (1978). Int. J. Cancer 21, 466.
21. Onions, D.O., Jarrett, O., Testa, N. et al. (1982). Nature 296, 156.
22. Jarrett, O., Goldner, M.C., Toth, S. et al. (1984). Int. J. Cancer 34, 283.
23. Rojko, J.L., Hoover, E.A., Mathes, L.E. et al. (1979). J. Natl. Cancer Inst. 63, 759.
24. Hoover, E.A., Rojko, J.L. and Olsen, R.G. (1980). In "Cold Spring Harbor Conference on Cell Proliferation," vol. 7, p. 86. Cold Spring Harbor, New York.
25. Hoover, E.A., Rojko, J.L., Wilson P.L. et al. (1981). J. Natl. Cancer Inst. 67, 889.
26. Rojko, J.L., Hoover, E.A., Mathes, L.E. et al. (1979). Cancer Res. 38, 3789.
27. Schaller, J.P., Mathes, L.E., Hoover, E.A. et al. (1978). Cancer Res. 38, 996.
28. Rojko, J.L., Hoover, E.A., Quackenbush, S.L. et al. (1982). Nature 298, 385.
29. Boyce, J.T., Hoover, E.A., Kociba, G.J. et al. (1981). Exp. Hematol. 9, 990.
30. Gasper, P.W. and Hoover, E.A. (1983). Exp. Hematol. 14, 153.
31. Kociba, G.J., Hoover, E.A., Sciulli, V.M. et al. (1981). In "Advances in Comparative Leukemia Research, 1981" (D.S. Yohn and J.R. Blakeslees, eds.), p. 211. Elsevier, New York.
32. Gasper, P.W. and Hoover, E.A. (1983). Leuk. Rev. Int. 1, 71.
33. Testa, N.G., Onions, D., Jarrett, O. et al. (1983). Leuk. Res. 7, 103.

FELINE ACQUIRED IMMUNE DEFICIENCY SYNDROME:
A FELINE RETROVIRUS-INDUCED SYNDROME OF PET CATS[1]

William D. Hardy, Jr.

Laboratory of Veterinary Oncology
Memorial Sloan-Kettering Cancer Center
and Sloan-Kettering Division
Graduate School of Medical Sciences
Cornell University
New York, New York

INTRODUCTION

In 1979 a new disease appeared in humans called acquired
immune deficiency syndrome (AIDS) (1,2). This syndrome was clinically very similar to a feline leukemia virus (FeLV)-induced
immunosuppressive syndrome that was first observed in 1969 (3).
The purpose of this chapter is to compare the etiologic and
therapeutic aspects of the human and cat acquired immune deficiency syndromes (see Tables I and II).

AIDS has occurred in over 10,000 patients to date and is
characterized by immunodysfunctions, opportunistic infections
and Kaposi's sarcomas (1,2,4). Most cases occur in homosexual or
bisexual men who are very active sexually, followed by intravenous drug users and Haitian immigrants to this country (1,4-6).

---

[1]Part of this work was funded by NIH grant CA-16599 and
grants from the Cancer Research Institute and the New York State
Department of Health, AIDS Institute.

TABLE I. Comparison of Immune Parameters in AIDS and FAIDS

AIDS	FeLV-FAIDS
1. Cellular Immunity	1. Cellular Immunity
a. Reduction in helper T lymphocytes but normal suppressor T lymphocytes	a. Reduction in numbers and functions of T lymphocytes
b. Lymphopenias common	b. Lymphopenias common
c. Cutaneous anergy	c. Cutaneous anergy
d. Reduced lymphocyte blastogenesis	d. Reduced lymphocyte blastogenesis
2. Humoral Immunity	2. Humoral Immunity
a. Impaired antibody response to	a. Impaired antibody response to
1. Sheep RBCs-low dose	1. New antigens
2. Synthetic polypeptide antigen	2. Hypergammaglobulinemia

Only 27% of the cases have occurred in women and 50% of these were intravenous drug users. However, AIDS occurs about equally in men and women in Zaire, Africa, and there is increasing evidence that AIDS is currently occurring much more frequently in heterosexual men and women in the United States (7,8).

AIDS is characterized by a defect in the cellular immune system. Low lymphocyte counts occur, often less than half the normal count (Table I) (2,4) and the helper T cell (OKT-4) subpopulation is greatly reduced, whereas the killer-suppressor T cell (OKT-8) subpopulation is much less reduced or is normal in numbers (2,4). B lymphocytes are less affected than T cells, although some B cell dysfunctions have been observed. Functional immune responses of lymphocytes are reduced as shown by cutaneous anergy and decreased lymphocyte blastogenesis (2,4).

TABLE II. Comparison of Secondary Intercurrent Disease
in AIDS and FAIDS

AIDS	FeLV-FAIDS
1. Lymphadenopathy	1. Lymphadenopathy
2. Pneumonia--Pneumocystis carinii	2. Pneumonia and upper respiratory diseases
3. Toxoplasmosis, mucosal Candida, Cryptococcosis	3. Toxoplasmosis
4. Skin sores and infections, Kaposi's sarcoma	4. Skin sores and infections
5. Viral diseases--herpesvirus, cytomegalovirus, hepatitis B virus	5. Viral diseases--feline infectious peritonitis

Approximately 60% of AIDS patients develop Pneumocystis
carinii pneumonia (Table II) (2). Other infections occur commonly
in AIDS patients such as herpes simplex virus, cytomegalovirus
and hepatitis B virus, fungi such as Candida and Cryptococcus,
protozoas such as Toxoplasma and bacteria such as the tubercu-
losis bacillus (1,5). Lymphadenopathy occurs in some patients
while most evidence fever, weight loss, fatigue, diarrhea and
general malaise (9). Approximately 90% of AIDS patients die
within 2 years from the time of diagnosis (10).

Epidemiological data suggested an infectious viral etiology
for AIDS (1). Immunosuppressive syndromes, similar to AIDS, have
been observed in mice and cats infected with murine and feline
retroviruses. Because a newly discovered human retrovirus, the
human T cell lymphotropic virus (HTLV-I), induced T cell leukemias that occurred frequently in the Caribbean (11,12) and since
numerous AIDS patients were Haitian immigrants to the United
States (6), several groups investigated the occurrence of HTLV-I

in AIDS patients (13,14). HTLV-I was apparently found in several
patients with AIDS (13,14) and antibody to HTLV-I was detected
in approximately 36% of patients (15) and in 12% of healthy
hemophiliacs (16). Recently, Gallo's group and Montagnier and
his colleagues, discovered a new HTLV subgroup (HTLV-III or
lymphoadenopathy-associated virus [LAV]) in approximately 86% of
AIDS patients (17-20). HTLV-III/LAV has been shown to be antigenically related to, but distinct from, HTLV-I, the isolate
used in previous seroepidemologic studies of AIDS patients (20).
Using HTLV-III, Gallo's group found that 88% of AIDS patients
have antibody to this new serotype of HTLV (19). The higher percent of HTLV-III seropositive AIDS patients in these recent
studies, compared to the previous studies that used HTLV-I, can
be explained by the unique antigens present in the immunosuppressive HTLV-III (20). Using morphologic and molecular biologic
criteria, HTLV-III has recently been shown to be in the subfamily
Lentivirinae of the family Retrovirinae.

Some animal retroviruses are know to cause immunosuppression
(21). In 1960, Old and his coworkers first demonstrated that
Friend murine leukemia virus (MuLV) impairs the ability of
infected mice to produce antibody to sheep erythrocytes (22). A
syndrome similar to human AIDS, termed the FeLV-induced feline
acquired immune deficiency syndrome (FAIDS), occurs in pet cats
infected with a contagiously transmitted feline retrovirus, the
feline leukemia virus (FeLV) (23-25). Many FeLV-infected pet cats
develop marked immunosuppression and subsequently develop various
opportunistic infectious diseases. Like HTLV-I, FeLV induces
mainly T cell leukemias although, more commonly, causes immunosuppression in pet cats and predisposes them to various opportunistic infections (Table III) (23). In fact, many more FeLV-
infected pet cats die of opportunistic infections than die of
lymphosarcoma. FeLV causes thymic atrophy in kittens and, in
adult cats, causes lymphopenias and granuloblastopenias which

TABLE III. Common Opportunistic Infectious Diseases
in FeLV-Infected Cats with FAIDS

Chronic stomatitis and gingivitis

Skin sores and recurrent abscesses

Viral infections: feline infectious peritonitis

Upper respiratory disease and pneumonias

Chronic generalized infections

---

lead to FAIDS (23,26). FeLV-infected cats with FAIDS commonly
develop feline infectious peritonitis, a coronavirus-induced
disease; chronic upper respiratory diseases and pneumonias;
chronic oral ulcers and gingivitis; chronic skin sores and
recurrent abscesses and chronic bacterial septicemias (Table
III) (23,25).

Similar to AIDS patients, many FeLV-infected pet cats develop
immune cell alterations characterized by a drastic reduction in
the numbers of lymphocytes and neutrophils (23) and immune cell
dysfunctions consisting of cutaneous anergy (27), reduced T cell
blastogenesis (28,29) and impaired antibody response to low numbers of sheep RBCs (22) or to a polypeptide synthetic antigen
(Table I) (30).

FELINE LEUKEMIA VIRUS

FeLV is a naturally occurring contagiously transmitted retrovirus of pet cats that causes both neoplastic and non-neoplastic
diseases (Table IV) (24). The virus induces immunity in about 40%
of exposed cats but causes immunosuppression in those cats that
become persistently infected (31).

TABLE IV.   FeLV Lymphoid and Hematopoietic Diseases

Cell type	Neoplastic diseases	Blastopenic diseases
Lymphoid cells	Lymphosarcoma	FAIDS (adults), thymic atrophy (kittens)
Myeloid cells	Granulocytic leukemia	Myeloblastopenia
Erythroid	Erythremic myelosis, erythroleukemia	Erythroblastopenia (nonregenerative anemia), pancytopenia

Virology

FeLV is a chronic leukemogenic retrovirus that induces lymphoid tumors after a long latent period. Chronic leukemia viruses lack oncogenes and induce monoclonal tumors. The FeLV genome contains the gag gene which encodes the internal viral structural proteins, the pol gene which encodes the viral reverse transcriptase and the env gene which encodes the envelope proteins (32). The FeLV envelope consists of two antigens, a major glycoprotein of 70,000 daltons (gp70), and the minor 15,000 dalton protein (p15E) component. There are three subgroups of FeLV (FeLV-A, -B and -C) which are distinguished by their gp70 envelope components (33,34). FeLV-A has been found in all infected pet cats either alone (50%), in combination with FeLV-B (49%) or with FeLV-B and FeLV-C (1%) (35,36). FeLV-B and -C are never found without FeLV-A. Although there is no clear association of any FeLV subgroup with any specific naturally occurring feline disease there may be immunosuppressive strains of FeLV which may be responsible for the immunosuppression observed in many FeLV-infected cats (37,38).

The four internal FeLV structural antigens, p15, p12, p27 and p10 are coded for by the gag gene and are produced in great

TABLE V.   Occurrence of FeLV in Healthy Pet and Stray Cats

Exposure environment	Percent FeLV-infected
Single cat household	
No known exposure to FeLV	1
Stray cats	
Unknown FeLV exposure	1
Multiple cat households	
Not exposed to FeLV	0
Exposed to FeLV	28

excess in the cytoplasm of infected cells. Detection of these antigens can be used to diagnose FeLV infection by an immuno-fluorescent antibody test of antigen containing leukocytes or by detection of soluble antigens in the plasma by an enzyme-linked immunosorbent assay (ELISA) (39,40).

Epidemiology

In multiple cat households, 28% of cats exposed to FeLV-infected cats become persistently, lifelong, infected, whereas 42% become immune and 30% become neither immune nor infected (Table V) (31). However, approximately 1% of cats living in single cat households or as stray cats are infected with FeLV (31). The prognosis for healthy FeLV-infected pet cats is poor. Eighty-three percent of such cats die within 3.5 years, most from the immunosuppressive effects of the virus (41). We have found that 12% of cats used as blood donors or chosen as potential blood donors were infected with FeLV (31). Infected cat plasma contains approximately 10^5 infectious FeLV per ml (42) and, as in humans who develop AIDS after blood transfusion, the spread of FeLV has occurred with as little as 10 ml of infected cat blood (31,42,43).

The transmission of FeLV among pet cats can be prevented by
the use of a test and removal program where all exposed cats are
tested for FeLV and all infected cats are removed (44). This
program can effectively stop the spread of FeLV in multi-cat
households throughout the world. Presently, there are HTLV-III
ELISA antibody test kits available to screen donated blood for
the presence of antibody to HTLV-III to prevent transfusion-
acquired HTLV-III transmission, but a routine viral antigen
diagnostic test for the virus, similar to that for FeLV, is not
presently available.

PATHOGENESIS OF FeLV INFECTION

The major route of FeLV transmission is via the saliva, which
may contain as many as 2×10^6 infectious FeLV per ml (3,43,45).
The virus penetrates the ocular, oral and nasal membranes and
replicates in lymphocytes in the lymph nodes of the head and neck
(46). Most FeLV infected cats became only transiently infected
and reject the virus at this early stage and develop immunity
(31). Twenty-eight percent of exposed cats become persistently
infected, and the virus spreads to the rapidly dividing cells of
the bone marrow where it replicates to high titers in erythroid
and myeloid precursor cells and enters the circulation in
infected leukocytes and as free virus in the plasma.

FeLV DISEASES

FeLV-induced diseases are the leading cause of death from an
infectious agent in pet cats (31). The virus can cause degenerative (blastopenic) or proliferative (neoplastic) diseases involving the cells in which it replicates (Table IV). For example,
thymic atrophy is an FeLV-induced degenerative disease of T
cells, and T cell lymphosarcoma is a neoplastic disease of

lymphocytes. FeLV rarely induces neoplastic diseases of erythroid cells, erythemic myelosis and erythroleukemia, whereas FeLV-induced degenerative erythroid diseases which include several types of anemias (erythroblastosis, erythroblastopenia and pancytopenia) (47,48) are much more common. FeLV also causes fetal abortions and resorptions (31,49).

FeLV-INDUCED FAIDS

Opportunistic Infectious Diseases

In 1969, we first observed the more frequent occurrence of opportunistic infections in FeLV-infected pet cats than in uninfected cats (3). Since then there have been numerous reports of the occurrence of various opportunistic infections occurring in FeLV-infected cats (31,49,50). FeLV-induced blastopenic diseases, such as lymphopenia, granulocytopenia and thymic atrophy, occur frequently in FeLV-infected cats (Table VI) (23). We found that 83% of infected healthy pet cats died within 3.5 years compared to only 16% of healthy uninfected cats living in the same households (41). In this study most of the FeLV-infected pet cats died of opportunistic infections rather than of leukemia. As in humans infected with HLTV-III, FeLV-infected cats may develop a lymphadenopathy syndrome (Fig. 1) before any opportunistic infectious disease occurs. The opportunistic infectious diseases that occur often in infected cats are chronic stomatitis and gingivitis, oral ulcers, recurrent nonhealing skin sores (Fig. 2), recurrent abscesses, various viral infections, upper respiratory diseases and pneumonias and chronic generalized bacterial infections (Fig. 3) (Table III) (23).

TABLE VI.   Immune Diseases and Alterations Induced by FeLV

---

1. Diseases

    a. Lymphoid depletion

       (1) Thymic atrophy--kittens
       (2) Lymphopenias--adults

    b. Myeloid depletion

       (1) Neutropenias-myeloblastopenias

    c. Immune complex glomerulonephritis

2. Immune alterations

    a. Deficient cell-mediated immunity

       (1) Decreased allograft rejection

       (2) Decreased lymphocyte blastogenesis

    b. Deficient antibody-mediated immunity

       (1) Decreased antibody responsiveness

    c. Complement deficiency

Thymic Atrophy

Prenatally or neonatally FeLV-infected kittens often develop
a runting syndrome characterized by retarded growth, opportunistic infections, thymic atrophy, lymphoid depletion and usually
die between 8 to 12 weeks of age from infections (23,26,27,51).
Anderson and her coworkers observed thymic atrophy in 32 of 97
(33%) experimentally infected kittens and we found that 12 of 14
pet kittens with thymic atrophy were infected with FeLV (23,26).

Lymphoid Depletion

As in human AIDS patients, both lymphoid hyperplasia (lymphadenopathy) and lymphoid atrophy occur in FeLV-infected cats (23,
51). In infected cats that do not have intercurrent or secondary
opportunistic infections lymphoid atrophy is the only lesion and

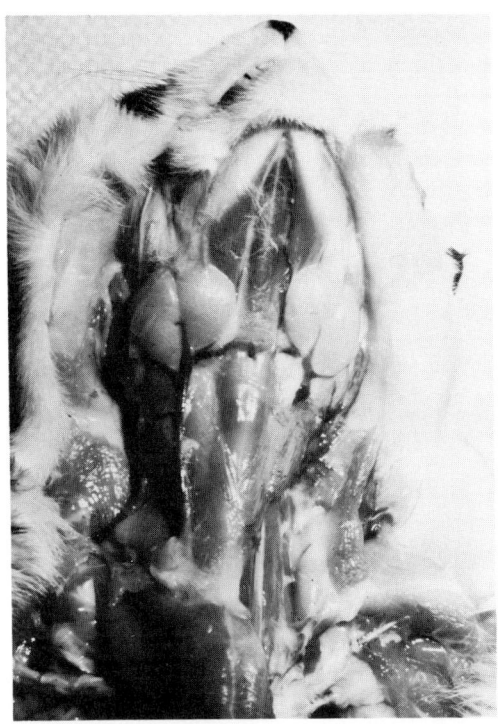

Fig. 1.   Enlarged submandibular lymph nodes in an FeLV-
infected pet cat with lymphadenopathy syndrome.

it is more pronounced in the T cell-dependent paracortical areas
even though there is a marked reduction of lymphocytes in all
areas of the nodes (51). Lymphoid depletion also occurs in
Peyer's patches and some infected cats develop chronic hemorrhagic enteritis which mimics feline distemper (31). Lymphoid
depletion diseases, similar to those observed in pet cats, has
also been observed in cats experimentally infected with FeLV
(26,51). In experimentally infected cats the death rate from
FAIDS is often as high as 50% and can be much more (26).

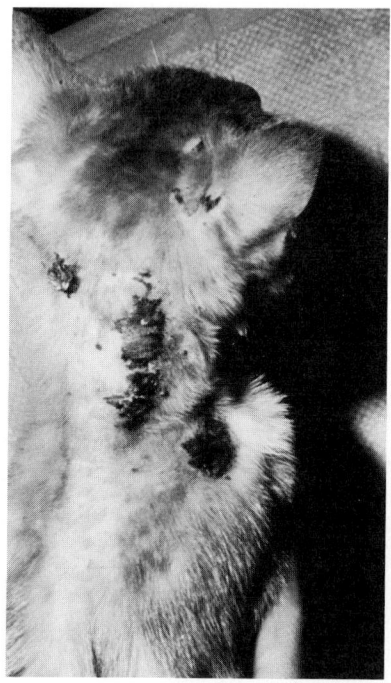

Fig. 2.   Chronic nonhealing skin sores of the neck of an FeLV-infected pet cat with FAIDS.

Neutropenias

FeLV grows well in the bone marrow cells and can induce either neoplastic or degenerative diseases (39). FeLV induces degenerative bone marrow diseases such as anemia, neutropenias or pancytopenias more often than neoplastic diseases (25). In both pet cats and experimentally infected cats, FeLV often causes neutropenias which result in death due to the increased susceptibility to opportunistic infections (23,52). FeLV induces a specific neutrophil disease syndrome called the FeLV-myeloblastopenia syndrome or panleukopenia-like (distemper) syndrome (53). The disease is characterized by a severe leukopenia (300 to 3000 mm^3) and, in some cats, a severe anemia. These cats also

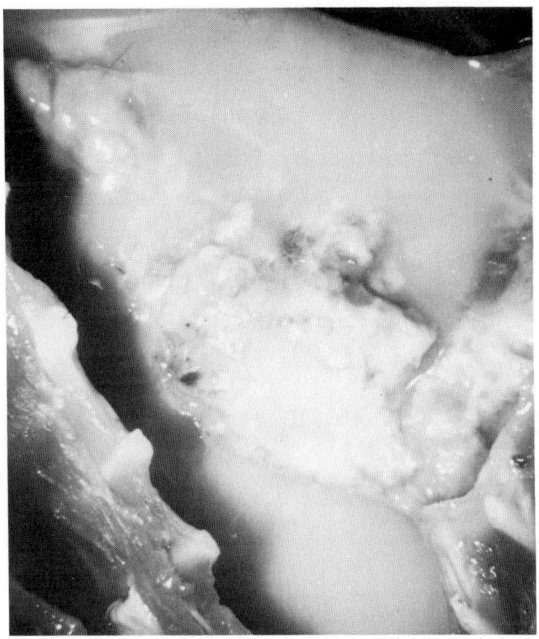

Fig. 3. Pyothorax and generalized septicemia in an FeLV-
infected pet cat with FAIDS.

develop severe gastrointestinal hemorrhaging in the late stages
of this disease and can often die acutely as a result of rapid
excessive blood loss.

T Lymphocyte Dysfunctions

Feline T lymphocytes respond to phytomitogen- and antigen-

induced blast transformation (28). However, unlike most other

animals, it is difficult to induce gross delayed hypersensitiv-

ity reactions to an intradermal antigen in cats (54,55). FeLV-

infected specific pathogen-free (SPF) kittens retained their skin

allografts longer than the uninfected control kittens indicating

a cutaneous anergy T cell dysfunction (27,28). Infected kittens

in this study also developed thymic atrophy signifying a gener-

alized T cell defect. FeLV may cause immunosuppression not only

by reducing the number of immune cells but by altering or
depressing their functional abilities (Table VI). Serum from most
FeLV-infected cats causes a 40 to 70% reduction in the mean lymphocyte blastogenic response to concanavalin A (29). An FeLV
envelope protein, p15E, present in FeLV-infected cat serum, is
responsible for this in vitro T cell depression (29,56). FeLV
p15E, but not the major viral structural protein p27, decreases
blast transformation by 45 to 92% (56). Thus a soluble FeLV protein, p15E, present in infected cat serum may be one factor
responsible for in vivo T cell immune dysfunctions.

B Lymphocyte Dysfunctions

MuLV-infected mice can produce antibody as well as uninfected
mice when the dose of the antigen is high but do not produce
antibody as well if the dose of antigen is low or near threshold
levels (21,57). This indicates a possible defect of the helper T
lymphocytes or macrophages in the infected mice (58).

The B cell response of FeLV-infected SPF and pet cats has
been evaluated using sheep RBCs, panleukopenia virus vaccine and
a synthetic polypeptide antigen as immunogens (23,27,30,59). Both
FeLV-infected SPF and pet cats are able to produce antibody to
large doses of sheep RBCs (23,27,59). Thus, we decided to determine if FeLV-infected pet cats were able to produce antibody to
low or threshold doses of sheep RBCs. We found that FeLV-infected
pet cats are less able (fourfold) to produce antibody to low numbers of sheep RBCs than uninfected cats and two of the five
infected cats (40%) were completely unresponsive. A similar study
of the humoral response of cats was done using the synthetic
multichain polypeptide (L-tyrosine-L-glutamic acid)-poly-DL-
alanine-poly-L-lysine, denoted (T,G)AL (30). The FeLV-infected
healthy cats were shown to have a markedly depressed humoral
response compared to six uninfected healthy pet cats from similar
households. These studies show that many FeLV-infected healthy

pet cats have B cell dysfunctions and this may be one reason for the high occurrence of opportunistic diseases in these cats. Similar B cell hyporeactivity has been found in human AIDS patients.

FeLV Circulating Immune Complexes

It is well known that circulating immune complexes (CICs) can cause immunosuppression. The life-long FeLV viremia in infected pet cats provides ideal conditions for the development of CICs. As many as 8×10^5 whole infectious FeLV per ml are present in the sera of viremic cats (43). In addition, FeLV structural antigens (FeLV gp70, p15E, p27, p15, p12 and p10) that become solubilized as a result of viral or infected cell lysis are present in infected cat serum (23). Six of 12 infected pet cats that we studied had CICs consisting of whole infectious FeLV complexed with cat anti-FeLV IgG (23,60). Day and her coworkers found that the CIC levels in nine FeLV-infected healthy cats were significantly higher than in 32 uninfected control cats (61). Snyder and his coworkers found that the CICs obtained from the plasma of three infected cats were composed of IgG heavy and light chains and FeLV gp70, p27, p15 and p12 (62).

Therapeutic Removal of Circulating Immune Complexes

CICs may act as specific blocking factors and inhibit the immune response (63). Jones and his coworkers were able to reverse the FeLV infection in some of cats by therapeutically removing FeLV CICs using ex vivo immunosorption on Staphylococcus aureus Cowan I columns (64,65). There was an enhanced antibody response to FeLV gp70 and free antibodies to gp70 appeared in the sera of cats that cleared their FeLV infection (66). Therapeutic removal of CICs may also be beneficial for human AIDS patients.

Mechanism of FeLV-Induced Immunosuppression

The mechanism by which FeLV induces immunosuppression is not fully understood. FeLV may lyse the cells in which it replicates such as lymphocytes, macrophages and neutrophils. The virus may also depress immune cell functions. In this regard, the p15E of the FeLV envelope has been shown to abrogate feline lymphocyte blastogenesis in vitro (56). In addition, FeLV CICs have been shown to occur in persistently infected cats and it is well known that CICs are immunosuppressive (61,62). Thus, the chronic viremia that occurs in FeLV-infected cats may cause immunosuppression by one or a combination of several mechanisms. FeLV-infected pet cats, specifically those with FAIDS, are an important naturally occurring animal model in which to study the mechanism of retroviral-induced immunosuppression and experimental therapy.

ACKNOWLEDGMENT

The author thanks Evelyn Zuckerman and Rachelle Markovich for excellent technical assistance.

REFERENCES

1. Center for Disease Control. (1982). N. Engl. J. Med. 106, 248.
2. Masur, H., Michelis, M.A., Greene, J.B. et al. (1981). N. Engl. J. Med. 305, 1431.
3. Hardy, W.D., Jr., Geering, G., Old, L.J. et al. (1969). Science 166, 1019.
4. Gottlieb, M., Schroff, R., Schanker, H.M. et al. (1981). N. Engl. J. Med. 305, 1425.
5. Mildvan, D., Mathur, V., Enlow, R.E. et al. (1982). Ann. Intern. Med. 96, 700.
6. Vieira, J., Frank, E., Spira, T.J. et al. (1983). N. Engl. J. Med. 308, 125.
7. Piot, P., Taelman, H., Minlangu, K.B. et al. (1984). Lancet 2, 65.

8. Brun-Vezinet, F., Rouzioux, C., Montagnier, L. et al. (1984). Science 226, 453.
9. Groopman, J.E., Salahuddin, S.Z., Sarngadharan, M.G. et al. (1984). Science 226, 447.
10. Mildvan, D., Mathur, U., Enlow, R. et al. (1982). MMWR 31, 249.
11. Catovsky, D., Greaves, M.F., Rose, M. et al. (1982). Lancet 1, 639.
12. Blattner, W.A., Kalyanaraman, V.S., Robert-Guroff, M. et al. (1982). Int. J. Cancer 30, 257.
13. Gallo, R.C., Sarin, P.S., Gelmann, E.P. et al. (1983). Science 220, 865.
14. Gelmann, E.P., Popovic, M., Blayney, D. et al. (1983). Science 220, 862.
15. Essex, M., McLane, M.F., Lee, T.H. (1983). Science 220, 859.
16. Essex, M., McLane, M.F., Lee, T.H. (1983). Science 221, 1061.
17. Popovic, M., Sarngadharan, M.G., Read, E. et al. (1984). Science 224, 497.
18. Gallo, R.C., Salahuddin, S.Z., Popovic, M. et al. (1984). Science 224, 500.
19. Sarngadharan, M.G., Popovic, M., Bruch, L. et al. (1984). Science 224, 506.
20. Schupbach, J., Popovic, M., Gilden, R.V. (1984). Science 224, 503.
21. Dent, P.B. (1972). Prog. Med. Virol. 14, 1.
22. Old, L.J., Clarke, D.A., Benacerraf, B. et al. (1960). Ann. NY Acad. Sci. 88, 264.
23. Hardy, W.D., Jr. (1982). In "Springer Semin. Immunopathol." (G. Klein, ed.), p. 75. Springer-Verlag, New York.
24. Hardy, W.D., Jr., Old, L.J., Hess, P.W. et al. (1973). Nature 244, 266.
25. Hardy, W.D., Jr. (1981). J. Am. Animal Hosp. Assoc. 17, 941.
26. Anderson, L.J., Jarrett, W.F.H., Jarrett, O. et al. (1971). J. Natl. Cancer Inst. 47, 807.
27. Perryman, L.E., Hoover, E.A. and Yohn, D.S. (1972). J. Natl. Cancer Inst. 49, 1357.
28. Cockerell, G.L., Hoover, E.A., Krakowka, S. et al. (1976). J. Natl. Cancer Inst. 57, 1095.
29. Cockerell, G.L. and Hoover, E.A. (1977). Cancer Res. 37, 3985.
30. Trainin, Z., Wernicke, D., Ungar-Waron, H. et al. (1983). Science 220, 858.
31. Hardy, W.D., Jr. (1980). In "Feline Leukemia Virus" (W.D. Hardy, Jr., M. Essex and A.J. McClelland, eds.), p. 33. Elsevier, North Holland.
32. Coffin, J. (1982). "RNA Tumor Viruses," 2nd Ed. (R. Weiss, N. Teich, H. Varmus, and J. Coffin, eds.), p. 261. Cold Spring Harbor Laboratory, New York.
33. Sarma, P.S. and Log, T. (1973). Virology 54, 160.

34. Jarrett, O., Laird, M. and Hay, D. (1973). J. Gen. Virol.
    20, 169.
35. Hardy, W.D., Jr., Hess, P.W., MacEwen, E.G. et al. (1976).
    Cancer Res. 36, 582.
36. Jarrett, O., Hardy, W.D., Jr., Golden, M.C. et al. (1978).
    Int. J. Cancer 21, 334.
37. Mackey, L.J., Jarrett, W., Jarrett, O. et al. (1975).
    J. Natl. Cancer Inst. 54, 209.
38. Onions, D., Jarrett, O., Testa, N. et al. (1982). Nature 296,
    156.
39. Hardy, W.D., Jr., Hirshaut, Y. and Hess, P. (1973). In
    "Unifying Concepts of Leukemia" (R.M. Dutcher and L. Chieco-
    Bianchi, eds.), p. 778. Karger, Basel.
40. Kahn, D.E., Mia, A.S. and Tierney, M.M. (1980). Feline Pract.
    10, 41.
41. McClelland, A.J., Hardy, W.D., Jr. and Zuckerman, E.E.
    (1980). In "Feline Leukemia Virus" (W.D. Hardy, Jr.,
    M. Essex and A.J. McClelland, eds.), p. 121. Elsevier, North
    Holland.
42. Francis, D.P., Essex, M. and Hardy, W.D., Jr. (1977). Nature
    269, 252.
43. Jaffe, H.W., Francis, D.P., McLane, M.F. et al. (1984).
    Science 223, 1309.
44. Hardy, W.D., Jr., McClelland, A.J., Zuckerman, E.E. et al.
    (1976). Nature 263, 326.
45. Gardner, M.B., Rongey, R.W., Johnson, E.Y. et al. (1971).
    J. Natl. Cancer Inst. 47, 561.
46. Rojko, J.L., Hoover, E.A., Mathes, L.E. et al. (1979).
    J. Natl. Cancer Inst. 63, 759.
47. Herz, A., Theilen, G.H., Schalm, O.W. et al. (1970). J. Natl.
    Cancer Inst. 44, 339.
48. Hoover, E.A., Kociba, G.J., Hardy, W.D., Jr. et al. (1974).
    J. Natl. Cancer Inst. 53, 1271.
49. Cotter, S.M., Hardy, W.D., Jr. and Essex, M. (1975). J. Am.
    Vet. Med. Assoc. 166, 449.
50. Essex, M., Hardy, W.D., Jr., Cotter, S.M. et al. (1975). In
    "Comparative Leukemia Research 1973" (Y. Ito and
    R.M. Dutcher, eds.), p. 483. Karger, Basel.
51. Hoover, E.A., Perryman, L.E. and Kociba, G.J. (1973). Cancer
    Res. 33, 145.
52. Hoover, E.A., Rojko, J.L. and Olsen, R.G. (1980). In "Viruses
    in Naturally Occurring Cancers" (M. Essex, G. Todaro and
    H. zurHausen, eds.), p. 635. Cold Spring Harbor Laboratory,
    Cold Spring Harbor, New York.
53. Hardy, W.D., Jr. and McClelland, A.J. (1977). Vet. Clin.
    North Am. 7, 93.
54. McCusker, H.B. and Aitken, I.D. (1967). Res. Vet. Sci. 8,
    265.
55. Aitken, I.D. and McCusker, H.B. (1969). Res. Vet. Sci. 10,
    208.

56. Mathes, L.E., Olsen, R.G., Hebebrand, L.C. (1978). Nature 274, 687.
57. Wedderburn, N. and Salaman, M.H. (1968). Immunology 15, 439.
58. Rose, N.R., Milgrom, F. and van Oss, C.J. (1979). In "Principles of Immunology," 2nd Ed., p. 3. MacMillan Publishing Co., New York.
59. Essex, M., Hardy, W.D., Jr., Cotter, S.M. et al. (1975). Infect. Immun. 11, 470.
60. Notkins, A.L., Mahar, S., Scheele, C. et al. (1966). J. Exp. Med. 124, 81.
61. Day, N.K., O'Reilly-Felice, C., Hardy, W.D., Jr. et al. (1980). J. Immunol. 126, 2363.
62. Snyder, H.W., Jr., Jones, F.R., Day, N.K. et al. (1982). J. Immunol. 128, 2726.
63. Sjogren, H.O., Hellstrom, I., Bansal, S.C. et al. (1971). Proc. Natl. Acad. Sci. 68, 1372.
64. Jones, F.R., Yoshida, L.H., Ladiges, W.C. et al. (1980). Cancer 46, 675.
65. Jones, F.R., Yoshida, L.H., Ladiges, W.C. et al. (1980). In "Feline Leukemia Virus" (W.D. Hardy, Jr., M. Essex and A.J. McClelland, eds.), p. 235. Elsevier, North Holland.
66. Snyder, H.W., Jr., Singhal, M.C., Hardy, W.D., Jr. et al. (1984). J. Immunol. 132, 1538.

VIROLOGY OF EQUINE RETROVIRUSES

C. J. Issel[1]
R. C. Montelaro[2]
L. D. Foil[3]

[1]Department of Veterinary Science,
[2]Biochemistry and [3]Entomology
Louisiana State University,
Baton Rouge, Louisiana

Two equine retroviruses have been recognized. One, characterized by investigators at Washington State University, has been
associated with equine sarcoids (1). This virus is separate and
distinct from, in my opinion, the more important equine retrovirus, equine infectious anemia virus (EIAV). This chapter will
be limited to a discussion of EIAV.

In the early 1900s, EIA was shown to be caused by a filterable animal virus (2). The early studies with EIAV did not, of
course, demonstrate its retrovirus character, but they demonstrated that the agent was found in the blood stream of infected
horses for long periods of time, probably for the life of the
individual, and the transfer of blood was the usual means by
which EIAV was transmitted. In the 1960s, studies were expanded
by Japanese scientists who analyzed the basic biology of the
virus (3). The major limitation in working with EIAV, even today,
is the difficulty in its cultivation. This is done usually by
either harvesting and culturing macrophages from infected horses
or harvesting macrophages from uninfected individuals which will
show cytopathic effects after EIAV is added. These cultures are

95

helpful if the donor horse happens to be free of the endogenous
equine herpes virus type 2 (EHV-2), and if a serum source can be
found which can effectively supplement the macrophage cultures.
It has been very difficult to obtain cultures and to maintain
donor horses that are free of EHV-2, and many laboratories have
not identified suitable serum donors to maintain good cultures.

The Japanese scientists also demonstrated in their studies
that various EIAV strains shared common antigens (4) and that
antigenic variation occurred with EIAV in chronically infected
horses (5). At about the same time, Dr. Leroy Coggins purified
antigens from the spleens of infected horses and used these antigens in agar gel immunodiffusion tests to accurately demonstrate
antibodies in naturally infected horses (6,7). The Japanese produced a vaccine that would protect against homologous virus challenge but would not usually protect horses challenged with a different serologic type of virus (8,9). As a result of these vaccine studies and the development of the immunodiffusion test
(thought to be a reliable indicator of natural exposure to EIAV),
research on EIAV in this country and in most other areas of the
world was pretty much terminated. An effective vaccine was not
immediately forthcoming, and a definitive serologic test to identify infected horses in nature was available. It was thought that
the spread of this virus could be controlled through local eradication within breeds or within defined geographic areas. Unfortunately, in many areas of the world and in certain areas of the
United States, the infection rate is too high for these types of
controls to be effectively applied (10).

Fortunately, our research team was organized just when most
other investigators had "quit" EIA. We have pursued EIA as a mul-
tidisciplinary venture and we are actively involved in both basic
and applied studies on EIAV. We are making substantial inroads
into understanding the nature of the virus-host-vector interactions, especially the antigenic variation.

Like many retrovirus infections, most infections with EIAV
are inapparent, i.e., the infected horse shows no outward signs
of disease, but his blood contains infective virus, a percentage
of which is in the form of infectious immune complexes (11). Once
these infected horses mount detectable immune responses, they are
thought to remain positive in the immunodiffusion test for life.
They are persistent virus carriers but the level of viremia is
quite variable. Horses most likely to have virus free in the
plasma (up to 10^6 infectious doses/ml) are those with acute EIA
or acute exacerbations in the chronic form of the disease. The
inapparent carrier, on the other hand, usually does not have
virus free in the plasma and may not even have one dose of virus
in 250 ml of blood (12). The chronic form of the disease is most
frequently diagnosed and is cyclic in nature. The cycles of fever
and associated disease are correlated with the release of virus
into the plasma. Antigenic variation of EIAV is thought to
account for these chronic bouts and immunopathology may be of
some importance. Clinical signs associated with chronic EIA
include severe depression, dependent edema, marked anemia, low
platelet counts and chronic weight loss.

The pathogenic mechanisms accounting for the anemia may be
diverse. For example, complement has been shown to coat erythrocytes in EIA probably as a consequence of viral attachment to red
blood cells (13,14). These virus-erythrocyte mixtures could then
be complexed with antibody and subsequently activate the normal
complement cascade. The erythrocytes coated with complement are
more fragile than normal and are more readily phagocytosed (15).
It is also possible that the oligosaccharides on the surface of
the erythrocytes may be similar to oligosaccharides on the surface of EIAV. Through a cross reaction, the EIAV may actually
stimulate immune factors against the red blood cell fraction.

A model proposed by Dr. Kono suggested that the antigenic
variation of EIAV was driven by immune pressures (5). When

infected with virus 1, the horse mounts immune responses to that
virus. Antibodies to the major group specific core protein, p26,
are detectable by an immunodiffusion test. The immune responses
include the production of type-specific neutralizing antibodies
which play a role in controlling virus multiplication. When
immune pressures bring the multiplication of virus 1 under control, novel antigenic variants can emerge and these can spread
and initate an acute attack. These are subsequently brought under
control by immune reactions involving neutralizing antibody and
cell-mediated immune responses (16,17). Again the mutant is
brought under control and then another variant emerges and the
cycle continues. It is quite possible for an individual horse to
have six or more febrile attacks over a 6 to 8 month period, each
attack being associated with a different antigenic variant
(5,18).

With that brief introduction to EIA, I would like to address
the topic of EIAV transmission. Since all infected horses harbor
virus in their blood stream, anything which transfers blood from
one individual to another can transfer the infection. Understanding the mechanical transmission of EIAV by blood-feeding insects
may be of extreme importance when AIDS viruses are documented to
be vector transmitted.

Man may be the best vector of EIAV in many cases, but in the
absence of human intervention EIAV is effectively transmitted
in a mechanical fashion by blood-feeding insects. During acute
disease or during periods of fever in the chronic form, a horsefly can very effectively transfer the virus, whereas mosquitoes
are very poor vectors (19). There have been some reports of
transplacental transfer, which would be expected with greater
frequency if the mare has acute disease or an exacerbation of
the chronic form during pregnancy (20). Neonatal infections are
usually severe and most transplacental transfers probably result
in abortion of the infected fetus. Venereal transfer is possible

since semen can contain EIAV especially if collected during an
acute episode, but no one has definitively shown that virus can
be transferred to healthy mares in this manner. Venereal transfer may require local trauma allowing semen to come in contact
with white blood cells. Contact transfer is also possible,
because acutely infected horses have virus in their secretions
and excretions (21). It is unlikely that contact transmission is
important in nature because it is very difficult to transmit EIAV
even if you tether an infected and an uninfected animal side by
side for prolonged periods during an acute episode.

We have studied vector transmission of EIAV with focus on the
mechanical transmission by tabanid species. The horsefly burden
on horses can be extensive. Thousands may feed on an individual
over a 24 hour period, exacting a remarkable blood loss not to
mention the stress induced by the painful bites. We have examined
vector biology in relation to EIAV transmission in a number of
ways. One way is to find out how far horses have to be separated
in the field in order to effectively break transmission. This has
been accomplished by using water-based paints to mark flies that
are feeding on four different horses at various distances (22).
The flies are then mechanically interrupted in their feeding and
released one foot from the host. The number of flies with different paint colors that return to individual horses are then monitored. If horses are separated by 120 feet, about 90% of the
horseflies will return to the original host. With 160 feet separation, over 99% of the flies would be expected to return to the
original host. States that have regulations concerning the identification and segregation of infected horses really need these
data to design effective control programs. A 200 yard segregation
is considered sufficient by most officials and our data confirm
it as effective. Another variable that affects transmission is
the host susceptibility or attractiveness to the vectors. We have
observed that while epidemics of EIA in adult sentinel horses

were in progress, foals of infected mares remained uninfected
(23). The tabanid (horsefly) burden of the foal is observed to be
lower than that of the mare, and the foals remained unattractive
to horseflies even when moved from the mare (24). In contrast,
a Shetland pony of similar size to the foal becomes much more
attractive to flies as it moves farther away from the adult
horse. The foal is apparently not perceived as an attractive host
for the horsefly and factors such as this are probably very significant in natural EIAV transmission.

EIA virus has a reverse transcriptase which prefers Mg^{++}
(25). The virus matures by budding from cytoplasmic membranes,
both into cytoplasmic vacuoles and extracellularly (26). A DNA
provirus is established and in culture, multiple copies of provirus are found in persistently infected cells (27). To date,
EIAV provirus has not been found in cells from uninfected horses
and we do not think endogenous EIAV sequences are present in
equine DNA. The virus is morphologically identical to the AIDS
virus (28,29). It contains 60S to 70S RNA composed of subunits
(30). It has a characteristic polypeptide composition analogous
to the polypeptides of other oncoviruses (31,32). As far as we
know, it is serologically unrelated to the other oncoviruses or
lentiviruses although data from Dr. Luc Montagnier's laboratory
show some serologic crossreactivity between EIA antiserum and the
AIDS virus major core protein (29).

The unique feature of EIA is the persistent nature of the
infection involving recurrent clinical symptoms and viremia,
i.e., the chronic form of the disease. To approach the molecular
basis of chronic EIA we have utilized a cell-adapted strain of
EIAV. This work expanded dramatically when we obtained the strain
of EIAV that Dr. Malmquist at the National Animal Disease Center
adapted for growth in equine dermal cell cultures (33). This
Wyoming strain was adapted through passage in equine macrophages,
fetal equine spleen cells and then in fetal equine dermal cells.

The virus can also be propagated in equine kidney cells and in
all equine fibroblastic cells tested to date (34). This virus
replicates in canine, feline and some mink cells, but produces no
cytopathology in these or in the equine cell cultures. We have,
however, observed cytopathology in fetal donkey dermal cells
infected with the cell-adapted strain of virus (McManus, J.J.,
Issel, C.J., Allgood, T. et al., manuscript submitted).

We have extensively characterized this isolate of EIAV but
know very little about wild strains of EIAV because of the
inability to cultivate them in vitro. There are two major glycoproteins, gp90 and gp45, and four major nonglycosylated components, p26, pp15, p11 and p9 (31). Others have suggested that
there were an acidic and a basic p10 but our procedures resolve
the p11 and p9. We have separated quantities of the major proteins for biochemical analysis and have characterized them fairly
extensively (32). It has been more difficult to purify large
amounts of gp90 and gp45, because they have been difficult to
separate from each other and from other cellular or serum
components.

The major core proteins have been studied by amino acid
analysis, isoelectric point determination, protease fragmenta-
tion and two-dimensional peptide mapping. Surface and internal
components have been determined by bromelin digestion studies of
intact virus. The virus has been characterized further by oligonucleotide fingerprinting of the vRNA, and reactivity against
monoclonal antibodies and serum from naturally infected horses.

The major glycoprotein gp90 has an apparent molecular weight
of 90,000 daltons in sodium dodecyl sulfate-polyacrylamide gel
electrophoresis (SDS-PAGE), but 74,000 daltons on guanidine gel
filtrations. This glycoprotein accounts for about 6% of the
labeled virion protein. The gp45 is very hydrophobic. On SDS-PAGE
it has a molecular weight of 45,000 daltons but aggregates on
guanidine hydrochloride gel filtration to yield a component with

an apparent molecular weight of greater than 100,000 daltons. The
major core components p26, pp15, p11 and p9 show very similar
molecular weights on both SDS-PAGE and guanidine hydrochloride
gel filtration analysis.

The gp90 is very heavily glycosylated and bromelin digestion
studies suggest it is the major surface component of the virion.
The gp45 is not as heavily glycosylated, is very hydrophobic, is
also on the virion surface and is likely to be a transmembrane
protein similar to p15E of murine leukemia virus.

The p26 is the major internal protein and the predominant
structural protein. It has an isoelectric point of 6.2. The phosphorylated protein pp15 has a variable isoelectric point. It is
probably also an internal component. The basic protein, p11, is
also internal, has negligible absorbance at 280 nm, stains red
with Coomassie blue and cannot be radioiodinated with the chlora-
mine T procedure because it lacks tyrosine residues. The p9 is
acidic. There are several other minor components that we have
identified reproducibly in all of our purified or radiolabeled
virus preparations.

By analogy with the model of the type-C oncoviruses, the
major surface component is gp90. The pp15 would have an important mantle or matrix role, p26 and p9 make up the core, p11
would associate with the RNA to form the ribonucleoprotein and
gp45 would be the transmembrane protein.

Our approach to determining the mechanisms of antigenic variation of EIAV has used the well-characterized prototype cell-
adapted strain in repeated passages in Shetland ponies to
increase its virulence. A high dose of the cell-adapted strain
is typically avirulent in first passage through at least 200
days post inoculation. The rationale for using the cell-adapted
strain was that wild strains of EIAV in nature are very difficult to cultivate in vitro; whereas with the cell-adapted strain,
we were hoping to recover all isolates in cell cultures assuming

that the mutants would retain their in vitro growth properties.
The cell-adapted strain became as virulent as the wild-type
Wyoming strain with seven passages in ponies and virus could be
reisolated from plasma through the seven passages. During febrile
episodes, viremia levels ranged to $10^{5.5}$ TCID$_{50}$/0.5 ml of plasma;
during afebrile periods, virus usually could not be demonstrated
free in the plasma (18). However, virus could be found in whole
blood from afebrile individuals where it probably was localized
intracellularly (18). During febrile episodes, we took plasma and
made dilutions of it in order to isolate the virus at its end
point in equine kidney cell cultures, thus "cloning" the predominant strain present during a febrile episode. To date we have
more than 100 isolates from different febrile episodes. We hope
that by comparing the isolates biochemically and antigenically
that some common features will be identified that may serve in
developing an effective immunogen.

The prototype cell-adapted strain produced no febrile
response in the first recipient (P1) through 200 days. However
at day 18, virus could be demonstrated in the plasma (P1-1),
which was inoculated into a second passage recipient (P2). The
first febrile peak was observed in the P2 recipient at 108 days
post inoculation. That individual subsequently had a number of
febrile episodes. We end-point diluted or "cloned" the viruses
from the plasma of recipient 2 at the first and sixth episodes
(P2-1 and P2-6). The plasma sample collected during the first
febrile episode was used to inoculate a third recipient who also
had a series of febrile episodes. Isolates from the first and
third febrile episodes (P3-1 and P3-3) were compared (35,36).

The SDS-PAGE electrophoretograms of the prototype, P1-1,
P2-1, P2-6, P3-1 and P3-3 essentially look identical although
by neutralization tests the isolates proved to be distinct. The
major core proteins p26, pp15, p11 and p9 migrate similarly
and few differences are observed in Coomassie blue stained

preparations in the higher molecular weight regions. If, however, the same virus preparations are transferred to nitrocellulose membranes and blotted using serum from naturally infected horses, the electrophoretic mobilities of gp90 and gp45 are observed to vary considerably. Obviously the horse recognizes the surface glycoproteins as important antigens, even though they constitute a minor percentage of virion proteins.

The two-dimensional peptide maps of virion proteins p26, pp15 and p9 are identical in all preparations. We have observed that p11 cannot be radioiodinated, so maps cannot be obtained by this procedure.

The two-dimensional peptide maps of gp90 comparing prototype and isolate P1-1 show a number of deletions after 18 days adaptation in a pony in the absence of detectable immune pressure. The isolate was passed through a second recipient and additional deletions and substitutions were evident. The peptide maps of gp90 of all isolates tested to date have dramatic changes. Many of the substitutions or deletions reproducibly occur at specific spots, suggesting a relatively low number of possible peptide combinations.

Oligonucleotide fingerprints have been performed on the prototype virus, P1-1, P2-1 and P2-6, and a series of isolates from sequential febrile episodes from a third passage recipient. A number of changes in the T1-resistant fragments are observed. These deletions and substitutions prove that genotypic changes are occurring in these isolates which have bona fide phenotypic changes.

Today, the control of EIA is based primarily on control of the movement of infected horses. Horse owners 10 miles distant will not come near a farm where an EIA-infected horse is housed. In my opinion, vaccine development for EIA should be a high priority item. The results of studies in Japan suggest that live virus vaccine preparations protect against homologous challenge

but not against heterologous challenge. A subunit vaccine might
be the best approach to ensure protection while not compromising
the only effective diagnostic test (the agar gel immunodiffusion
test) available for the disease today. We hope to document the
extent of antigenic variation that can occur with EIAV. By identifying those antigenic domains that are conserved and those
which are unique, we hope to identify antigenic sites which will
offer some protection. If influenza virus is an accurate model,
there may be hope of identifying some epitopes with cross-
protective value.

REFERENCES

1. Cheevers, W.P., Roberson, S.M., Brassfield, A.L. et al.
   (1982). Am. J. Vet. Res. 43, 804.
2. Valle, J. and Carree, H. (1904). C. R. Acad. Sci. 139, 311
   (original not seen).
3. Kono, Y. and Yokomizo, Y. (1968). Natl. Inst. Anim. Health Q
   (Tokyo) 8, 182.
4. Nakajima, H., Norcross, N.L. and Coggins, L. (1972). Infect.
   Immun. 6, 416.
5. Kono, Y., Kobayasi, K. and Fukunaga, Y. (1973). Arch. Gesamte
   Virusforsch. 41, 1.
6. Coggins, L. and Norcross, N.L. (1970). Cornell Vet. 60, 330.
7. Norcross, N.L. and Coggins, L. (1971). Infect. Immun. 4, 528.
8. Kono, Y., Kobayashi, K. and Fukunaga, Y. (1970). Natl. Inst.
   Anim. Health Q (Tokyo) 10, 113.
9. Kono, Y. (1973). In "Proc. 3rd Int. Conf. Equine Infectious
   Diseases," p. 242. Karger, Basel.
10. Issel, C.J. and Adams, W.V., Jr. (1979). J. Am. Vet. Med.
    Assoc. 174, 286.
11. McGuire, T.C., Crawford, T.B. and Henson, J.B. (1972).
    Immunol. Commun. 1, 545.
12. Coggins, L. and Kemen, M.J. (1976). In "Proc. 4th Int. Conf.
    Equine Infectious Diseases," p. 14. Karger, Basel.
13. Sentsui, H. and Kono, Y. (1976). Infect. Immun. 14, 325.
14. Sentsui, H. and Kono, Y. (1981). Arch. Virol. 67, 75.
15. McGuire, T.C., Henson, J.B. and Quist, S.E. (1969). Am. J.
    Vet. Res. 30, 2091.
16. Kono, Y., Sentsui, H. and Murakami, Y. (1976). Vet. Micro-
    biol. 1, 31.
17. Shively, M.A., Banks, K.L., Greenlee, A. et al. (1982).
    Infect. Immun. 36, 38.

18. Orrego, A. (1983). Ph.D. dissertation. Louisiana State University, Baton Rouge, Louisiana.
19. Issel, C.J. and Foil, L.D. (1984). J. Am. Vet. Med. Assoc. 184, 293.
20. Kemen, M.J., Jr. and Coggins, L. (1972). J. Am. Vet. Med. Assoc. 161, 496.
21. Kono, Y., Fukunaga, Y. and Kobayashi, K. (1973). Natl. Inst. Anim. Health Q (Tokyo) 13, 182.
22. Foil, L.D. (1983). J. Med. Entomol. 20, 301.
23. Issel, C.J., Adams, W.V., Jr. and Foil, L.D. (1985). Am. J. Vet. Res. 46, 1114.
24. Foil, L., Stage, D., Adams, W.V., Jr. et al. (1985). Am. J. Vet. Res. 46, 1111.
25. Archer, B.G., Crawford, T.B., McGuire, T.C. et al. (1977). J. Virol. 22, 16.
26. Gonda, M.A., Charman, H.P., Walker, J.L. et al. (1978). Am. J. Vet. Res. 39, 731.
27. Rice, N.R., Simek, S., Ryder, O.A. et al. (1978). J. Virol. 26, 577.
28. Weiland, F., Matheka, H.D., Coggins, L. et al. (1977). Arch. Virol. 55, 335.
29. Montagnier, L., Dauguet, C., Axler, S. et al. (1981). Ann. Virol. (Inst. Pasteur) 135E, 119.
30. Cheevers, W.P., Archer, B.G. and Crawford, T.B. (1977). J. Virol. 24, 489.
31. Parekh, B., Issel, C.J. and Montelaro, R.C. (1980). Virology 107, 520.
32. Montelaro, R.C., Lohrey, N., Parekh, B. et al. (1982). J. Virol. 42, 1029.
33. Malmquist, W.A., Barnett, D. and Becvar, C.S. (1973). Arch. Gesamte Virusforsch. 42, 361.
34. Klevjer-Anderson, P., Cheevers, W.P. and Crawford, T.B. (1979). Arch. Virol. 60, 279.
35. Montelaro, R.C., Parekh, B., Orrego, A. et al. (1984). J. Biol. Chem. 259, 10539.
36. Payne, S., Parekh, B., Montelaro, R.C. et al. (1984). J. Gen. Virol. 65, 1395.

BOVINE LEUKEMIA VIRUS
AS AN INDUCER OF BOVINE LEUKEMIA

A. Burny,[1/2] C. Bruck,[1] Y. Cleuter,[1]
D. Couez,[1] D. Gregoire,[1] R. Kettmann,[1/2]
M. Mammerickx,[2/3] G. Marbaix,[1] D. Portetelle[1/2]
and L. Willems,[1/2]

[1]Department of Molecular Biology, University of
Brussels; [2]Faculty of Agronomy, Gembloux;
[3]National Institute for Veterinary Research,
Brussels, Belgium

I will divide my chapter into four parts. One quarter will
be about molecular biology, tumor induction and host-virus relationships; one quarter will be about immune responses; and the
remainder will be about the relatedness of human T cell lymphotropic virus (HTLV) and bovine leukemia virus (BLV), about characteristics of the various HTLV isolates, about a possible model
for AIDS induced by BLV in rabbits and a few words about transmission and host range.

On Christmas Eve, 1978, I received a telephone call from
Robert Gallo. He said, "We think we are following something
important. Would you send us all the BLV reagents you have?
Because we are afraid we are following an infection by BLV."
This chapter will show that, indeed, Gallo was following an
infection related to BLV.

Bovine leukemia was described for the first time a century
ago by a Polish veterinarian. It seems to have originated on the
shores of the Baltic Sea. At that time, Americans were importing
cattle from that part of the world. When the importation stopped,

around 1900, a good strain of cattle which would be improved upon
had been imported. Most cattle in the United States were selected
further from that original breed, and today it is sometimes difficult to find in the United States a herd that is not infected
by BLV.

Leukemia induction in cattle by BLV is in many ways comparable to disease caused by HTLV. The systems are quite inter-
changeable, although the cell target is a B lymphocyte in the
case of BLV and a T lymphocyte in the case of HTLV. There is good
evidence that the most efficient agent of transmission of BLV
from animal to animal is the needle of the veterinarian. Following transmission, infection either takes or does not take. The
frequency of each is unknown but may depend on the size of the
virus infection. If enough virus is used, I think that no animal
is resistant to infection whatever its genetic background.

When the virus takes in cattle there are four possible consequences. First, there is a chronic infection that may last
for years. Some infections have been followed for as long as
20 years. Second is persistent lymphocytosis involving high numbers of circulating lymphocytes persisting for a very long time—
years. Third is persistent lymphocytosis followed by development
of the tumor phase of the disease. Since this sequence occurs in
20 to 85% of tumor cases that have been analyzed, persistent
lymphocytosis has been considered as a kind of preleukemic state.
Fourth is direct onset of a tumor without prior development of
persistent lymphocytosis. That happens in 15 to 70% of tumor
cases.

BLV can also infect sheep, and it has been found in sheep in
a number of countries. The disease in sheep is much the same as
it is in cattle, except that persistent lymphocytosis never
occurs in sheep. When the number of circulating lymphocytes
increases, it is because tumor cells are proliferating, and the
animal will die within a very short time.

Goats are another species which can be experimentally infected with BLV. Nobody knows if infection by BLV can occur naturally in goats. Among 25 goats that were infected in Belgium, in the United States and in Holland, two died of tumor 10 years after infection, and footprints of the virus could be demonstrated in the tumor after a very long period of incubation. Hybridization experiments in liquid using a BLV probe have shown no hybridization to DNA of normal bovine cells, sheep cells or goat cells. Therefore, the virus apparently does not originate in the cow, sheep or goat but comes from somewhere else and is now adapted to these ruminants. When the same probe is used to look at tumor cells, significant hybridization does occur and less hybridization occurs with DNA in cells obtained from cases of persistent lymphocytosis. The proportion of cells infected varies from animal to animal and from one stage of disease to another during the development of persistent lymphocytosis. Hybridization of cDNA from BLV to DNA extracted from circulating cells of individuals with persistent lymphocytosis and cleaved by EcoRI yields a smear of hybridiation. Many cells are infected, and the disease is polyclonal. If the DNA is restricted by an enzyme that cuts more than once into the provirus, internal fragments are obtained and appear as well-identified bands; and flanking sequences, that are not well-defined, are barely visible in restriction maps (Fig. 1). Therefore, the integration sites are quite variable from one cell to the other. If tumor cells are studied, several different types of results can be obtained. In some cases, tumors consist of cells from a single clone; in others, cells arise from a mixture of clones. In each of the three animal species tested, it is, to date, unclear whether it is the single cell clones that are the rule and mixed clones the exception or the reverse.

A very puzzling result was obtained when provirus genome expression was studied first by liquid hybridization and later by

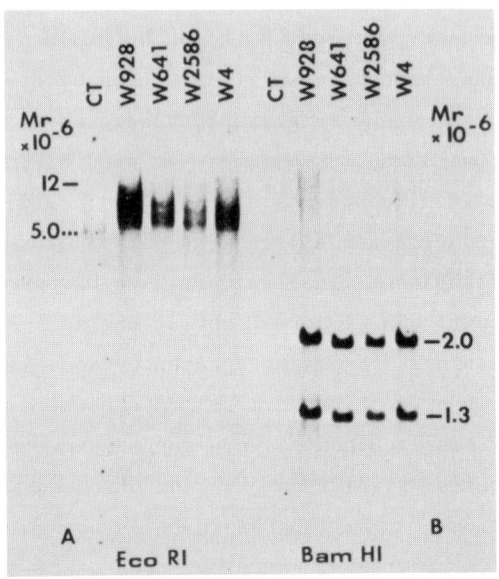

Fig. 1. Hybridization patterns of BLV[^{32}P]cDNA or DNA
restriciton fragments from leukocytes of animals in persistent
lymphocytosis. 20 µg each of leukocyte W928, W641, W2586 and W4
and calf thymus (CT) DNAs were exhaustively digested by either
EcoRI (A) or BamHI (B) and electrophoresed on a 1% agarose gel.
Only fragments larger than 0.5×10^6 were detected on these gels.
After the restriction fragments were transferred to nitrocellulose sheets, they were soaked in the prehybridization mixture at
65°C and hybridized for 24 hours with 5×10^6 cpm of BLV[^{32}P]cDNA
per ml. This probe was separately prehybridized with 3 mg of calf
thymus DNA per ml. The last washing was performed in 45 mM NaCl/
4.5 mM Na citrate. Autoradiograms are shown.

dot-blot analyses. There was no viral expression whatsoever in
the tumor cells when the cells were taken from a well-developed
tumor (Fig. 2). We thought then that we were looking at a fully
developed tumor in which a number of cells would no longer be
proliferating, and we were not therefore surprised at the result.
Later, when the technique became available, we ran dot-blot
hybridization with exactly the same result: no expression whatsoever in the total RNA extracted from tumors from cows or from
sheep, but very nice hybridization with control cells that

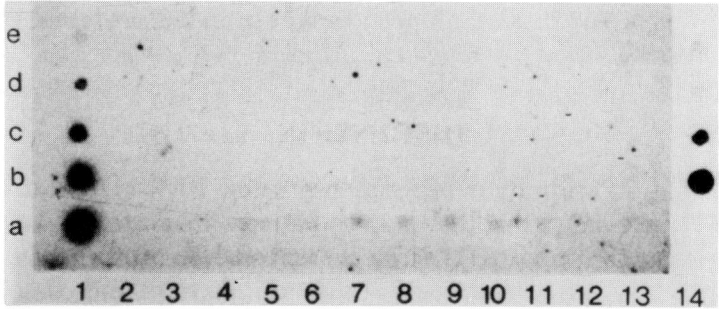

Fig. 2. Dot-blot assay of total RNA from leukocytes of a
normal animal (lane 2) or animals in persistent lymphocytosis
(lanes 3, 4 and 5) and from tumors of several other animals
(lanes 6-13). In lanes 2 to 13, 1:5 dilutions were tested, from
2 μg (a) to 3.2 ng (e) of total RNA. BLV 35S genomic RNA (lane
1) and total RNA from BLV-infected FLK cells (a BLV-producing
fetal lamb kidney cell line used in previous studies [lane 14])
were taken as positive controls. Also, 1:5 dilutions were
tested, from 2 ng (a) to 3.2 pg (e) of viral RNA in lane 1 and
from 360 ng (b) to 3 ng (e) of FLK total RNA in lane 14. The
dot-blot preparation was hybridized with the complete cloned
[32]P-labeled BLV proviral DNA and processed as described in the
legend to Figure 1. Lane 3 corresponds to animal 12, lane 4 to
animal 2586, lane 5 to animal 2587, lane 6 to animal 120, lane 7
to animal 96, lane 8 to animal 106, lane 9 to animal 104, lane 10
to animal 3168 and lanes 11, 12 and 13 to three tumors of animal
15.

produced the virus. Therefore, either the tumor cells are not

taken at the right time or there is indeed no expression of the

provirus once the tumor cell has become a tumor cell. This would

imply that the virus would be necessary to initiate the process

but not necessary once the process is underway.

It was possible that the virus was acting through a position

effect. We cloned the flanking sequences, we did hybridization

experiments with DNA from a number of tumors and with DNA from

calf thymus as a control. In the tumor from which the provirus

was cloned, two fragments were seen corresponding to the two

chromosomes, one that integrated the provirus and one that did

not. In all other tumors, we got the same kind of profile showing

provirus integrated at different places in the bovine genome and
not expressed. This is really a puzzling result, because, if the
provirus is integrated at many places, it is hard to believe that
it would stimulate or inhibit a given gene or two.

We then looked at a number of hamster-bovine cell hybrids.
In these hybrids, the provirus was not integrated in the same
chromosome. The provirus clearly gets into the cell. It is integrated at many possible different places; there is induction of
a tumor, but no expression of the proviral information (Fig. 3).

To be sure that the provirus was not expressed in the tumor
cell, we tried to grow tumor cells in tissue culture and looked
at them for proviral expression when the cells were fully proliferating. In one case, using tumor cells from a bovine tumor,
the restriction profile of the tumor that killed the animal was
identical to the restriction profile of the cells growing in culture. The profile was not the same as that of DNA extracted from
the blood of the animal. In a similar experiment using sheep
cells, which grow in culture more easily than do bovine cells,
what was growing in vitro had the same restriction profile as
what was growing in the tumor of the sheep. The search for viral
RNA expression in the cultured cells gave the following results:
1) the bovine tumor cells expressed very little viral RNA and
2) sheep cells did not show any viral expression. These data further support the earlier finding that BLV virus is necessary to
initiate transformation but then is dispensable once a critical
event has occurred. So far we have not seen provirus expression,
but we have not done much to try to induce expression. The RNA
from these cells does not appear to be more methylated than RNA
in expressing cells. During the stage of lymphocytosis, RNA can
be found in cells put in culture. Somewhere in the animal there
is viral expression, perhaps in the bone marrow or the spleen or
perhaps in cells that are not in the lymphocyte lineage. At any

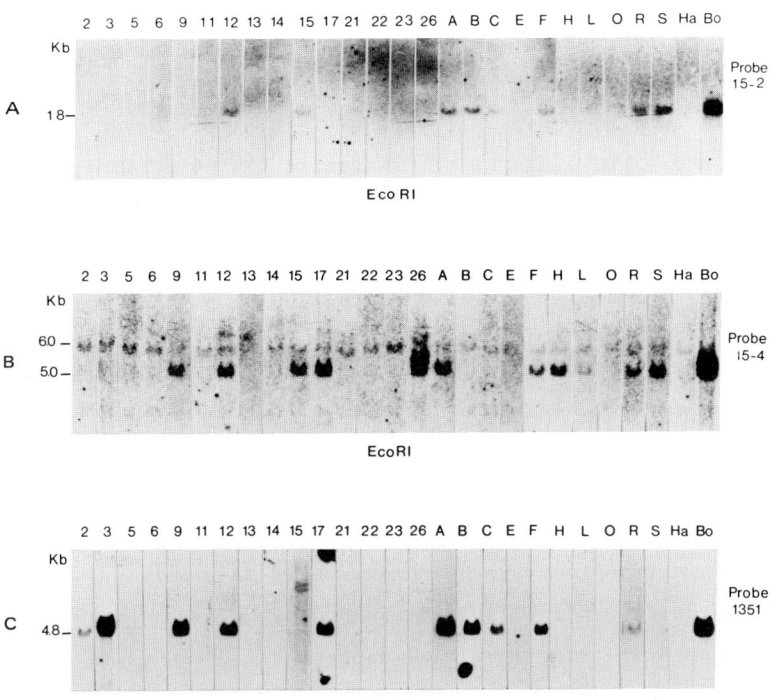

Fig. 3.   Restriction analysis of hamster × bovine hybrid DNAs. (A) Ten μg each of normal parental hamster cell DNA (lane Ha), normal parental bovine DNA (lane Bo) and 25 hamster × bovine hybrid DNAs (lanes 2 through 5) were digested to completion by EcoRI and were treated as described in the legend to Figure 1, except that depurination of the DNA before denaturation was performed. The filters were hybridized for 48 hours with 0.007 μg (10^9 cpm/μg) of ^{32}P-labeled probe 15-2 per ml. Autoradiography was carried out after a 5 day exposure. (B) Same as in (A), but with ^{32}P-labeled probe 15-4 (0.007 μg/ml, 10^9 cpm/μg). Exposure time was 10 days. (C) Same as in (A), but with ^{32}P-labeled probe 1351 (0.010 μg/ml, 3×10^8 cpm/μg). Exposure time was 3 days. (The molecular weights of all native DNAs were above 50 kb, as estimated by electrophoresis in 0.8% agarose gels with λ phage DNA as the molecular weight marker.)

rate, BLV antigens continuously stimulate the immune system of
the infected host.

The structural relationship of BLV with HTLV-I was studied in
experiments carried out in collaboration with Ray Gilden, Nancy
Rice and Robert Stephens at Frederick. The envelope glycoprotein
of HTLV-I and the comparable glycoprotein of BLV have 32% homology and there are a number of base pairs that are identical in
the two. For the transmembrane protein, the homology is much more
striking, reaching 50%. If BLV is compared to HTLV, to Moloney
murine leukemia virus and even to Rous sarcoma virus, there is
good homology, particularly at the carboxylic end of the protein.
At a number of places, the amino acids are exactly the same. A
study, recently published by Snyderman and coworkers, shows that
in viruses that exert an immunosuppressive effect, an amino acid
sequence is conserved. This sequence is present in BLV transmembrane protein.

The order of genes in BLV provirus is gag, pol, env, followed
by a region originally called leuk and now called lor. There is
an open reading frame that expands over 924 nucleotides with a
strongly conserved region in the 5' end. The protein synthesized
there has an apparent molecular weight of 31,000, and the RNA
that carries the information for the protein is a 2.1 kb RNA. The
RNA carries the information from that region if spliced around
the 5' end of the env gene and again in the gag region. The messenger RNA has a coding capacity for a protein that is indeed
much longer than the 31,000 dalton protein that is observed.
These viruses are also peculiar in having the env-lor messenger.
The env-lor putative protein is encoded by a messenger RNA that
is 5000 bases long.

All animals infected with BLV react with very strong immunological responses against the invading virus. The reaction
against the glycoprotein antigen occurs very early, within a few
days, after infection. gp51 is the major envelope glycoprotein

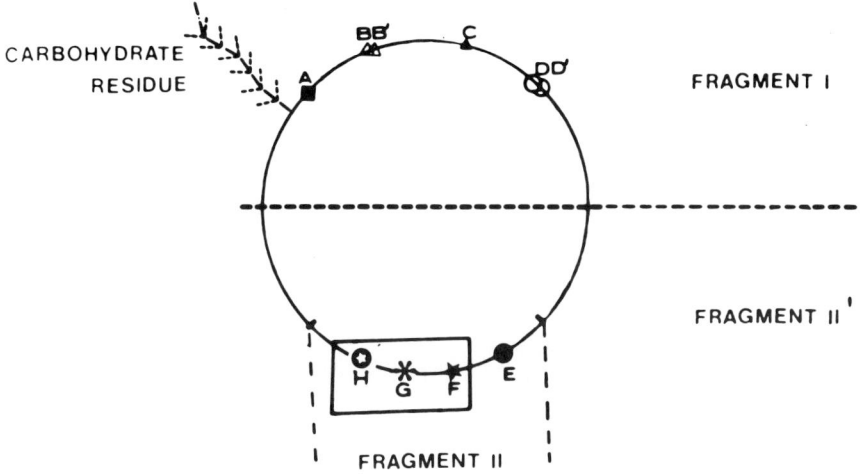

CARBOHYDRATE
RESIDUE

FRAGMENT I

FRAGMENT II'

FRAGMENT II

Fig. 4. Model for the location of the epitopes recognized by mouse monoclonal antibodies on the BLV gp51 molecule.

and p24 being the major internal protein. The anti-GP antibody titer correlates quite well with the antigen titer. To test for the presence of antibody, gp51 was purified to homogeneity and used to induce monoclonal antibody production in mice. Eight antigenic sites, A to H, could be distinguished on the glycoprotein gp51 (Fig. 4). Two determinants, B and B', are very close to each other but are not identical. Similarly, F, G and H are three antigenic sites that are very close to each other. This was ascertained by showing that there was steric interference among the three determinants in ELISA assays. The ELISA test that we designed has a very high sensitivity. Monoclonal antibodies against site E are attached to the plastic well, and tissue culture fluid (we do not purify the glycoprotein any more) is used as a source of glycoprotein. Pools of up to 85 to 90 sera are taken from infected animals and tested for the presence of antibody to glycoprotein. If one animal is infected, even with an

early infection, it can be detected by this ELISA test. The test
will detect both IgM and IgG antibody.

Infected cattle develop antibodies against F, G and H. They
apparently do not make antibodies to other antigenic sites of the
glycoprotein. Sheep also make antibodies against F, G and H; in
addition, they react against the other epitopes of the glycoprotein. F, G and H are the critical sites of the virus. Both infectivity and syncytia induction reside in F, G and H. Monoclonal
antibodies to F, G and H will only react with the determinants if
the protein is glycosylated. If the glycoprotein is deglycosy-
lated or produced in the presence of tunicamycin, neither monoclonal antibodies nor bovine sera (they are directed against F, G
and H) will recognize the proteins without the sugar moieties.
Although glycosylation is mandatory, the antibodies are reacting
to conformational epitopes that depend on glycosylation of the
glycoprotein rather than the sugar moieties directly. So far,
competition does not occur using sugars in the radioimmunoassay
or the ELISA test.

F, G and H were compared from various cell types infected
with BLV (Fig. 5). The cells used included fetal lamb kidney
(FLK) cells (the original cell used by Van Der Maaten to propagate the virus) and a bat line (BL) designed by Robert Callahan
in George Todaro's laboratory. In these cells, the three epitopes
are present and they are present in about the same extent as they
are in the in vitro system.

We looked at two virus isolates from Van Der Maaten. VdM 7290
behaved as FLK-BLV, whilst VdM 7628 practically lacked the F epi-
tope. G and H were present. An isolate of Mark Mammerickx, my
colleague working in Brussels at the Veterinary Research Institute, has F but G was practically abolished and H was very much
reduced. So far, we have seen a number of these variations. Never
has a virus been isolated that lacked F, G and H. At least one of

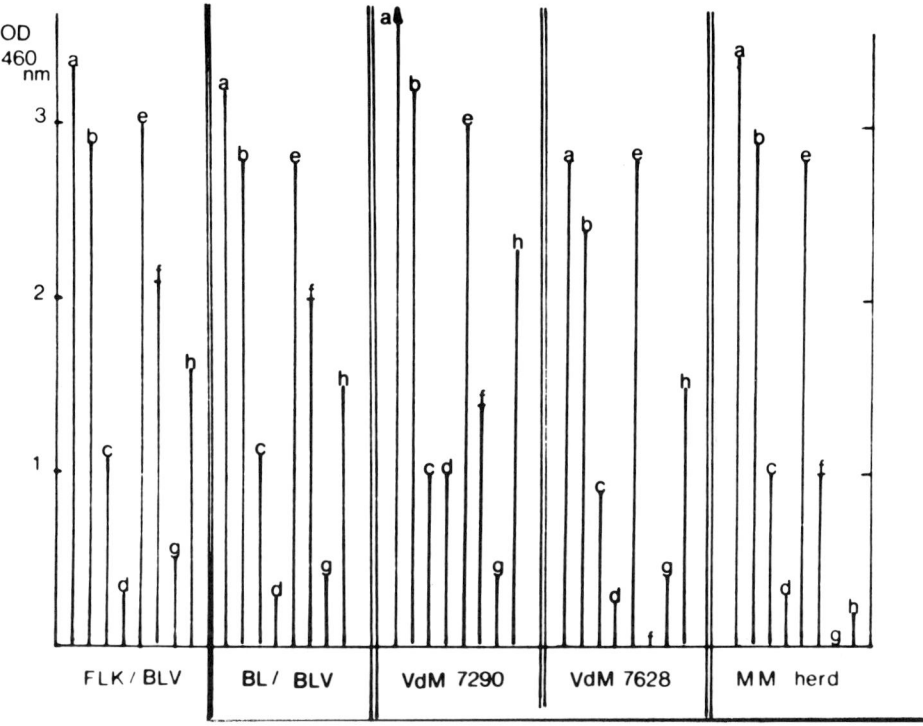

Fig. 5. Comparison of the epitopes A to H distinguished on the glycoprotein (gp51).

these was always present. This, we think, means that a successful vaccine may be developed.

Some recent data on the virus were obtained by L. Thiry and S. Sprecher in Brussels to whom we gave reagents. Electron microscopic studies done by W. Feremans of lymphocytes from a prodromal AIDS patient show production of virus particles just as beautifully illustrated by Luc Montagnier, Francois Barre, J. C. Chermann and by Robert Gallo 2 years ago, and by Jay Levy and their coworkers. Budding of the virus can be seen. These tissues were then studied with our BLV reagents, including monoclonal or monospecific polyclonal antibodies, raised against BLV p24 or BLV

gp51. Samples from two Zairian AIDS patients were studied and
gave comparable results. Lymph nodes of patients were put in culture; reverse transcriptase activity and antibody reactivities
were measured. Polyclonal antibodies directed against BLV p24
recognize antigenic determinants in the homogate of the lymphocytes put in culture; the reactivity goes up and then goes down.
After 15 days in culture, there is no reactivity detectable. The
same pattern is obtained when blood of the patient is put in culture. If polyclonal antibody against gp51 is used, the reactivity
goes up and then down. But if fresh lymphocytes are fed to the
culture, the reactivity keeps up. If the supernatant of the culture is filtered and used to reinfect new cells, the reactivity
is sustained. When cells that were producing virus were irradiated and normal lymphocytes were seeded into the culture, reactivity could be detected by antibody directed against purified
p24 or gp51 protein of BLV.

Walter Feremans, an electronmicroscopist working in the
Faculty of Medicine in Brussels, observed multivesicular bodies
in the cells of these AIDS patients. These multivesicular bodies
were visualized by immunogold reaction using either the polyclonal antibody against p24 or the polyclonal antibody against
gp51. Two monoclonals against gp51 and one monoclonal against p24
gave the same type of reaction.

The possibility of mimicking an AIDS reaction in experimental
animals with BLV seems very strong. The ruminants and other animals that naturally develop tumors from BLV do not show immunodeficiency syndrome. However, experimental infections of chimpanzees, macaques, pigs and rabbits are successful.

The rabbit results are especially interesting. The animals
are infected intravenously using infected tissue culture cells or
cells from infected animals; they show ups and downs in antibody
titers and suddenly the antibody titer drops to zero. It looks
like the cells that have been producing the antibody are killed

by the virus. Concurrently, the animal loses weight, has diarrhea and is leukopenic. At that time when the antibody titer falls to zero, the average immunoglobulin concentration remains quite constant and the animal dies within a few days. These rabbits seem to be suffering from a syndrome mimicking an immune deficiency syndrome induced by BLV and not requiring any previous immunosuppressive agents.

I think that the best transmission experiments were done by German veterinarians. They had two experimental stables, and put an infected animal in the middle of each stable. The door in the first stable was on the left and the door in the second was on the right. In the first stable, propagation of the virus went from left to right and in the second stable, propagation went from right to left. Propagation followed the veterinarian who came in and stuck a needle in every animal, one after the other. The veterinarian's needle seems to be a good mode of transmission. Two years ago, Martin Van Der Maaten put lymphocytes in the uterus or the vagina of a recipient cow and showed that this also could be a route of infection. In nature, bulls have not been identified as transmitters of BLV since there are not normally infected lymphocytes in the semen. However, in experimental conditions, British investigators have been able to transmit the virus through the semen after manipulation of the seminal vesicles. In this case they may have increased significantly the level of infectious lymphocytes in the semen.

Ticks, insect vectors and the like do not seem to contribute to transmission in temperate climates, but their role in tropical conditions is unknown.

LENTIVIRUSES

Ashley T. Haase

Department of Microbiology
University of Minnesota
Minneapolis, Minnesota

HISTORICAL PERSPECTIVE

In the 1930s, two French investigators at the Pasteur
Institut inoculated sheep with scrapie and discovered the long
incubation periods of slow infections. In that same decade, German sheep introduced into Iceland caused epidemics in sheep,
called locally visna and maedi, for wasting and shortness of
breath. Visna and maedi were shown to have the same long incubation periods as scrapie, and led Sigurdsson at the Institute of
Experimental Pathology in Iceland to formulate the concept of
slow infections. It is now abundantly clear that the agents of
visna and maedi are nearly indistinguishable, and that they are
retroviruses. In this chapter, I will discuss what is known about
these sheep retroviruses as prototypes for slow virus infections
caused by conventional viruses.

DESCRIPTION OF THE DISEASES AND THEIR PATHOLOGY

Visna is a paralytic disease of sheep that first affects the
hind quarters of the animal. The paralysis is a consequence of
demyelination in inflammatory foci. Inflammatory infiltrates are

also present in the lungs. Most of the retrovirus diseases in
sheep in Iceland and elsewhere are predominantly pulmonary infections. In this country the disease is called progressive pneumonia. During the Icelandic epidemics, about 100,000 sheep suc-
cumbed to maedi and visna. Heroic eradication programs in which
650,000 animals were slaughtered largely freed Iceland of these
diseases.

VIROLOGICAL ASPECTS

    Sigurdsson was the first to isolate the causative agent of
visna and maedi in tissue cultures derived from sheep choroid
plexus cells. Visna virus is directly lytic in tissue culture.
It causes the fusion of cells, with formation of polykaryocytes.
These degenerate and retract so that the cells have a starshaped
appearance. Small, round degenerating cells are also produced as
a direct cytopathic effect of the virus. The causative agents of
visna-maedi belong to the family of retroviruses. Common characteristics include morphology and morphogenesis, polyploid RNA
genome and replication by reverse transcription. Distinctive
features include a large gapped linear DNA, and replication in
tissue culture from extrachromosomal DNA. Serological tests with
visna virus P30 define a subfamily of lentiviruses comprised of
visna, maedi, PPV and CAEV. These viruses differ from oncogenic
retroviruses, the third retrovirus subfamily, the spuma viruses
and unclassified agents such as equine infectious anemia virus.
    The extrachromosomal replication of the lentiviruses may hold
the explanation for a number of unusual aspects of their replication: 1) the dependence of transcription on the extent of early
DNA synthesis, 2) the lack of endogeneous sequences in sheep
cells and 3) their resistance to interferon. This latter infer-
ence relies on the following line of reasoning: In tissue culture
the predominant form of visna DNA is a gapped linear duplex of

about 9.5 kbp. Circular forms of DNA are relatively rare; and, if these are the preferred topological precursor for integration, as a number of lines of evidence suggest, treatments such as interferon that inhibit formation of circular DNA and integration would predictably not affect the growth of visna virus.

PATHOGENESIS

In infected sheep choroid plexus cells, the entire growth cycle of visna virus is completed in 3 or 4 days. In animals, infection evolves over months or years. What accounts for the novel time scale of the slow infection?

This issue can be addressed in experimental models that mimic what happens in nature. Virus inoculated intracerebrally will replicate in choroid plexus, ependyma and brains of sheep and then spread by the bloodstream to infect many organ systems, particularly the lungs and reticuloendothelial system. Animals mount both a cellular and humoral immune response, usually within a matter of weeks or months, and immunity to virus is sustained throughout the course of the disease. With the advent of neutralizing antibody, there is a sharp decrease in the amount of cell-free virus that can be detected. Nevertheless, most animals become persistently infected. Lymphocytic infiltrates in the lungs and central nervous system lead to cumulative tissue lesions and paralysis, interstitial pneumonitis and death. This animal model poses, in addition to the slow evolution of infection, two questions: 1) How does the virus persist in the face of that immune response? 2) What is the mechanism of tissue damage?

We have developed a unifying hypothesis to answer these questions which posits that the genome is introduced into the cell in a stable fashion, but that later steps in the life cycle are curtailed. This is analogous to lysogeny or pseudolysogeny, where the reductions in virus-specific RNA and viral antigens allow the

virus to satisfy two logical preconditions for slow and persistent infections: 1) that there must be some way for the virus to
survive and escape detection and destruction by host defense
mechanisms and 2) that there must be a mechanism for the host to
survive the destructive consequences of acute infection exemplified by cytopathic effects seen in tissue culture.

There are some very clear predictions of this model that we
have tested by in situ hybridization experiments. In tissues
infections are focal, and virus genomes can be demonstrated in
foci. In subjacent sections virus-specific RNA (Fig. 1) and
virus-specific antigens can also be detected. The number of
copies of virus-specific RNA is reduced by about two orders of
magnitude in cells of infected animals compared to what is seen
in infected tissue culture cells (a permissive system). We attribute persistence and slowness to this restriction in virus gene
expression.

Tissue damage occurs in inflammatory foci, but we have only
recently defined the antigens that incite inflammation, and some
of the important cellular targets. To do so, we have had to
develop some new technology that warrants a brief description
because of its general utility.

In situ hybridization experiments are effective in finding
virus genes in a few cells in tissues. However, only a small portion of the tissue can be examined. In order to screen whole
brains of infected animals, we embedded whole coronal sections of
brain in carboxymethylcellulose. The frozen block was covered
with a piece of clear tape, a section was cut from it and transferred to the clear tape. After fixation and pretreatments, the
section was hybridized to a probe containing both ^{35}S and ^{125}I.
The ^{125}I gamma radiation with amplifying screens produces a
strong signal on x-ray film. The darkened area on the x-ray film
can then be used as a guide to where virus genes are located in
the section. This area is then studied under the microscope,

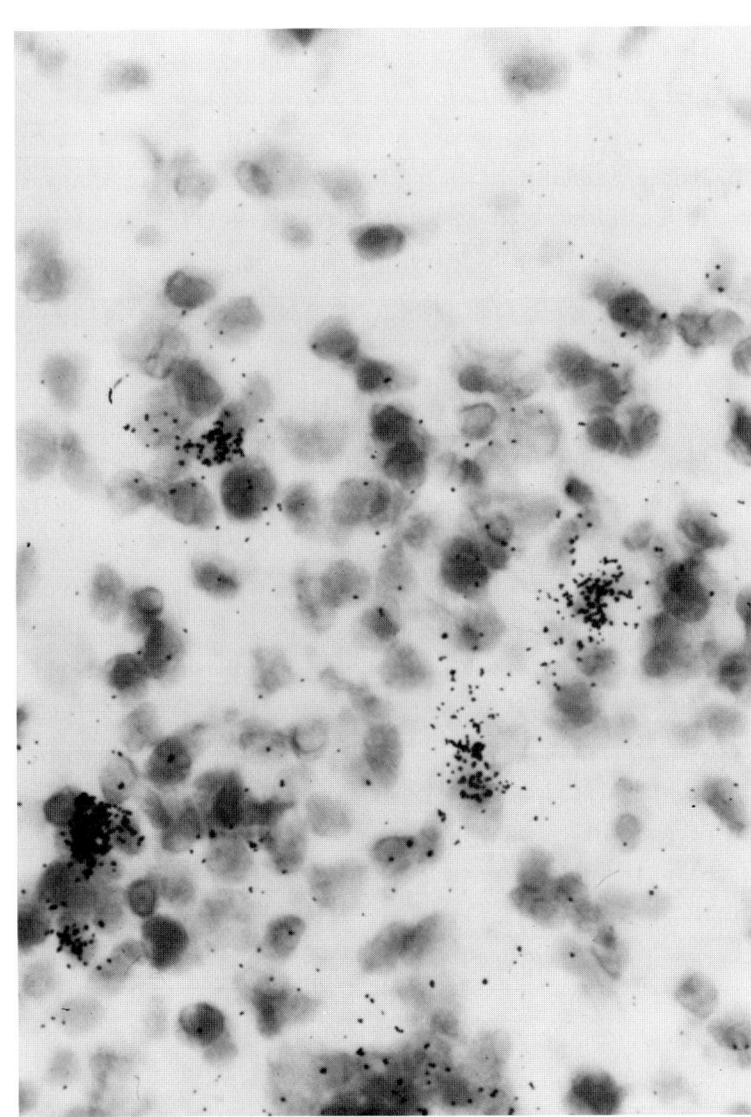

Fig. 1. Demonstration of visna virus RNA in brain by in situ hybridization.

after coating the section with nuclear track emulsion, developing
it and staining. With nuclear track emulsions, ^{125}I and ^{35}S give
good resolution in microradioautographs, and efficient grain
development. We call this technique a combined macroscopic-
microscopic assay, or hybridization tomography. It allows imaging
of virus genes in multiple planes in whole organs or whole
animals.

Using these techniques with visna, virus-specific RNA was
found to be distributed around the ventricles (Fig. 2). There is
a perfect correspondence between the inflammatory response and
the level of virus gene expression. In areas showing no virus-
specific RNA, there are only background levels of silver grains.
Modest levels of virus-specific RNA are seen in areas where there
are a few inflammatory cells next to infected cells. The areas
with the densest inflammatory collection correspond to the highest levels of virus RNA. In collaboration with Petursson and his
collaborators at the Icelandic Institute of Experimental Pathology, we have been able to demonstrate for the first time virus-
specific antigens in these inflammatory foci. Thus, in accord
with previous interpretations, visna is an immunopathological
disease, with virus-specific antigens as targets. Because the
extent of virus gene expression is restricted, and is correlated
with inflammation, the pace at which pathological damage accumulates in response to inflammation is slow.

The cellular targets of the inflammatory response can also be
ascertained now by the simultaneous detection assay developed in
conjunction with Michel Brahic at the Pasteur Institut. In this
assay both virus genes and antigens are visualized in the same
cell. The first step involves reacting the cell with specific
antibody to a protein, and then visualizing the reaction immuno-
cytochemically by depositing diaminobenzidine at the sites of
antigen accumulation. This polymeric product withstands the subsequent stringent procedures used for in situ hybridization to

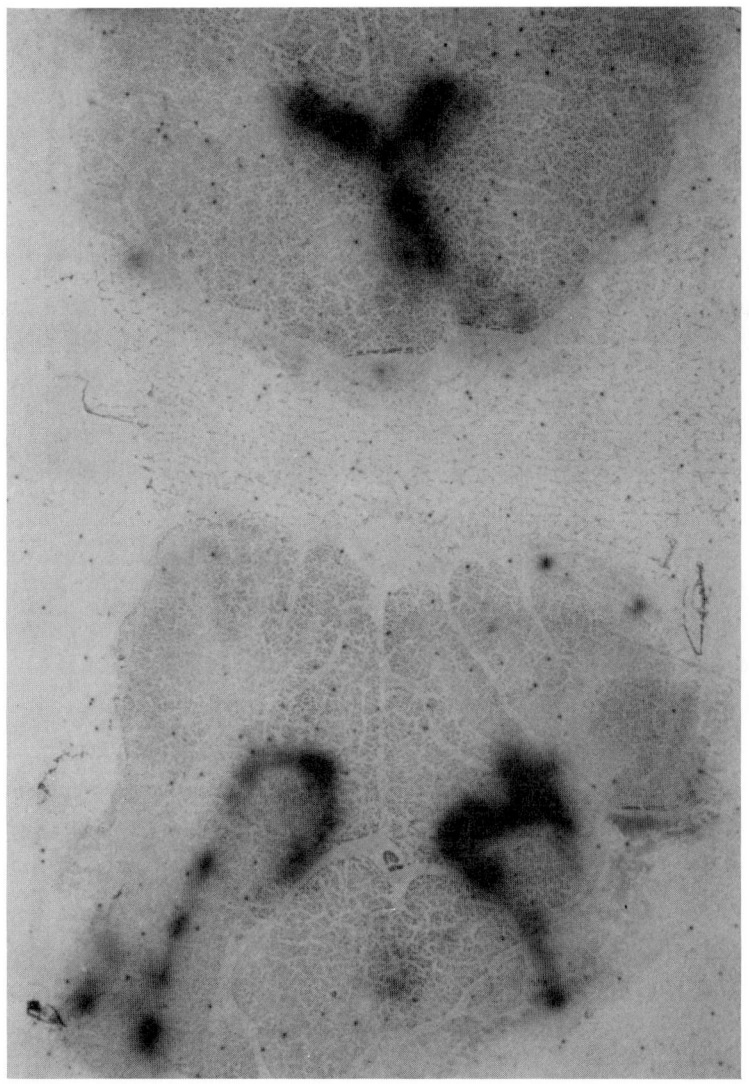

Fig. 2. Detection of visna RNA by hybridization tomography.

identify viral genes. In the radioautograph, silver grains
identify cells with virus-specific RNA, and the brown DAB stain
identifies cells that have antigen as well. In our experiments,
we used the assay to identify oligodendrocytes, cells responsible for maintaining the myelin sheaths in the central nervous
system. Tissues were first reacted with antibody against sheep
oligodendrocytes. In situ hybridization was then performed with
virus-specific probes. Oligodendrocytes were found containing
virus-specific RNA in the nucleus. Other oligodendrocytes did
not have viral RNA, and cells of other types were found that did
contain virus-specific RNA. Thus, the oligodendrocyte is not the
only cellular target for the immunopathological process in visna,
but it is clearly one of the cellular targets. It thus seems reasonable to attribute demyelination in visna to the inflammatory
response directed against the cell that maintains myelin.

PROSPECTUS: THE MOLECULAR BASIS FOR RESTRICTED GENE EXPRESSION
IN ANIMALS

How gene expression is restricted in animals at the level
of RNA accumulation is presently unanswered. Since the virus in
tissue culture is produced from extrachromosomal templates, and
viral production is related to the number of genes, or to the
extent of early DNA synthesis, we have looked for gene dosage
effects in a pulmonary model of visna. Sheep were intubated, and
virus was injected into the right upper lobe through a broncho-
scope. Pulmonary alveolar macrophages were collected by lavage,
and in situ hybridization was performed to quantitate virus-
specific nucleic acids. Even though most of the cells are not
infected, a large number of infected cells can be detected with
this kind of single cell assay. The number of copies of virus-
specific DNA peaks within the first day of infection just as in
tissue culture. The peak levels of RNA occur at day 3, and then
subsequently decline. Even though the kinetics parallel those

found in tissue culture, the number of copies of RNA is less than 100. Thus, the same kind of restriction occurs in alveolar macrophage as in choroid plexus and glial cells. However, the results of these experiments were not consistent with a simple gene dosage model. The number of copies of viral DNA did not correlate in every instance with the number of copies of RNA. We are currently examining other possibilities such as tissue-specific regulatory elements (enhancers), transactivation and integration in vivo.

OVERVIEW OF SIMIAN AIDS[1]

Preston A. Marx

California Primate Research Center
University of California Davis
Davis, California

Simian AIDS (SAIDS) is an AIDS-like disease that occurs in rhesus monkeys (<u>Macaca</u> <u>mulatta</u>) at the California Primate Research Center. The current outbreak is characterized by persistent lymphadenopathy and opportunistic infections, such as noma (necrotizing gingivitis), generalized cytomegalovirus infections and candidiasis (1). No lymphomas or central nervous system diseases have occurred during the 9 year history of this current outbreak. This is a spontaneous disease which has developed in six or seven species of the macaque genus of Old World monkeys (Table I). In all cases to date, a type D retrovirus has been associated with the disease.

Of the type D retroviruses, Mason-Pfizer moneky virus (MPMV) has been known for the longest amount of time. It is the prototype D retrovirus. It was first found in a rhesus monkey with a breast carcinoma in 1970 (2). The SAIDS group of viruses was identified in 1984. These include SAIDS/D (New England) from the

[1]This research was supported by grants 19900 by the State of California, P51 RR00169-122 from the National Institutes of Health, N01-CA37467-01 from the National Cancer Institute, R01-A120573-01 from the National Institute of Allergy and Infectious Diseases and special appropriations from Syntex, Inc.

TABLE I. Macaque Species Affected by Spontaneous SAIDS

Macaque species	Common name	Disease observed	Primate center location
M. mulatta	Rhesus	SAIDS	California
M. arctoides	Stump-tailed	SAIDS/lymphoma[a]	California
M. mulatta	Rhesus	SAIDS/lymphoma	New England
M. nemestrina	Pigtailed macaque	SAIDS/RF[b]	Washington
M. nigra	Celebes black macaque	SAIDS/RF	Oregon
M. cyclopsis	Taiwanese-rock macaque	SAIDS/lymphoma	New England
M. fascicularis	Crab-eating macaque	SAIDS	New England
M. radiata	Bonnet macaque	SAIDS[c]	California

[a]SAIDS in association with lymphomas. Stump-tailed macaques are no longer kept at the California Center. SAIDS was identified retrospectively by examination of clinical histories (1). Lymphomas have not occurred in the group of rhesus macaques currently experiencing SAIDS at the California Primate Research Center.

[b]SAIDS in association with retroperitoneal fibromatosis (RF).

[c]Only a few SAIDS-like cases have been observed, more information is needed on this species.

New England Primate Research Center (NEPRC), SAIDS/D (California)
from the California Primate Research Center (CPRC), SAIDS/D
(Washington) from the Seattle, Washington Primate Research Center
(WPRC) and SAIDS/D (Oregon) from the Oregon Primate Research Center (OPRC). SAIDS/D New England and SAIDS/D California appear to
be very similar to each other; however, differences in restriction endonuclease maps have been found (Marx, P.A., unpublished
data). SAIDS/D Washington appears to be different from SAIDS/D
New England and SAIDS/D California; all are different from MPMV
when compared by restriction endonuclease mapping and antigen
characteristics. Since some of the clinical syndromes observed in
Oregon and in Washington are similar, the Oregon isolate may be
similar to the Washington isolate.

Studies of monkey retroviruses are about 80 years behind
avian studies and some 100 years behind equine studies. We have
only been examining this problem for 1 year and do not yet all
agree exactly which diseases are induced by these different isolates. The clinical syndromes are somewhat different at each center and may even involve additional new agents. What we do know
is that we are dealing with a closely related family of type D
retroviruses that are found in quite a few species of the macaque
monkeys.

Most of the monkeys in California are housed outdoors in
half-acre corrals. Because of the good weather in Davis, California, the monkeys can live outdoors year around. Each corral is
composed of a stable family group. About 80 to 100 monkeys live
in each corral and there is no movement between corrals. The
animals are born, reach maturity and live quite a long life (some
for 20 years) in a particular corral. The outbreak of SAIDS at
the CPRC has been confined to one corral (North Corral #1) where
a group of rhesus monkeys has been living together for about
9 years.

The type D retrovirus isolations were done in collaborative studies with the Infectious Diseases Branch of the National Institute of Neurological and Communicative Disorders and Stroke (NINCDS) (3,4). The virus was obtained from an animal with naturally occurring disease in North Corral #1. A tissue homogenate (spleen, bone marrow, lymph node and liver homogenate) from this animal was inoculated intravenously into two juvenile rhesus monkeys at the NINCDS. This was one of the very first transmission experiments, and a tissue cocktail was used because we did not know which particular tissue contained the virus. The recipient animals developed SAIDS. A sample of whole blood from one of these animals was divided in half. Half of the sample was inoculated into two additional rhesus monkeys at the CPRC, and the other half went into a number of different tissue culture systems. It turned out that the SAIDS retrovirus was relatively easy to isolate. We grew the virus in a number of species of cells, including rhesus monkey kidney cells which were ideal for our use since the virus would be growing in the host species of origin and its pathogenicity might best be preserved for future transmission experiments. The virus was characterized by electron microscopy, showing it to be a type D retrovirus (3). Radioimmunoassays showed that the SAIDS retrovirus was a new type D retrovirus which was partially related to MPMV (3,4). In transmission studies at the CPRC, fatal disease was induced in four of nine animals that were inoculated intravenously with the virus grown in rhesus monkey cells (3).

Previously, the prototype D retrovirus, MPMV, was believed to be a nonpathogenic retrovirus. Don Fine, working with MPMV in the early 1970s (5), inoculated newborn rhesus monkeys with MPMV and was able to induce an immunosuppressive type disease in many, though not all, of the animals inoculated. At that time, however, researchers were searching for tumor-inducing agents, not immunosuppressive diseases, and it was not clearly established that

MPMV was indeed pathogenic. Since we also considered MPMV to be probably a nonpathogenic strain of retrovirus, we thought at first, that we had isolated MPMV from our animals with SAIDS. We were pleased to find out that the SAIDS virus was different from MPMV, because, if SAIDS was a new disease, it had to involve some new agent. It is now clear, however, that MPMV is also a member of the SAIDS group in that, under the right circumstances, it also induces a SAIDS-like disease. It is also clear that there are a number of related type D retroviruses that are involved to one extent or another with the simian AIDS disease. Curiously, MPMV has not been re-isolated from SAIDS cases at any of the primate centers. It may be that MPMV was a "one-time only" recombinant that arose in the rhesus monkey with the breast carcinoma. It is also interesting to note that this rhesus with the breast carcinoma had been previously irradiated (2).

The virus isolated from tissue culture was clearly a type D retrovirus showing a cylindrical nucleoid (Fig. 1A). If cut in cross-section, a slightly eccentric core is seen (Fig. 1B). The buds have a completed ring form when still attached to the membrane (Fig. 1C). Larry Arthur at the Frederick Cancer Research Facility performed sensitive, competitive radioimmunoassays comparing the various SAIDS viral isolates. Among those studied were MAC-1 (a type C macaque endogenous virus), squirrel monkey retrovirus (a type D retrovirus isolated from the squirrel monkey and also an endogenous virus), SAIDS/D California, SAIDS/D New England, SAIDS/D Washington, MPMV and PO-1-Lu (the endogenous type D virus of the Langur monkey). The major core proteins of the various viruses were compared. Using ^{125}I-labeled p27 of MPMV and anti-MPMV p27, the very same competition was obtained with all macaque D viruses, indicating that the viral core antigens are very closely related. Langur virus and squirrel monkey virus gave a different competition curve. MAC-1 did not compete. In another assay using MPMV gp70 glycoproteins, differences were found. In

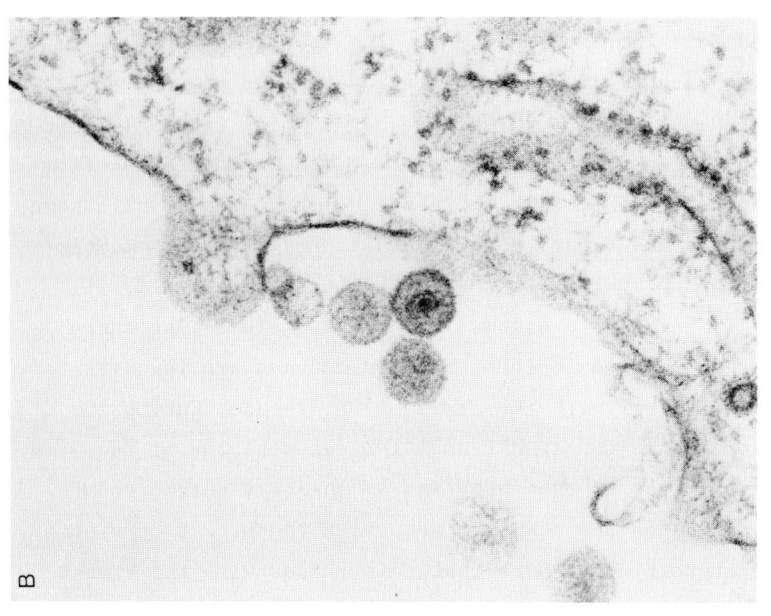

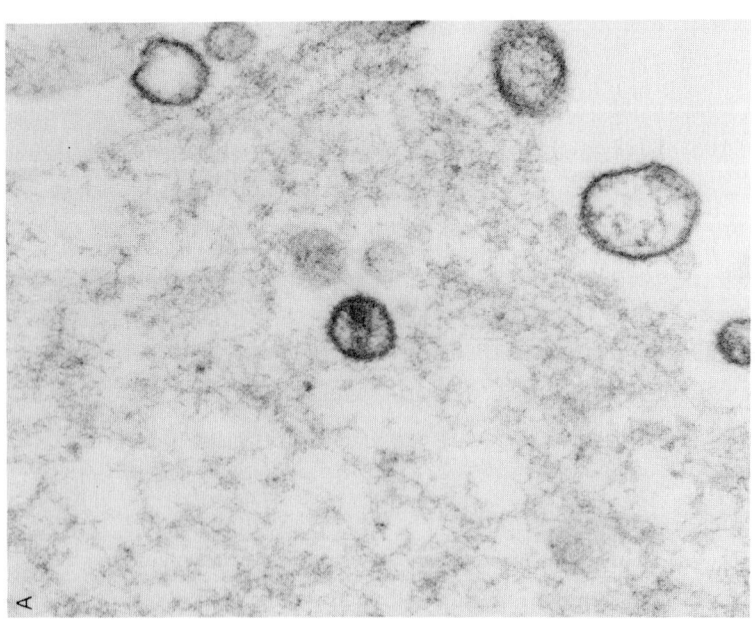

Fig. 1. SAIDS type D retrovirus showing typical type D morphology. (A) Cylindrical nucleoid.
(B) Cylindrical nucleoid in cross-section. (C) Budding virus with the completed ring in the bond
(80,000x).

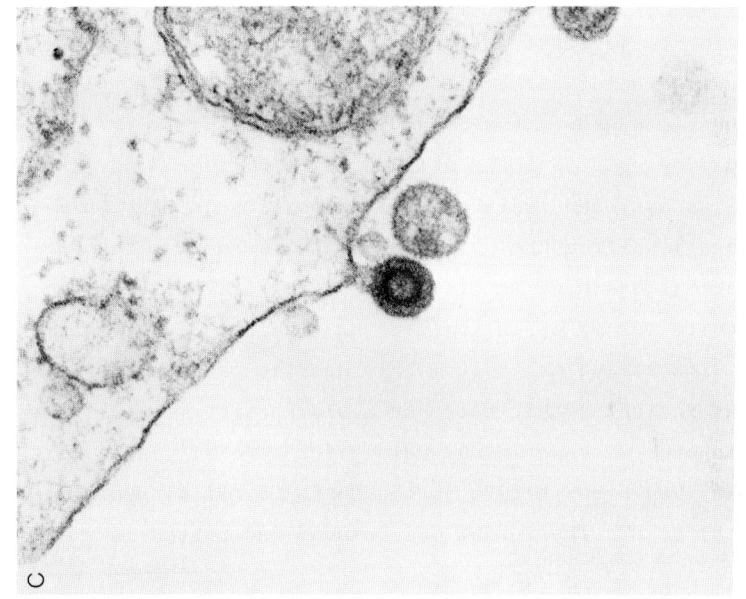

Fig. 1C

this gp70 assay, the same slopes were obtained when SAIDS/D
California and SAIDS/D New England were tested, but this slope
differs from the slope of MPMV or SAIDS/D Washington gp70.

SAIDS/D Oregon has not yet been tested, but there are some
indications that it will be similar to SAIDS/D Washington.

In other assays, the SAIDS virus-infected tissue culture was
shown not to be contaminated with known type C viruses, human T
cell lymphotropic virus type I (HTLV-I) or HTLV-III.

The macaques are social animals. Social activities range from
mutual grooming to aggressive fights with biting. Regarding the
natural transmission of SAIDS, it must be emphasized that virus
has been found in blood, tissues and in saliva. A salivary gland
from an animal dying of SAIDS contained numerous type D particles. The virus has been isolated from the saliva of many animals
with SAIDS and also from the saliva of at least one healthy carrier. That animal has high levels of virus in saliva (1.6×10^6
infectious units per ml of saliva). We have been able to transmit
the disease with saliva taken from this healthy carrier. We have
evidence that indicates that this particular healthy carrier has
been spreading the disease in our colony for several years. This
animal (17636) was born in 1976 in the North Corral #1 where its
mother died of SAIDS. The infant was removed and raised in a
nursery and travelled through the indoor colony until 1981, when
it went back into North Corral #1. It remains there today,
healthy and still shedding virus.

This animal's movements were associated with two cases of
SAIDS in the first location, 12 cases in the second, eight cases
in the third and 12 cases in the fourth. The epidemiologic work
was done by Nicholas Lerche. These results were shown to be statistically significant, and this disease pattern did not appear
in association with movements of other animals through the
colony. Even today, saliva taken from this animal can be used to
transmit the disease. Therefore, this disease can be transmitted

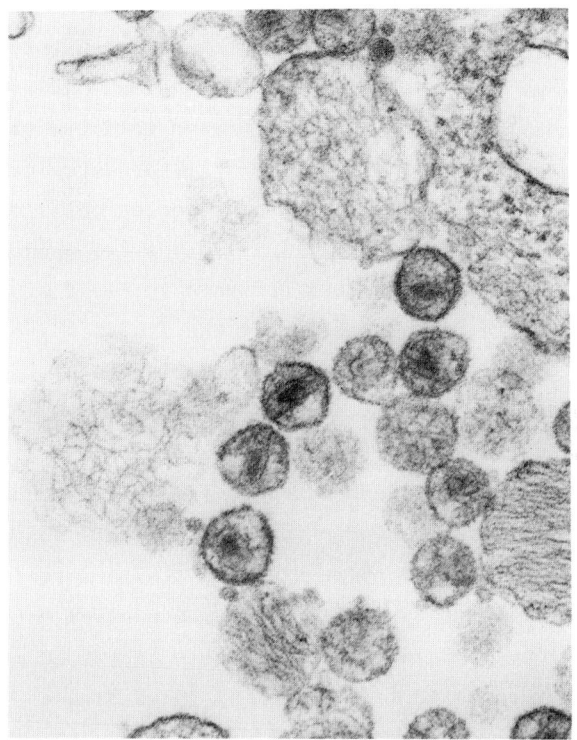

Fig. 2. SAIDS type D retrovirus obtained from the saliva of
a healthy carrier (80,000×).

by both sick and healthy animals. Figure 2 shows the type D
retrovirus isolated from the saliva of 17636.

In our studies, we can readily distinguish SAIDS/D California
from SAIDS/D Oregon. We have begun to use a new nomenclature
which we feel is more meaningful than the geographic designations
(e.g. California, New England, etc.). SAIDS/D California is named
SAIDS retrovirus type 1 (SRV-1) and the Oregon isolate is SAIDS
retrovirus type 2 (SRV-2). The previous nomenclature (Cal, NE, WA
and so forth) was helpful in some ways but does not indicate
which virus isolates are related to each other.

The SAIDS type 2 is the isolate from the OPRC. SRV-1 was compared by restriction mapping with SRV-2 and MPMV. This work was

done by Martin Bryant at CPRC with a clone of SRV-1 and SRV-2
which he used to probe infected Raji cells. We cultured the virus
in rhesus monkey cells for inoculation studies, but, for other
studies, the Raji cell line is a very good cell line for growing
SAIDS retrovirus for in vitro purposes. It produces characteristic syncytia and makes recognition of infected cells very easy.
With double digest of Sph/EcoRI, SRV-1 gives two bands, type 2
gives three and MPMV, which does not have an EcoRI site, has one
band. We, therefore, easily show that the isolates are different.
This type 1, type 2, etc. nomenclature will help us to eventually
sort out the different isolates.

Further studies showed that the antigens of SRV-1 and SRV-2
also differ. Differences were detected in a radioimmunoassay
using the MPMV p10 as the competing antigen (data not shown).

In the Oregon colony, there had been a high mortality rate
observed among the Macaca nigra, the Celebes black macaque. There
is a small colony of Celebes monkeys there (about 80 monkeys),
and mortality rates have varied from 5% to as high as 50% in
some years. Since the Oregon Center was having problems similar
to ours, we attempted to isolate type D virus from the Celebes
macaque. We received 11 coded blood samples, and we isolated
peripheral blood mononuclear cells from them and cocultured them
with Raji cells. The type 2 SAIDS virus was isolated from seven
of the group. We decoded the experiment, examined the clinical
records and found that health problems were present only in the
virus-positive group and not in the virus-negative group. The
kinds of health problems that were found were persistent diarrhea, lymphadenopathy, anemia and retroperitoneal fibromatosis
(which is a characteristic lesion that occurs in association with
the SAIDS at the Oregon Center and also occurs in association
with SAIDS in Washington). This is the clinical reason why we
suspect that SRV-2 may be the same as the SAIDS/D Washington
isolate. We also found abdominal masses indicative of retroperi-

toneal fibromatosis present in the animals with virus. In the
animals that were negative for virus, there were no abdominal
masses and the health status included only transient splenomegaly
and lymphadenopathy.

We, therefore, found that there was an association of SAIDS
type 2 virus with the unhealthy group of Celebes macaques at the
OPRC. Transmission studies cannot be done in Celebes monkeys
because captive colonies are small. There are some transmission
studies using this isolate inoculated into rhesus monkeys which
are in progress.

Table II summarizes the subtypes of viruses that are associ-
ated with particular species. In $\underline{M}$. $\underline{mulatta}$, there is SAIDS-like
disease definitely associated with experimentally inoculated
MPMV. As reported by Fine et al., MPMV induced a SAIDS-like
disease (5). We have confirmed this observation. The virus does
not appear to be naturally occurring in captive macaque populations in the United States. Two type D endogenous viruses have
been found, one in the squirrel monkey ($\underline{Saimiri}$ $\underline{sciureus}$) (6),
and another in the Langur monkey ($\underline{Presbytis}$ $\underline{obscurus}$) (7).
Neither is associated with disease. SRV-1 is associated with
SAIDS in the rhesus monkey at the CPRC (3,4). A similar virus is
found in the Taiwanese-rock macaque ($\underline{M}$. $\underline{cyclopsis}$) and the crab-
eating macaque ($\underline{M}$. $\underline{fascicularis}$). SRV-2 is associated with SAIDS
plus retroperitoneal fibromatosis in the Celebes macaque ($\underline{M}$.
$\underline{nigra}$) at the OPRC (Marx, P.A. et al., in press). A similar agent
is present in pig-tailed macaque ($\underline{M}$. $\underline{nemestrina}$) (8).

TABLE II. Distribution of Type D Retroviruses Among Nonhuman Primates

Species	Common name	Virus name	Disease association
Macaca mulatta	Rhesus	Mason-Pfizer monkey virus[a]	SAIDS-like disease
Saimiri sciureus	Squirrel monkey	Squirrel monkey retrovirus	None (endogenous virus)
Presbytis obscurus	Spectacled langur	PO-1-Lu	None (endogenous virus)
Macaca mulatta	Rhesus	SAIDS/type 1[b] retrovirus	SAIDS
Macaca cyclopsis	Taiwanese-rock macaque	D/New England	SAIDS[c]
Macaca fascicularis	Crab-eating macaque	D/New England	SAIDS[c]
Macaca nemestrina	Pig-tailed macaque	SAIDS-D/Washington	SAIDS/RF
Macaca nigra	Celebes black macaque	SAIDS type 2[d] retrovirus	SAIDS/RF

(continued)

TABLE II (continued)

---

^aMason-Pfizer monkey virus (MPMV) is not currently found in captive rhesus colonies. Only one or possibly two isolations of MPMV have been reported.

^bSAIDS type 1 retrovirus and D/New England have different restriction endonuclease maps.

^cLymphomas have been seen in association with SAIDS in these macaques.

^dClinical features of SAIDS/retroperitoneal fibromatosis suggest that D/Washington and SAIDS type 2 retrovirus may be the same virus.

143

ACKNOWLEDGMENT

I thank my coworkers at the University of California.

REFERENCES

1. Henrickson, R.V., Maul, D.H., Osborn, K.G. et al. (1983).
   Lancet 1, 388.
2. Chopra, H.C. and Mason, M.M. (1970). Cancer Res. 30, 2081.
3. Marx, P.A., Maul, D.H., Osborn, K.G. et al. (1984). Science
   223, 1083.
4. Gravell, M., London, W.T., Hamilton, R.S. et al. (1984).
   Lancet 1, 335.
5. Fine, D.L., Landon, J.C., Pienta, R.J. et al. (1975). J.
   Natl. Cancer Inst. 54, 651.
6. Heberling, R.L., Barker, S.T., Kalter, S.S. et al. (1977).
   Science 195, 289.
7. Todaro, G.J., Benveniste, R.E., Sherr, C.J. et al. (1978).
   Virology 84, 189.
8. Stromberg, K., Benveniste, R.E., Arthur, L.O. et al. (1984).
   Science 224, 289.

SIMIAN RETROVIRUS

Ronald Desrosiers

New England Region Primate Research Center
Southborough, Massachusetts

The New England Regional Primate Research Center (NERPRC) houses over 700 macaques of three species: Macaca mulatta (the rhesus monkey), Macaca fascicularis (the cynomolgus monkey) and Macaca cyclopis (the Taiwanese rock macaque). Around 1980, scientists at the NERPRC began to notice an unusual number of deaths in the macaque colony, especially among the M. cyclopis. Fully one third of the animals in this group died in 1980 and another third died in 1981. These animals once numbered as many as 100 in our colony and bred well in the past, but we now have less than 50 of this particular species.

M. cyclopis are endangered in the wild and we have probably the largest breeding colony in the world. In December 1979, 13 M. cyclopis were placed together in one gang cage, cage 43. As a striking example of the severity of the problem, all 13 animals were dead by 16 months after placement, with the median time to death being 8 months. These 13 animals shared a similar disease pattern that included opportunistic infections, diarrhea and severe weight loss. Figure 1B shows one of these 13 animals just prior to death; his appearance contrasts sharply with the healthy M. cyclopis of our cology (Fig. 1A). This disease has since been better characterized by Letvin, King and their colleagues as an acquired immunodeficiency syndrome of macaque monkeys (1,2).

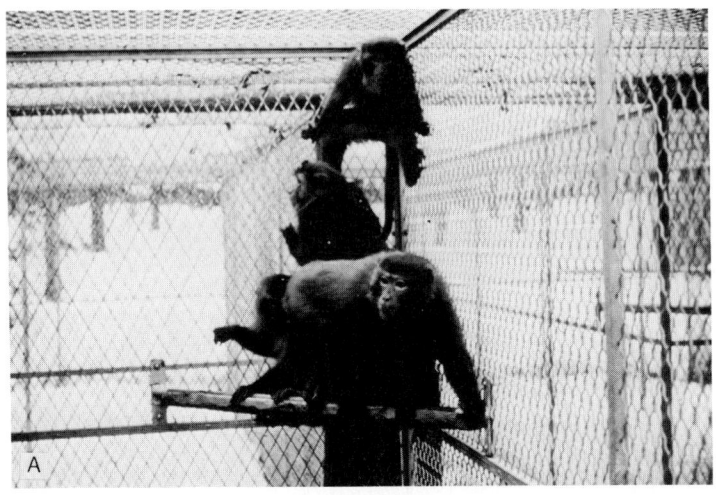

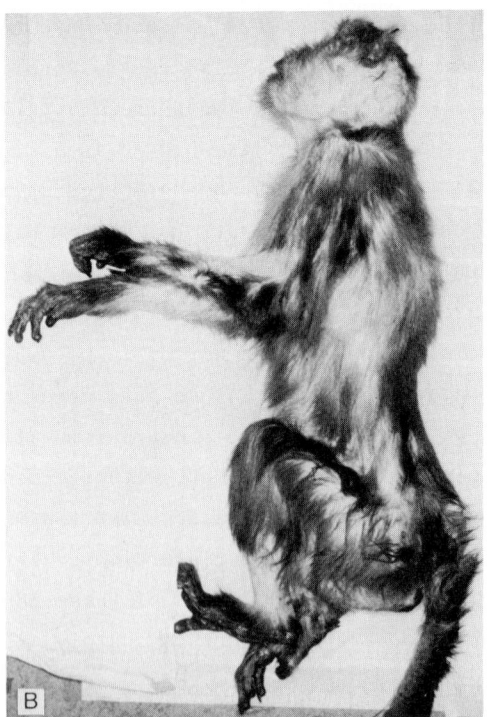

Fig. 1.   (A) Normal breeding colony. (B) Animal prior to death.

Over the last year and a half or so, type D retrovirus has been isolated from 17 macaques of the NERPRC colony (3). Most isolations were made by systematic co-cultivation of peripheral blood lymphocytes with Raji cells. Type D retrovirus was readily isolated from macaques with the naturally occurring immunodeficiency syndrome. Four of the 17 animals from whom virus was obtained clearly had the immunodeficiency syndrome, with opportunistic infections (cytomegalovirus [CMV], cryptosporidiosis, trichomoniasis, candidiasis) and markedly depressed T cell blastogenic responses. Although three other animals (398, 134 and 67) had near normal T cell blastogenic responses at the one time of testing, necropsy findings were consistent with the immunodeficiency syndrome. These seven animals have all died subsequent to virus isolation.

Attempts to isolate type D retroviruses from 97 healthy macaques of the NERPRC colony have not been successful (3). It thus appears that type D retrovirus can be readily isolated from animals with the immunodeficiency disease but not from apparently healthy animals. However, these results can say nothing about whether the virus is the cause of the disease, since the state of immunodeficiency, as with CMV, could allow opportunistic replication or reactivation of latent virus.

Type D retroviruses have also been isolated from macaques with less severe forms of illness. Isolates were obtained from nine animals which remain alive and healthy as long as 510 days after isolation (3). It is not clear at this time whether these nine animals had less severe forms of the immunodeficiency disease, whether they had other forms of illness or whether this may perhaps represent primary infection with the type D retrovirus.

Type D retrovirus in our colony has been isolated from three species: M. cyclopis, M. mulatta and M. fascicularis; although

the M. cyclopis are the least numerous, nine of the 17 isolates
were obtained from M. cyclopis.

We have cloned DNA from one of the D/New England isolates,
D398. Restriction maps were derived and compared to Mason-Pfizer
monkey virus (MPMV) restriction maps (3). The genomes are 8.1 to
8.2 kb pairs in length and the long terminal repeats for each of
these viruses are about 350 base pairs. Thirteen of 28 restriction endonuclease sites align when these two related viruses are
compared. This corresponds to a sequence homology of about 90%.
Although the overall sequence homology is about 90%, there are
areas where there is a strikingly reduced homology. For example,
in the presumed pol region, there is a series of eight restriction endonuclease sites that are not conserved (Fig. 2).

We further examined homology of MPMV and the D/New England
isolate by hybridization under varying degrees of stringency (3).
We used an assortment of cloned DNAs: cloned DNA from gibbon ape
leukemia virus (GaLV [provided by Ed Gelmann]), cloned DNA from
type D retrovirus of squirrel monkeys (provided by Stuart Aaron-
son), cloned DNA from MPMV, from the D/New England clone 398 and
from a cloned herpes virus DNA fragment of about the same size.
The viral DNA of each clone was excised with the appropriate
restriction enzyme, giving similar size DNA fragments. These
fragments were Southern blotted and hybridized under various
degrees of stringency to the ^{32}P-labeled D398 fragment. Approximately equal hybridization was obtained between MPMV and D398
using 30% formamide at 49°C. As the hybridization stringency was
increased using 40% formamide, 50% formamide and 60% formamide,
the ability of the MPMV DNA to hybridize to D/New England DNA
progressively decreased. Sixty percent formamide at 49°C represents about 10 to 15°C below the meling temperature (TM) of
homologous hybrid. Only very weak hybridization was obtained with
the squirrel monkey type D, even under lower hybridization stringency. We have found that approximately 100 times more squirrel

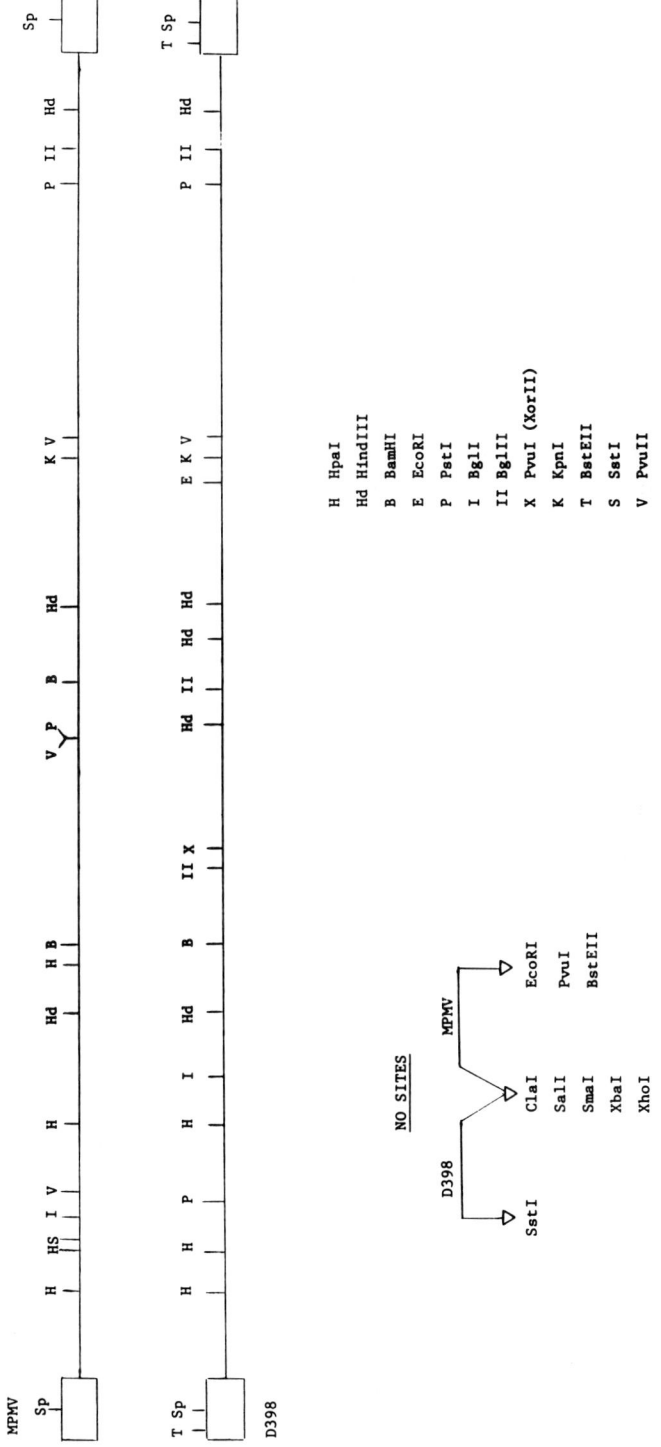

Fig. 2. Comparison of restriction enzyme maps of type D retrovirus isolate (D398) with MPMV.

monkey type D DNA is required than macaque type D DNA to give
approximately equal intensity in the autoradiogram. Significant
homology was not detected to the GaLV DNA or to the herpes virus
DNA.

Significant hybridization was also not detected between D398
DNA and cloned DNA from human T cell lymphotropic virus (HTLV)-I,
-II and -III kindly provided by Robert Gallo (Desrosiers, R.,
C. Butler and F. Wong-Staal, unpublished observation). This was
true even when 100 times more of the HTLV DNA was loaded onto the
gel and the hybridization was done under very low stringency,
about 50°C below the TM of homologous hybrid.

We next looked across the genome for areas having strongest
and weakest homology between MPMV and the D/New England. Under
conditions of very high stringency (60% formamide at 49°C), the
weakest homology was localized to the env and pol regions.

We have also compared a number of the isolates from the
NERPRC colony for strain variability. We have taken Hirt supernatant replicative intermediate DNA from infected cells and
digested with a number of enzymes. We compared DNA from MPMV-
infected cells with DNA from cells infected with D398 (derived
from a M. cyclopis), D114 (from M. fascicularis) and D225 (from
M. mulatta). All the D/New England isolates were easily distinguished from MPMV. However, even after examination of 30 restriction endonuclease sites, we have not been able to distinguish any
of the four D/New England isolates that have been looked at in
greatest detail. It thus appears that a single strain of type D
retrovirus is infecting three different species of macaques in
our colony.

This lack of variability is somewhat surprising, I think,
especially when one considers the variability that can occur
among type D retroviruses and the variability that can occur
among other retroviruses, such as GaLV (4). Unfortunately, not
much work has been done to compare the various type D isolates

from the several United States primate centers. Larry Arthur et
al. (manuscript submitted) have found that the p27 products from
the New England, California and Seattle isolates competed as
effectively as MPMV in a radioimmune competition assay for p27.
However, gp70 products from the same isolates were easily distinguished from MPMV in a competition assay with gp70. These competition assays measuring antigenic relatedness between MPMV and
D/New England agree quite well with the DNA homology studies
described above in which the region of greatest divergence, not
surprisingly, is the envelope region. Antigenic relatedness was
not detected between the type D retroviruses and HTLV.

In order to monitor disease induction, 13 naive rhesus
macaques have been inoculated with retrovirus D/New England (5).
A number of parameters have been varied. These include the age
of the animal at the time of inoculation (from 1 day to 12 months
old), the particular isolate used (including D398, D184 and
D225), the type of cells in which the virus was grown and the
amount of virus (up to greater than 10^9 infectious units) that
each animal received. The first animals of this study are still
alive $1\frac{1}{2}$ years following inoculation. All of the inoculated
macaques became infected. This was proven by our ability to
reisolate the virus from peripheral blood lymphocytes long after
experimental infection. Some of the animals were sporadically
viremic, and virus could be isolated from cell-free plasma as
long as 6 months after experimental infection. However, even
after a year and a half of follow-up, we have not observed any
lymphomas, any leukemias or anything that looks like the naturally occurring immunodeficiency disease.

The parameters followed for the inoculated animals included
clinical status, ability to isolate virus, hematologic values,
immunologic status and lymph node biopsies. Occasional diarrhea
was noted in the infected macaques and there was also transient
lymphadenopathy. One of the most striking features in all the

inoculated animals was a persistent neutropenia. T cell blastogenic responses to four different stimulants dipped transiently
during the first month after inoculation but returned to normal
and remained normal for the course of the experiment. This sort
of transient decrease in T cell blastogenic responsiveness is
not unusual after viral infection and is, in fact, seen following
infections with a number of viral agents. Opportunistic infections were not observed. Two of the animals, one 1 day old and
one 1 month old at the time of inoculation, died during the
course of this study. Both had a terminal diarrhea illness, and
thymic atrophy was noted at necropsy.

In summary, type D retrovirus has been readily isolated from
macaques with a spontaneous immunodeficiency syndrome. However,
experimental infection of naive macaques with D/New England has
not induced the immunodeficiency syndrome. Unfortunately, sufficient numbers of M. cyclopis are not available to determine
whether they may be more susceptible to disease induction by
type D retrovirus. Also, we do not yet know the extent of type D
retrovirus in our macaque colony. If infection were confined
primarily to the disease population, this would provide strong
evidence for a causative role of type D retrovirus in disease.
If, however, the rate of infection in our macaque colony is high,
as with CMV, it would not be surprising to recover the virus with
high frequency from immunodeficient animals. In this scenario,
type D retrovirus could play an important role in the pathogenesis of disease without being primarily responsible for the
immunodeficiency. Serologic screening has provided evidence for
prior infection with an HTLV-related virus among at least some
NERPRC macaques with lymphoproliferative and immunodeficiency
disorders (6). The recent isolation of HTLV-related viruses from
immunodeficient macaques and from one macaque with lymphoma will
allow us to study the interaction of these retroviruses with
type D retrovirus in the disease process (Daniel, M.D. et al.,
manuscript submitted).

REFERENCES

1. Letvin, N.L., Eaton, K.A., Aldrich, W.R. et al. (1983). Proc.
   Natl. Acad. Sci. USA. $\underline{80}$, 2718.
2. King, N.W., Hunt·, R.D., Letvin, N.L. et al. (1983). Am. J.
   Pathol. $\underline{113}$, 382.
3. Desrosiers, R. et al. (1985). Virology, in press.
4. Trainor, C., Wong-Stall, F. and Reitz, M. (1982). J. Virol.
   $\underline{41}$, 298.
5. Letvin, N.L., Daniel, M.D., Sehgal, P.K. et al. (1984).
   J. Virol. $\underline{52}$, 683.
6. Homma, T., Kanki, P.J., King, N.W., Jr. et al. (1984).
   Science $\underline{225}$, 716.

SIMIAN ACQUIRED IMMUNE DEFICIENCY SYNDROME

John Sever

National Institute of Neurological
and Communicative Disorders and Stroke
National Institutes of Health
Bethesda, Maryland

TRANSMISSION OF SAIDS

Our first studies were performed in collaboration with
investigators from the California Primate Research Center at
Davis, California. The inocula for these experiments consisted of
tissue materials from monkeys which contracted simian acquired
immune deficiency syndrome (SAIDS) at Davis. SAIDS was not occurring in our colony at the National Institutes of Health (NIH).
The inoculation of rhesus monkeys at NIH with various tissue
homogenates from Davis-diseased animals resulted in the transmission of the disease to these animals. Subsequently parallel
experiments were done at Davis and NIH. Filtered serum and plasma
from SAIDS animals transmitted the disease. Subsequently a retrovirus with type D morphology was isolated from SAIDS tissues at
both Davis and NIH, and fatal SAIDS was transmitted to monkeys at
both laboratories. Both groups reported that SAIDS (California)
can be transmitted by tissue homogenates, plasma and serum or by
the retorvirus grown in a variety of tissue cultures.

ELECTRON MICROSCOPY—MORPHOLOGY OF SAIDS AND AIDS RETROVIRUSES

In addition to the SAIDS (California) virus, we also worked
with human T cell lymphotropic virus type III (HTLV-III) which
was received from Dr. Robert Gallo (National Cancer Institute,
NIH) and with lymphadenopathy-associated virus (LAV) received
from Drs. Chermann and Montagnier (Pasteur Institut, Paris,
France).

We have studied the morphology of the retroviruses associated
with SAIDS and AIDS. The electron microscopy (EM) studies were
performed by Dr. Michael Lecatsas (University of Pretoria, South
Africa) while he worked with us at the NIH. His studies of the
SAIDS (California) virus were on virus grown in tissue culture in
low passage rhesus monkey bone marrow fibroblast cultures. Examination of thin sections of infected cells gave evidence that few
"A" type particles were present in the cytoplasma of cells. Thin
sections of virions which had budded from cellular membranes had
cores of various shapes, usually dots, eccentric wedges or bars.
Examination of thin sections of HTLV-III infected cells also
showed virions with cores of variable shapes similar to those of
SAIDS virus. Based on a series of studies, Dr. Lecatsas proposed
a model to account for the variable core shapes seen in electron
micrographs. Briefly, during the process of viral maturation, the
virion core condenses to form a cylinder. According to his postu-
late, the shape of the core seen in electron micrographs will
vary with the plane through which virions are cut. Thus, the core
can have the appearance of a closed circle, triangle, target or
bar. If the plane of sectioning is through the edge of the virus,
there will be no core at all. These studies provided evidence
that the cores of the AIDS and SAIDS retroviruses are cylindrical
in shape. The insight gained from the morphological studies of
AIDS and SAIDS retroviruses was applied to screening various

tissue specimens from animals and man for the presence of similar retroviruses.

SAIDS VIRUS IN SALVIA, URINE AND PAROTID GLAND

In a study of transmission of SAIDS, animals were inoculated with a pool of serum from an animal with advanced SAIDS. Virus was isolated in vitro from the saliva of one recipient animal 14 weeks after inoculated and in terminal SAIDS. In another study, a normal animal developed SAIDS 17 weeks after it was caged with an animal inoculated with SAIDS virus. SAIDS virus was also isolated in tissue culture from the saliva of this animal. In addition, samples of saliva and urine studied by EM showed characteristic virus particles with typical SAIDS retrovirus morphology. SAIDS virus was also isolated from the urine of diseased animals. Isolations were made from the urine of animals which had been inoculated with serum pool A or with the tissue suspensions that came from Davis. SAIDS virus was isolated from animals in both early and late stages of disease. SAIDS was transmitted to healthy rhesus monkeys by inoculating them with saliva from diseased animals. Also, virus was isolated from the urine of an animal which had been infected with saliva. This isolation was made in human diploid fibroblast cells. An animal inoculated with this isolate also experienced symptoms of SAIDS. Thus, transmission was successful using either the tissue culture-passed virus isolated from urine or the virus taken directly from saliva. Furthermore, electron microscopic studies of thin sections of the parotid glands from an animal inoculated with saliva and dying of SAIDS showed characteristic SAIDS virus.

AIDS VIRUS IN PAROTID GLANDS, PROSTATE AND TESTES

Finally, we used EM to study samples from human patients with AIDS. Characteristic bar-shaped viruses were seen in samples of parotid glands, prostates and testes taken from AIDS patients at autopsy.

PATHOGENESIS OF
RETROVIRUS INFECTION

PATHOGENESIS OF ACQUIRED IMMUNE DEFICIENCY SYNDROME

Donald Francis

Center for Infectious Diseases
Centers for Disease Control
Atlanta, Georgia

One of the most impressive things about AIDS is what a
miserable disease it is. Over the last dozen years I have worked
around the world with many horrible bugs that have caused many
horrible diseases like smallpox, hemorraghic fever and cholera,
but seldom have I worked with a disease as bad as AIDS. It ranks
well up with those three I mentioned above.

There are some unique aspects of AIDS that have made it a
remarkably difficult disease to understand and treat. First, it
has an extremely long incubation period compared with the standard infectious diseases with which we are accustomed to working.
Second, AIDS concerns the groups which are unique in terms of
their lifestyles, their individual fears and anxieties, their
political abilities and their readiness to blame researchers and
others for publicizing their disease. Last are the politics of
AIDS—both classic Washingtonian politics and maybe less classic
scientific politics—which have made this so difficult a problem.

I will discuss the pathogenesis of AIDS in terms of disease
progression. This involves the inexorable loss of immune abilities, and this loss opens the gates of defenselessness, allowing
for the development of opportunistic infections. Instead of
describing again the published reports on loss of T cell

161

function, abnormalities in B cell activities and so on, I want to stress other pieces of the natural history puzzle that are starting to fit together. There is a fair amount of unpublished data that are being considered as we try to fit the virologic and epidemiologic puzzle pieces together. They are starting to give a glimmer of what AIDS really is, of what the natural history of the disease is, how it is transmitted and what happens to people who are affected.

The agent which is the cause of AIDS was first discovered in 1983 by Francoise Barre, Jean-Claude Chermann and Luc Montagnier. They named the initial isolate lymphadenopathy-associated virus (LAV). A year later, it was rediscovered by Robert Gallo and his group and named human T cell lymphotrophic virus type 3 (HTLV-III). Several months later, it was "rediscovered" by Jay Levy and his group and called AIDS-associated retrovirus. In the middle of all this, we also "rediscovered" it. Using standard scientific experiments, we compared our isolates to the initial French isolates and reported that it was LAV-like. The final name of this virus has not been agreed upon. I suspect it will be neither LAV nor HTLV-III. Until a name has been agreed upon by those involved in the disease, we are trying to respect the great work of all who have been working with it and refer to the virus as LAV/ HTLV-III or HTLV/LAV. That is rather cumbersome, and you will find that most people start talking about "the AIDS virus" quite rapidly.

This chapter will deal first with transmission, then the establishment of infection in the host, then disease outcome and finally describe where we are in terms of epidemiology. Some recent work on transmission has been done by Paul Feorino in our laboratory involving transfusion-associated AIDS patients. To date there have been 22 donor-recipient sets or transfusion-associated cases identified by local state health departments and reported to us. We investigate such cases, find the names of the blood donors, interview all donors, bleed the donors, do helper: suppressor ratios and other tests on the blood. In each set, essentially, there has been a high risk donor, defined as an individual who belongs to a risk group. However, some individuals do not give a history indicating membership in a high risk group, for example, two out of this group denied risk group membership but had abnormal helper:suppressor ratios. The remainer were gay men, except one who was an intravenous drug user and another who was a gay intravenous drug user.

The purpose of this study was to examine high risk donors at various times. The presumption was that high risk donors transmitted disease when they donated blood. We examined them from 1 to 4½ years after their donation to see if their lymphocytes were still infected. One high risk donor was found per set for 20 individuals. There was one child who received three transfusions, and two were from gay men; both were infectious. There was another individual who had transfusions from three infectious donors.

Virologically, out of the 25 high risk individuals, 22 had virus which could be cultured from their lymphocytes in primary lymphocyte cultures. The technique used was that of Francoise Barre and Jean-Claude Chermann, using phytohemagglutinin (PHA)-stimulated human lymphocytes. After 3 days of PHA stimulation, the cultures are co-cultivated with the suspect specimen and followed for the appearance of reverse transcriptase (RT), examined by electronmicroscopy (EM) and by fluorescence antibody (FA) for expression of LAV/HTLV-III antigens. Most of these appear relatively quickly, in about 7 days. We follow them for 3 weeks before calling them negative. All of the cultures which were positive were EM positive, FA positive and RT positive.

The essence of this study is that there are individuals who have been documented to transmit disease by blood donation and who, from 12 to 52 months after donation, have remained

infectious. Of this group, interestingly, all were healthy at the
time of donation and the majority of them are still healthy. Two
of them have developed AIDS, one has had apparent chronic lymphadenopathy, and four others have had lymphadenopathy detectable
only by physical examination.

Transmitters may be the equivalent of the carrier as seen in
hepatitis B. To whom do they give their virus? It is remarkable
that those who get AIDS belong to groups which have remained the
same over 3 years of disease with cases increasing from 6 to
6000. Cofactors may be involved in disease susceptibility. It is
hard to sort those who are going to come down with disease from
those who will not; everyone is probably susceptible if appropriately exposed to enough virus. I think the reason certain people
are infected is that they have the right kind of contact for
disease transmission. It seems that the AIDS virus is a relatively difficult virus to transmit. The groups involved in AIDS
are like the groups involved in hepatitis B virus infection. But
some differences are found. About 6% of acute hepatitis B
patients in the United States are health care workers, yet we
still have not documented a nosocomial case of AIDS, despite
literally hundreds of instances of people being stuck with needles used for taking blood from lymphadenopathy and AIDS patients
in hospitals. That could imply that a cofactor is needed for susceptibility to the disease. It also could be that the amount of
virus in these individuals is low. For example, in hepatitis B
with an e antigen-positive individual, one finds virus titers
that are 9 or 10 logs of chimpanzee infectious doses per ml.
Electronmicroscopic examinations of serum from these people show
full virions. AIDS virions cannot be seen in the plasma of AIDS
patients or implicated blood donors. Thus, there appears to be a
much lower amount of virus in AIDS compared to hepatitis B; it is
cell associated to an extent although it is certainly in plasma

as indicated by the observation that hemophiliacs who receive a plasma concentrate derivative get this disease.

So, although there could be a cofactor, I would suspect that the appropriate form of exposure is responsible for recipients of blood, people who share blood, drug users, hemophiliacs, transfusion recipients or sexual contacts being infected.

Another point in transmission that distinguishes AIDS from hepatitis B is that the group having no known risk factors has remained, fortunately, remarkably small for AIDS. Most of the individuals categorized in this group are dead or refused to give histories.

This contrasts with hepatitis B. The hepatitis virus is also difficult to transmit, but the sources of at least 20 to 30% of hepatitis B cases in the United States cannot be determined.

Since 1978, we have been following a cohort of men in San Francisco studying hepatitis B virus infections. Over the last 6 years, gay men who came to the sexually transmitted diseases clinic were bled and entered into various studies, a prevalence study, an incidence study and then a vaccine study. The cohort consists of 6875 men. Right now 2% of these men have AIDS. In this cohort the transmission of hepatitis B virus is very different from the transmission of AIDS. Twenty-nine percent a year have gotten hepatitis B virus infection; 13% a year have gotten LAV/HTLV-III. Thus, the overall transmission rate is much lower for AIDS virus infection than for hepatitis B virus. So, I would claim that AIDS is a more difficult disease to transmit than hepatitis B virus and that is why it is restricted to these groups.

How is AIDS transmitted to these groups? I'll refer to a hepatitis B study that we did in Denver with a cohort of men that we were following for the same reasons as the San Francisco group. This work was done by Drs. Reiner and Judson at the Denver City Clinic several years ago. This study showed that gay men are

frequently exposed to blood during anal intercourse. A group of
antigen-positive individuals who were identified at the clinic
were given an anoscopic examination. Of 22 men, 13 had visible
lesions; 10 of these were HBSAG positive. The lesions are oozing,
bloody, serous lesions in the rectum and anus, usually multiple.
It is more difficult to get blood from other areas where there
are not lesions.

Jerry Groopman noted in his article in Science that the AIDS
virus can be cultured from saliva and peripheral blood lymphocytes of healthy homosexual men. Virus can come into the mouth
by various means. With chewing, plasma is pumped up between the
teeth in what is called intracravicular fluid. If there is virus-
free material in plasma, it could be pumped up into the mouth.
Although there is virus in saliva which may provide a means of
AIDS transmission, there is no bus-acquired or restaurant-
acquired AIDS and so it is unlikely that the virus is aerosolized
in any way. But presumably, other means like heavy kissing,
toothbrush or gum sharing might transmit infection. So far, sis-
ters of gay men who kiss their brothers, dentists and so on have
not gotten AIDS.

How does infection become established? It appears that the
AIDS virus preferentially infects lymphocytes. In vitro, there is
good viral replication only if lymphocytes are stimulated prior
to or after inoculation. It is not known whether such stimulation
is necessary in real life for establishing an infection. Inflammatory disease of the lower bowel in gay men and proctitis are
extremely common (i.e., 13 of 22 men discussed above). Therefore,
virus that was deposited on inflammed anus or rectum would certainly find adequate numbers of lymphocytes to infect.

In our chimpanzee studies, four chimpanzees have been
infected with prototype LAV strain. Three animals were initially
"immunostimulated" either with human lymphocytes (one animal) or
a killed bacterial vaccine (two animals). After this, lymphocytes

were removed, infected with virus in the laboratory and
reinjected. Infection occurs readily, and ELISA positivity and
seroconversion occur within a few weeks. Subsequently, additional
animals have been infected without preinoculation immunostimula-
tion.

What proportion of infected people develop AIDS? To determine
this we must first observe the follow-up patients long enough to
ensure that those who are going to develop the disease have done
so. Although the incubation period for AIDS may extend longer as
we observe this infection longer, presently it appears to be
between 2 and 3 years.

In one study, serologically identified individuals in San
Francisco were evaluated; in another study, individuals who
donated blood were evaluated. Both groups were followed to determine how many of them have come down with AIDS. Of the 6875 men
in the San Francisco cohort, 500 were randomly selected for
follow up, and remarkably we found 360 of them 5 to 6 years after
they had visited the clinic. We bled these people, took their
lymphocytes and serum and tested them. Using the p25 RIP, 21 were
seropositive at the time of their first bleed in 1978 to 1979 and
222 are positive now.

We also looked at a totally different group: 23 high risk
donors who were seropositive following donation of blood and who
therefore presumably were infectious at the time that they
donated. Ten percent of individuals in this group who were presumably infectious several years ago have come down with AIDS.

What has happened in the United States with this disease? As
it stands now, the outbreak is large. It started a couple of
years ago with six cases reported by Dr. Gottlieb in Los Angeles.
Now 6400 cases have been reported in the United States. The rates
continue to go up; at this time next year there will be 12,000
cases. The sexual contact among gay men has decreased, but the

numbers in other groups will go up and the tragedy will probably
continue for a long while.

AIDS started in the coastal areas of the United States, in
New York City, California, then Miami and then Texas. It has
clearly spread into essentially all of the United States.

The Venn diagram shows the distribution of cases among risk
groups and cases which overlap. There are three gay hemophiliacs,
few gay Haitians. The Haitians are being investigated in detail
now with Haitian interviewers. Patients do not say they are gay,
but Haiti was an important place for gay men in New York to
visit; therefore, some of these people might have been passive
homosexual partners for financial gain even though they are not
actually homosexuals.

The mortality from AIDS is high. Essentially everyone meeting
the definition of AIDS, as supplied by the Centers for Disease
Control, dies of the disease.

When the 1978 serum specimens for the San Francisco cohort
were tested, 22 individuals were positive. Sixty-two percent of
the group were positive in 1984. Steve McDougle, Bruce Evatt and
Dr. Gomperts in Los Angeles looked at 14 hemophiliacs whose blood
was available from 1978. Of these, all of whom are heavy users of
concentrate material, 100% had been infected by 1984.

In summary, AIDS appears to be transmitted by blood and by
sexual activity. The virus is relatively dificult to transmit,
but there is effective transmission within groups that share
blood or share sex with each other. The epidemic is large in the
United States; now there are literally hundreds of thousands of
people who are infected with this virus. And tens of thousands
will die of AIDS over the coming years.

AVIAN LEUKOSIS VIRUS-INDUCED CANCER: THE INDUCTION
OF ERYTHROBLASTOSIS BY PROVIRAL INSERTIONS
INTO OR NEW TRANSDUCTIONS OF c-erbB[1]

H. L. Robinson
B. D. Miles
S. E. Tracy

Worcester Foundation for Experimental Biology
Shrewsbury, Massachusetts

For the past several years it has been realized that avian
leukosis viruses (ALV) cause cancer by mutating host genes that
are critical to normal growth and development. Host genes that
can be mutated to cancer-inducing genes are termed proto-
oncogenes. ALV can mutate proto-oncogenes to oncogenes by the
integration of proviral DNA into a proto-oncogene. ALVs can also
mutate proto-oncogenes to oncogenes by the incorporation of
sequences from a proto-oncogene into a viral genome. This latter
phenomenon is referred to as viral transduction of host
sequences. This chapter describes the induction of erythroblastosis by proviral insertions into the proto-oncogene c-erbB and the
induction of erythroblastosis and angiosarcomas by viral transductions of c-erbB. C-erbB is a proto-oncogene of high interest
since it represents sequences at the 3' end of the gene that
encodes the receptor for epidermal growth factor (EGF).

---

[1]This research was supported by Public Health Service
research grants RO1-CA27223 and RO1-CA23086 and core grant P30
12708 from the National Institutes of Health and by the W. J.
Tannenberg Fund.

169

RETROVIRAL GENOME: INTEGRATED PROVIRUS

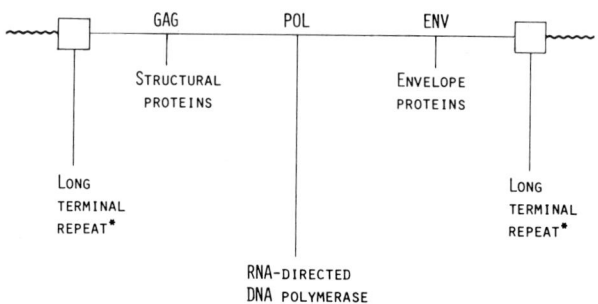

Fig. 1.   Proviral DNA of an avian leukosis virus. The open
squares represent the long terminal repeat sequences of proviral
DNA.

Figure 1 shows the genetic organization of the DNA of a
typical ALV provirus. The provirus contains three protein-coding
genes: gag, pol and env. These protein-coding sequences are
flanked by the long terminal repeat (LTR) sequences that form the
boundaries between proviral and host sequences. The LTRs contain
signals that are important for the reverse transcription of viral
RNA to DNA, the integration of proviral DNA and the control of
the transcription of integrated proviral DNA. The ALVs I work
with do not contain oncogenes. Infections by these viruses cause
cancer only if a provirus becomes inserted into a proto-oncogene
or if a virus transduces sequences from a proto-oncogene.

We obtain ALV-induced tumors by inoculating $\sim 1 \times 10^6$ infectious units of virus intravenously into a series of day old
chicks (Fig. 2). Most of the chicks become persistently viremic.
In a typical experiment, disease begins to occur at 2 to 3 months
after infection with between 20% and 50% of the infected chicks
developing cancer within the next year. As chickens become

Oncogenicity Tests

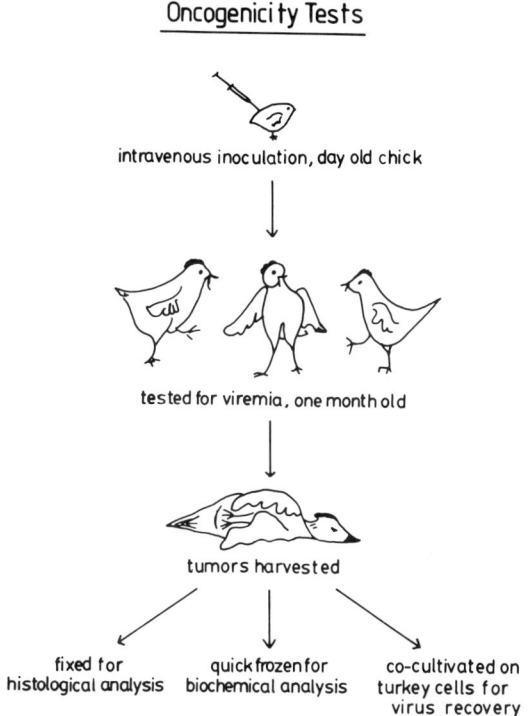

intravenous inoculation, day old chick

tested for viremia, one month old

tumors harvested

fixed for   quick frozen for   co-cultivated on
histological analysis biochemical analysis   turkey cells for
                                              virus recovery

Fig. 2.   Protocol for the induction of tumors.

diseased, moribund birds are sacrificed and tumor and control
tissues harvested for histologic as well as biochemical analyses.
The histologic analyses are used to diagnose the tumor. The biochemical analyses are designed to test tumor DNAs for proviral
insertions into or new transductions of proto-oncogene sequences.

ALV-induced erythroblastosis is caused by proviral insertions
into or viral transductions of the 3' half of the gene for the
EGF receptor. Erythroblastosis-inducing insertions or transductions result in the expression of a truncated form of the EGF
receptor. This truncated receptor includes the transmembrane and
cytoplasmic domains of the receptor protein. Host sequences
encoding the transmembrane and cytoplasmic domains of the EGF

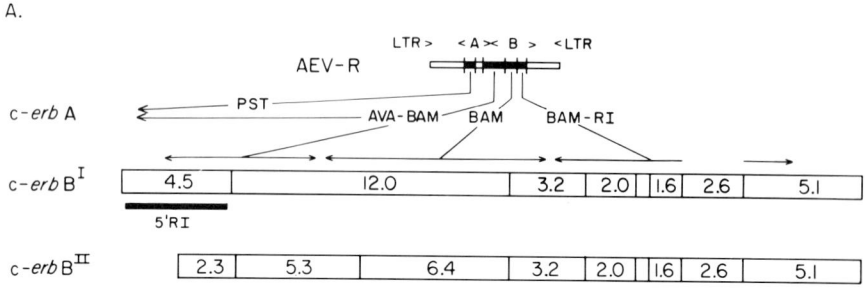

Fig. 3. Restriction endonuclease sites and probes used to identify viral and c-erbB sequences. Boxes indicate EcoRI fragments of the indicated cellular DNAs. The numbers indicate fragment sizes in kb. Heavy lines indicate probes used to detect c-erbA, c-erbB and proviral sequences.

receptor are referred to as c-erbB since these sequences were first identified by virtue of their homology to transduced sequences (v-erbB gene) in two closely related avian erythroblastosis viruses (AEV), AEV-R and AEV-ES4.

Chickens carry two different alleles of the EGF receptor gene (Fig. 3). The erbB regions of these two alleles are referred to as c-erb^I and c-erb^{II}. Both c-erbB^I and c-erb^{II} occupy about 20 kb of chromosomal DNA. Within that 20 kb are a series of small exons that contain ∿2000 bases of protein-coding sequences. To identify c-erbB sequences that had sustained proviral insertions or viral transductions, DNAs from cases of erythroblastosis were analyzed on Southern blots for novel c-erbB sequences that hybridized with probes for the 5', mid or 3' regions of the v-erbB gene of AEV-R. Each of the DNAs used as a probe contained sequences found in several of the exons of c-erbB. Consequently

each hybridized with several of the EcoRI fragments of chromosomal c-erbB sequences (see Fig. 3).

DNAs extracted from 21 cases of erythroblastosis were
analyzed for proviral insertions into or new transductions of
c-erbB. Ten of these cases of erythroblastosis were found to have
a proviral insertion in c-erbB and 10 were found to have one or
more new transductions of c-erbB. In the remainder of this chapter I am going to describe the insertions, the transductions,
speculate as to how the insertions might have led to the transductions and describe the disease potential of the new c-erbB
transducing viruses.

Each of the 10 erythroblastosis-inducing proviral insertions
occurred in the most 5' EcoRI fragment of c-erbB^{I} or c-erbB^{II}.
Seven of these were found just upstream of sequences that were
transduced in AEV-R while three occurred just within sequences
that were transduced by AEV-R. Figure 4 shows an example of an
insertion that occurred in the erythroleukemia in chicken 4888.
This insertion occurred in c-erbB^{II}. The schematic (Fig. 4,
panel C) maps the EcoRI and the SacI restriction endonuclease
sites in this insertion. The autoradiographs (Fig. 4, panels A
and B) present some of the data that were used to map the insertion. Panel A displays novel EcoRI fragments in the erythroleukemia in chicken 4888. Two novel fragments, 1.9 kb and 0.8 kb in
size, hybridized with the probe for the 2.3 kb EcoRI fragment of
c-erbB as well as with the probe for sequences at the 5' end of
v-erbB (AVA-BAM probe). These fragments did not hybridize with
probes for the mid or 3' regions of the c-erbB gene of AEV-R.
Thus these novel fragments represent the 5' and 3' junctions of
an erythroblastosis-inducing insertion. Hybridization of the blot
of EcoRI-digested DNA with a probe for viral LTR sequences also
revealed the two junction fragments. This result suggests that
both of the junctions contain LTR sequences. The sum of the sizes
of the two junction fragments is equal to the size of one LTR

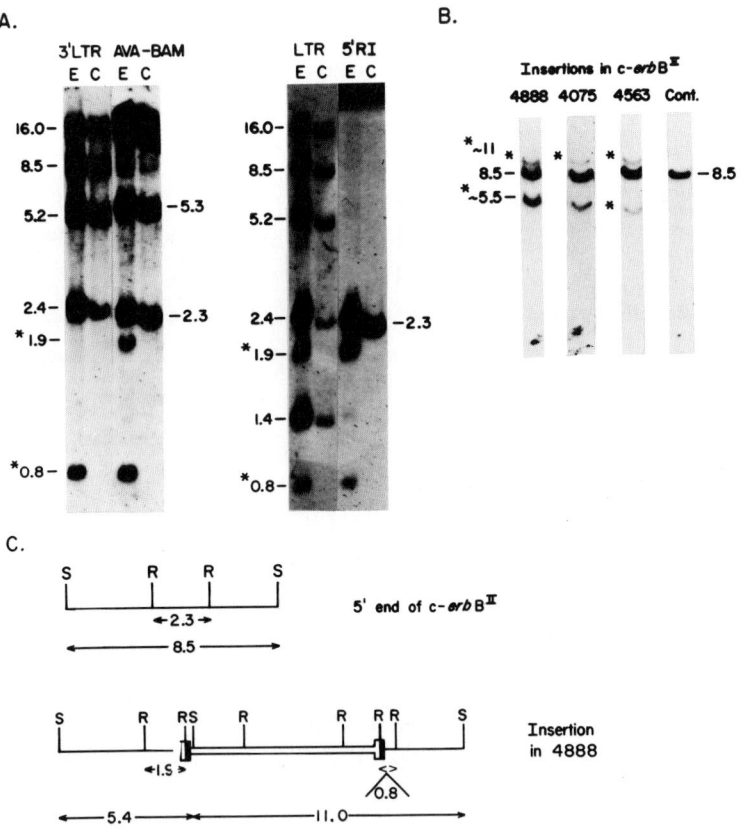

Fig. 4. Mapping of a proviral insertion in c-<u>erb</u>B^{II}.

Fig. 4.   (A) EcoRI fragments of the proviral insertion in chicken
4888. Data are presented from two blots. One blot was hybridized
with the 3' LTR probe and then the AVA-BAM probe. The second blot
was hybridized with the LTR and then the 5' RI probe. In between
hybridizations, probes were melted from the blots. Lanes designated E contain DNA from the erythroleukemia (bone marrow). Lanes
designated C contain DNA from a normal tissue. Sizes of fragments
are indicated in kb. Asterisks indicate novel fragments. (B) SacI
fragments of the proviral insertions in c-erbB in chickens 4888,
4075 and 4563. The blot was hybridized with the 5' RI probe.
Lanes designated 4888, 4075 and 4563 contain DNA from the erythroleukemias (bone marrow) in the indicated chickens. The lane
designated Cont contains DNA from an uninfected K28 chicken. Each
of the ~11 and ~5.5 kb tumor-associated fragments is of a
slightly different size. (C) Restriction endonuclease map of the
insertion in chicken 4888. Only the most 5' EcoRI fragment of
c-erbB^{II} is included in this map. Data for the mapping was taken
from panels A and B as well as from data on tumor-associated KpnI
fragments. R, EcoRI site; S, SacI site; ——, cellular sequence;
===, proviral sequence; [ ], proviral LTR.

(EcoRI cleaves once within the ∿300 bp LTR) plus the sequences
in the 2.3 kb EcoRI fragment of c-erbB[II]. Therefore the erythroblastosis-inducing insertion in chicken 4888 appears to have not
been associated with rearrangements or deletions in adjacent host
sequences. Hybridization of the same blot with a probe for
sequence 3' to the EcoRI site in the LTR revealed only the novel
0.8 kb fragment. This fragment therefore represents the 3'junction of proviral and host sequences. Panel B presents Southern
blot analyses of SacI-digested DNAs of the erythroleukemia in
chicken 4888 as well as of the erythroleukemias in chickens 4075
and 4563. SacI was used in these digests because the one SacI
site in the inducing provirus serves as a marker for sequences
that signal the packaging of viral RNA into virions. If this SacI
site is retained in an insertion, then the tumor should have two
novel SacI fragments. If this SacI site was deleted, the tumor
should have only one novel SacI fragment. Each of the three
tested erythroleukemias displayed two novel SacI fragments. Thus,
most erythroblastosis-inducing proviruses appear to have retained
sequences that encode the packaging of RNA into virions.

Restriction endonuclease mapping of the nine other erythroblastosis-inducing proviral insertions indicated that these
insertions were similar to the one that had occurred in chicken
4888. From these maps, we can conclude that erythroblastosis-
inducing proviral insertions occur at the 5' end of c-erbB. We
can also conclude that most erythroblastosis-inducing insertions
are proviruses that have retained both LTRs as well as sequences
that signal the packaging of RNA into virions. And, finally, we
can conclude that most erythroblastosis-inducing insertions are
proviruses that are in the same transcriptional orientation as
c-erbB.

The new c-erbB transducing viruses were recognized as novel
EcoRI fragments with sequences hybridizing with probes from the
5', mid and 3' regions of the v-erb gene of AEV-R. These novel

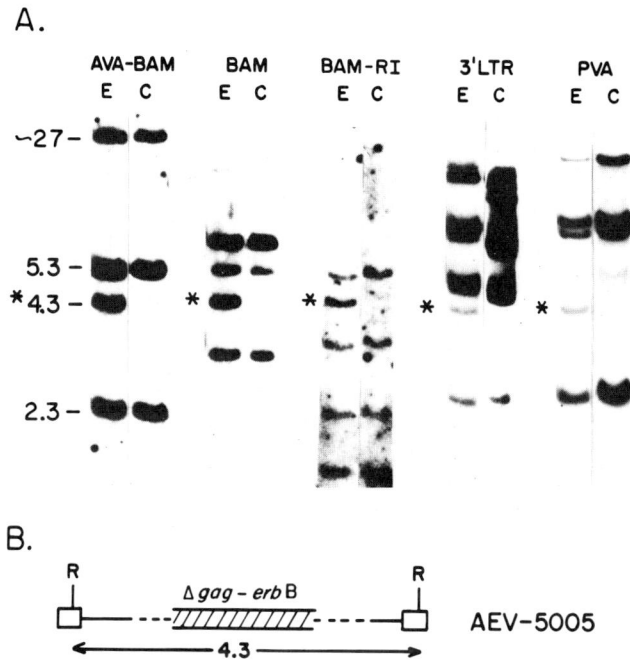

Fig. 5. EcoRI fragment of transduced c-erbB sequences in chicken 5005. (A) Autoradiographs of Southern blot analysis of EcoRI-digested DNAs from chicken 5005. Lanes designated E contain tumor DNA (bone marrow), and lanes designated C contain control DNA (bursa). Hybridization probes are indicated above each pair of lanes. Numbers indicate sizes of fragments in kb. The asterisks indicate the fragment of transduced c-erbB sequence. (B) Possible organization of the genome of AEV-5005. R, EcoRI site; [ ], proviral LTRs; [///], transduced sequence. Both AEV and AEV-H have an EcoRI site near the 3' boundary of transduced c-erbB sequences. This site is not portrayed in the schematic since we could not detect a novel PVC-related fragment in EcoRI-digested 5005 tumor DNA.

EcoRI fragments ranged from 2 to 5 kb in size. Since the exon sequences observed in these novel fragments reside in over 20 kb of chromosomal DNA, these fragments appeared to represent reverse transcripts of c-erbB mRNAs.

Figure 5 shows Southern blot analyses of sequences present in a transducing virus that originated in chicken 5005. This transduction appears to have recombined viral gag sequences with

A.

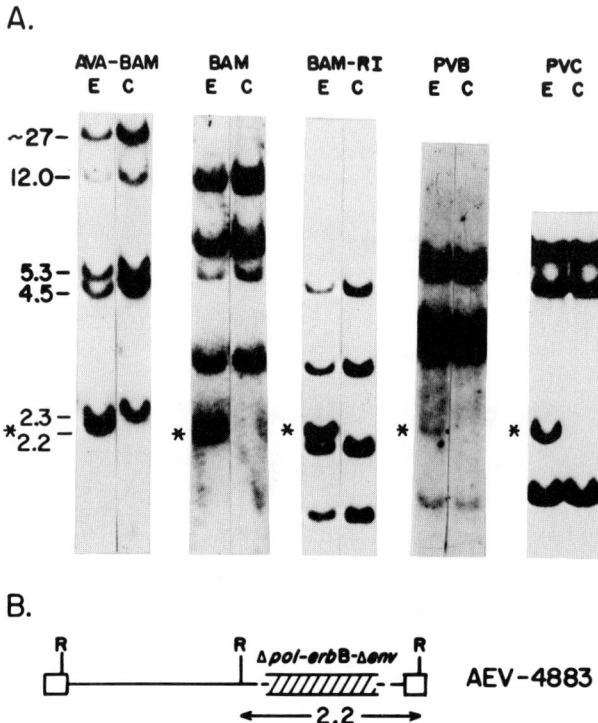

B.

Fig. 6. EcoRI fragment of transduced c-erbB sequences in chicken 4883. (A) Autoradiographs of Southern blot analysis of EcoRI-digested DNA from chicken 4883. Lanes designated E contain tumor DNA (bone marrow) and lanes designated C contain control DNA (bursa). Hybridization probes are indicated above each pair of lanes. Sizes of fragments are given in kb. Asterisks indicate the fragment of transduced c-erbB sequence. (B) Possible organization of the genome of AEV-4883. R, EcoRI site; [ ], proviral LTR; [///], transduced sequence.

c-erbB sequences (Fig. 5, panel B) since the novel 4.3 kb EcoRI fragment hybridized with probes for the 5', mid and 3' regions of the v-erbB gene of AEV-R as well as with proviral LTR and gag sequences (Fig. 5, panel A).

Figure 6 presents a transduction that originated in chicken 4883. In this transduction, the recombination of viral and c-erbB sequences appears to have joined the viral pol gene with c-erbB

TABLE I.   Induction of Rapid-Onset Erythroblastosis
by Filtered Homogenates of Tumors Containing
Candidate Transductions of c-erbB

Tumor homogenate	No. with erythroblastosis/ no. inoculated
4920	1/8
4883	4/6
5009	2/7
4890	5/5
5040	4/7
5005	4/6

Homogenates (10%, wt/vol) of tumors (spleens) with candidate transductions were passed through 0.22 µm filters and inoculated intravenously into 1-week-old (K28 × 15_1) × K28 chickens. Erythroblastosis occurred between 2 and 6 weeks post inoculation.

sequences (Fig. 6, panel B) since the novel 2.2 kb fragment hybridized with probes for the 5', mid and 3' regions of v-erbB as well as with probes for viral pol and env sequences (Fig. 6, panel A).

To prove that we indeed had new c-erbB transducing viruses, we prepared homogenates of the erythroleukemias that exhibited candidate transductions. These homogenates were filtered and inoculated intravenously into 1-week-old chicks and the inoculated chicks observed for disease. Every single filtered homogenate induced rapid-onset erythroblastosis (Table I). DNAs were isolated from these erythroleukemias. In each case the induced tumor was associated with the same novel erbB fragment that was present in the inducing homogenate (Fig. 7). Thus the novel fragments that appeared to contain spliced forms of c-erbB sequences did indeed represent new c-erbB transducing viruses.

The preferred model for transduction of a host gene by a retrovirus starts with a proviral insertion upstream of and in the same transcriptional orientation as the sequence to be

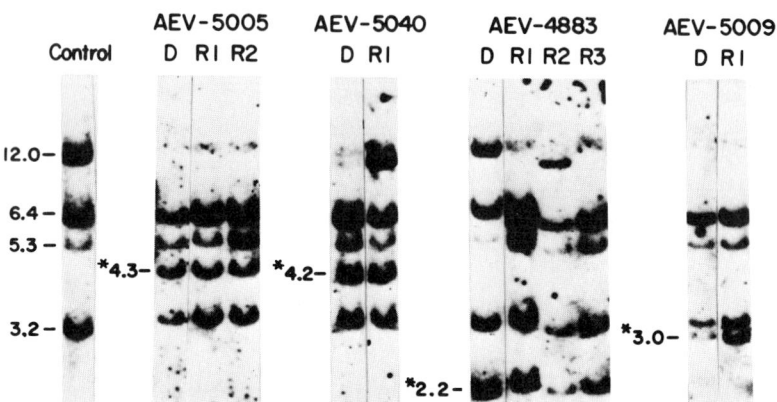

Fig. 7. EcoRI fragments of transduced c-erbB sequences in erythroblastosis induced by tumor homogenates. DNAs from erythroleukemias (bone marrow or spleen) induced by filtered tumor homogenates were EcoRI digested and analyzed for fragments that hybridized with the BAM probe. The viruses indicated over the lanes designate the AEV that originated in the donor tumor (D) and was present in the tumors of recipient chicks (R1, R2, etc.). The control lane displays DNA from a bird that was heterozygous for c-erbB^I and c-erbB^{II}. Numbers with asterisks indicate the sizes in kb of EcoRI fragments of the new AEVs, whereas numbers without asterisks indicate the sizes of EcoRI fragments of c-erbB^I and c-erbB^{II}.

transduced (Fig. 8a). If the 5' LTR of such a provirus initiated a transcript that terminated in host sequences (either by reading through the 3' LTR or as a consequence of the deletion of the 3' LTR), then a 5' viral-3' host transcript would contain the U5 region of the viral genome, sequences for the packaging of viral RNA into virions and host sequences (Fig. 8b). If this 5' viral-3' host RNA were co-packaged into a virion with the RNA of a replication competent helper virus (Fig. 8c), then the 5' viral-3' host transcript would be available for recombination with 3' viral sequences during the next round of infection. Such recombinations are thought to occur relatively frequently during the reverse transcription of viral RNA into proviral DNA. Once a provirus containing the newly transduced sequences had formed

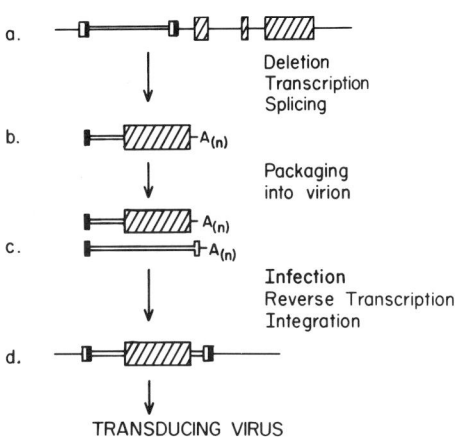

TRANSDUCTION OF A HOST GENE
BY A RETROVIRUS

Fig. 8. Model for the transduction of a host sequence by a
retrovirus. The line represents chromosomal DNA with the hatched
boxes representing exon sequences and the open barbell a proviral
insertion. The filled ends on the barbell represent the 3' ends
of the LTR sequences and thus give the orientation of the provirus with respect to the chromosomal sequences.

(Fig. 8d), its transcripts would be able to be packaged into
infectious virus particles by proteins expressed by replication
competent helper viruses.

We think that c-erbB undergoes a high frequency of transduction in RAV-I-induced erythroblastosis because erythroblastosis-
inducing proviral insertions represent the first step in the
transduction of a host sequence (Figs. 4 and 8a). In other series
of retrovirus-induced tumors that have been shown to be associated with proviral insertions in proto-oncogenes, there has not
been a high frequency of the transduction of the target proto-
oncogene (Table II). However, in these tumors the inducing insertions have not had the correct position, orientation or sequence
content for read through transcripts to initiate transduction.

TABLE II.   Transduction of Proto-oncogene Sequences
by Retroviruses

| Virus | Target proto-oncogene | Cancer-inducing proviral insertions | | | Viral trans-ductions |
		Position	Orienta-tion	Packaging signals	
ALV	c-myc	Upstream	Same	Deleted	1/75
REV	c-myc	Upstream	Same	Deleted	None
MoLV	c-myc	Upstream	Opposite	Present	None
FeLV	c-myc	Upstream	Same	?	7/32
ALV	c-erbB	Upstream	Same	Present	10/21
MMTV	int-1	Upstream	Opposite	Present	None
		Downstream	Same	Present	
	int-2	Upstream	Opposite	Present	None
		Downstream	Same	Present	

ALVs, avian leukosis viruses; REVs, reticuloendotheliosis viruses; MoLV, Moloney murine leukemia virus; FeLV, feline leukemia viruses; MMTV, mouse mammary tumor viruses. Only the most frequent position, orientation and pattern of deletion is given for the insertions associated with each of the series of viral-induced tumors. Viral transductions are given as the number of tumors with a transducing virus/the number of tumors tested for a transducing virus.

As we began to pass the new c-erbB transducing viruses in culture as well as in chickens, we rapidly came to appreciate that these viruses had disease potentials that were different from those reported for AEV-R and AEV-ES4. The new AEVs were like AEV-R and AEV-ES4 in that they caused erythroblastosis. The new AEVs however were unlike AEV-R and AEV-ES4 in that they did not appear to cause transformation of cultured cells or to cause fibrosarcoma. As we attempted to develop assay conditions in which we could see transformation of fibroblasts by the new AEVs, one of our cocultivations was found to contain a low number of cells that grew into colonies when suspended in soft agar. These

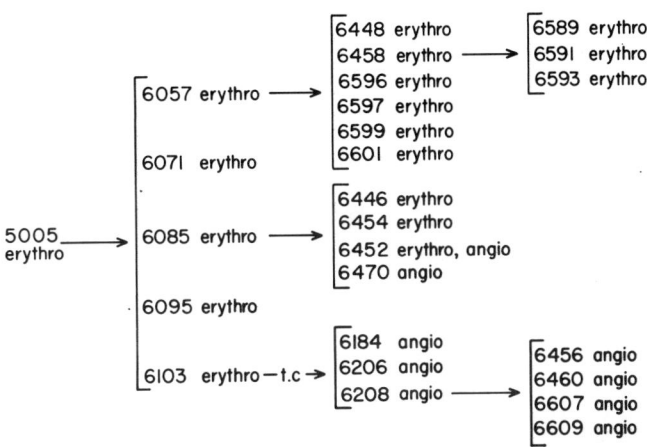

Fig. 9. Disease potential of the c-erbB transducing viruses originating in chicken 5005. Numbers refer to individual chickens. →, use of a tumor homogenate or serum for a virus stock; —t.c→, use of medium harvested from the cocultivation of a tumor with chicken embryo fibroblasts as a virus stock.

colonies were picked, cocultivated with fibroblasts and a virus stock harvested. When this stock was inoculated back into chickens, it did not cause erythroblastosis. Rather, it caused angiosarcoma (Fig. 9).

Further passage of this angiosarcoma-inducing virus using both filtered spleen homogenates of chickens with angiosarcoma or the culture medium of subsequent cocultivations of angiosarcomas and fibroblasts was associated with the induction of rapid onset angiosarcoma (Fig. 9). Analysis of the DNAs present in the tumors induced by the angiosarcoma virus on Southern blots revealed that these tumors were associated with a novel c-erbB-related EcoRI fragment that was similar in size to the novel c-erbB-related EcoRI fragment observed for the erythroblastosis-inducing virus that originated in chicken 5005 (Figs. 5, 9 and 10). Therefore, we feel that the angiosarcoma-inducing transduction of c-erbB that originated in chicken 5005 is closely related

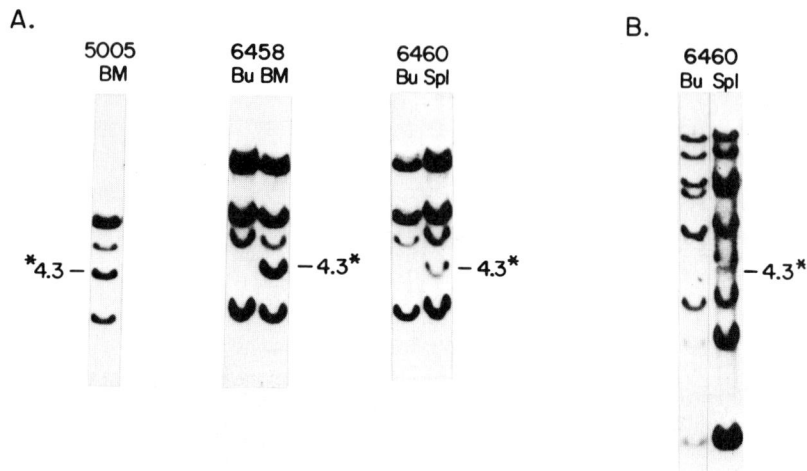

Fig. 10.   Novel c-erbB and viral sequences in AEV-5005- and AAV-5005-induced tumors. Shown are autoradiographs of a Southern blot of EcoRI-digested DNAs. Blots were hybridized with the BAM probe for v-erbB sequences (A) or with a probe for viral LTR sequences (B). The numbers over the lanes indicate the chickens from which the DNA was prepared. BM, DNA from an erythroleukemia (bone marrow); bu, DNA from normal tissue (bursa); spl, DNA from an angiosarcoma (spleen); *4.3, 4.3 kb, tumor-associated EcoRI fragment.

to the erythroblastosis-inducing transduction of c-erbB that also originated in chicken 5005.

The next several figures present histologic evidence that the c-erbB transducing virus that we now designate avian angiosarcoma viruses-5005 (AAV-5005) induces angiosarcoma. The lesions induced by the angiosarcoma viruses are hemorrhagic lesions caused by abnormal growth of endothelial cells (Figs. 11 and 12). The abnormal endothelial cells are frequently associated with areas of abnormally growing spindle-shaped cells (Fig. 13). These regions of the tumors have an appearance that is not unlike that of Kaposi's sarcomas. Some areas of the angiosarcoma display

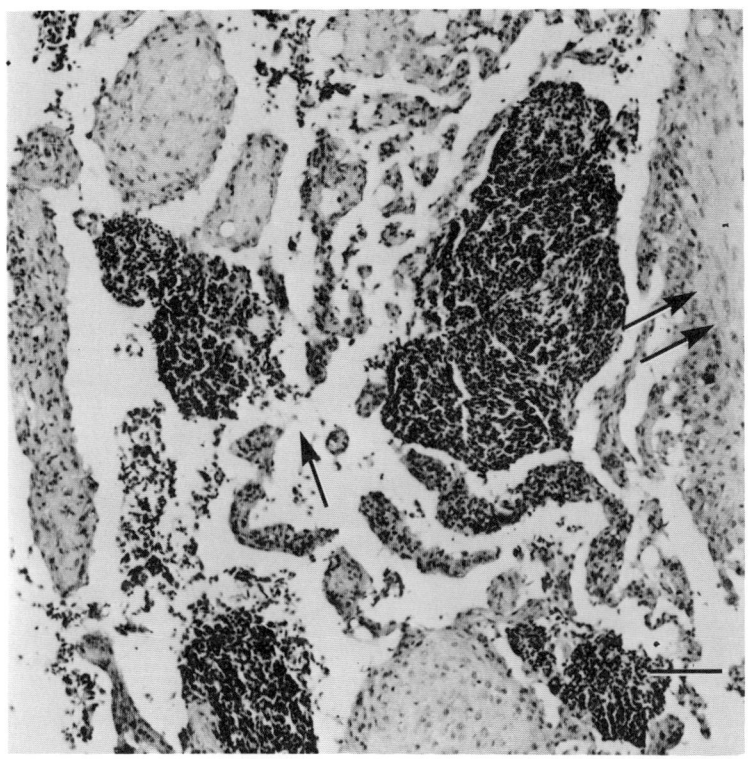

Fig. 11. Pathological patterns in AAV-5005-induced angiosarcoma. The micrograph shows an angiosarcoma composed of freely
anastomosing vascular channels (single arrow). A spindle cell
component is seen at the periphery of the lesion (double arrows).
Bar, 40 μm.

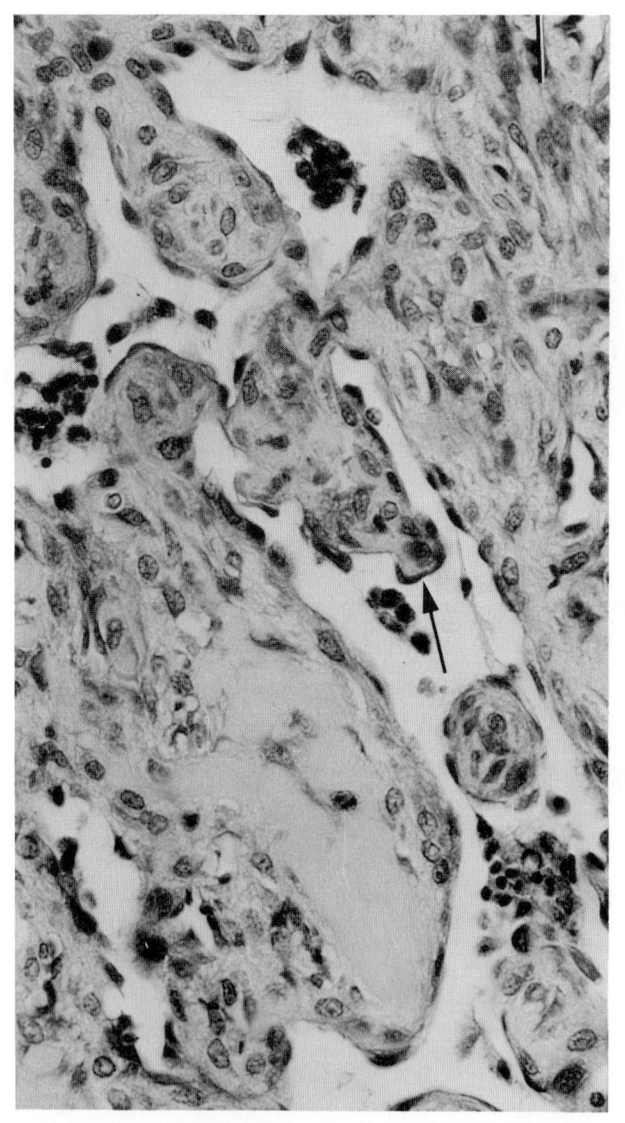

Fig. 12. Pathological patterns in AAV-5005-induced angiosarcoma. The micrograph shows intravascular tufted papillary projections lined by hyperchromatic, atypical endothelial cells (arrow). Bar, 20 μm.

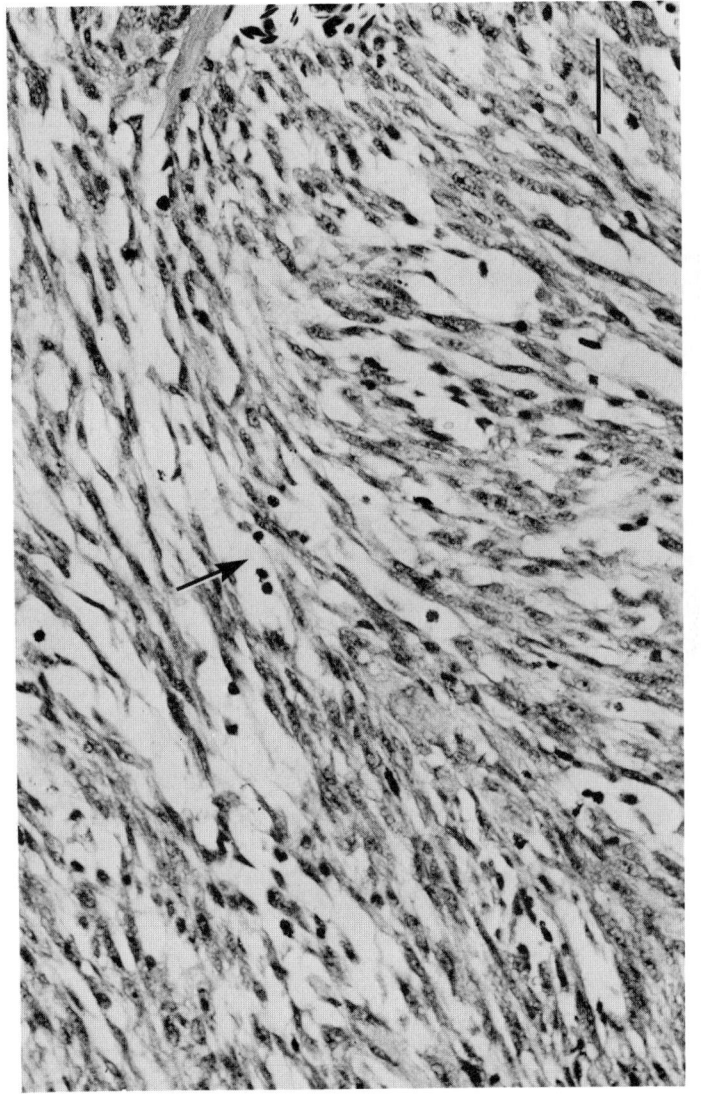

Fig. 13. Pathological patterns in AAV-5005-induced angiosarcoma. Some tumors showed a prominent spindle cell component. These tumors contained slit-like spaces that contained erythrocytes (arrow). Bar, 20 μm.

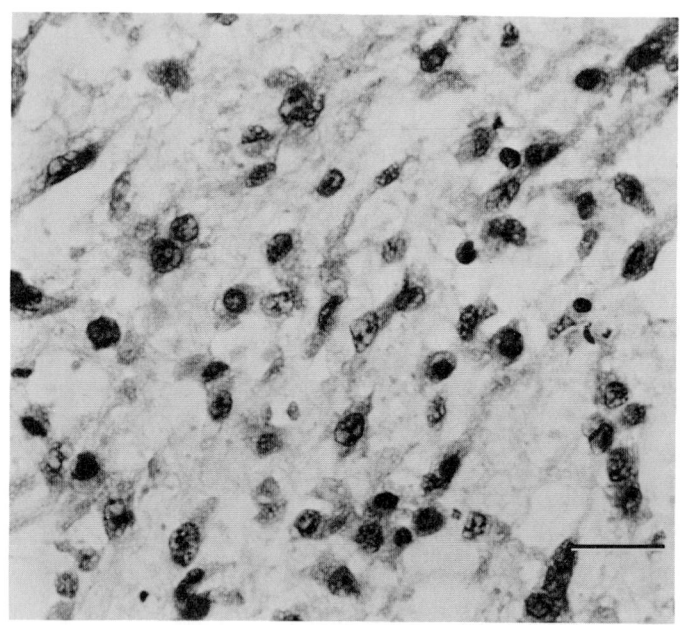

Fig. 14. Pathological patterns in AAV-5005-induced angiosarcoma. The micrograph shows a portion of tumor composed of
immature mesenchymal elements. The tumor cells are large and
polyclonal and are embedded in an abundant extracellular matrix.
Bar, 20 μm.

cells which are mesenchymal in appearance (Fig. 14). Interestingly, antiserum to factor VIII, a protein that is produced by
endothelial cells, reacts with areas of the angiosarcomas that
contain endothelial-like cells but not with areas of the angiosarcomas that contain more spindle-shaped or mesenchymal-appear-
ing cells (Fig. 15). Thus the endothelial cells that cause these
tumors appear to be dedifferentiating to cells with the morphological characteristics of fibroblastic and mesenchymal cells.

    In our work with the new c-erbB transducing viruses we have
been struck by the remarkable disease specificity of these
viruses. These viruses are defective viruses that are packaged

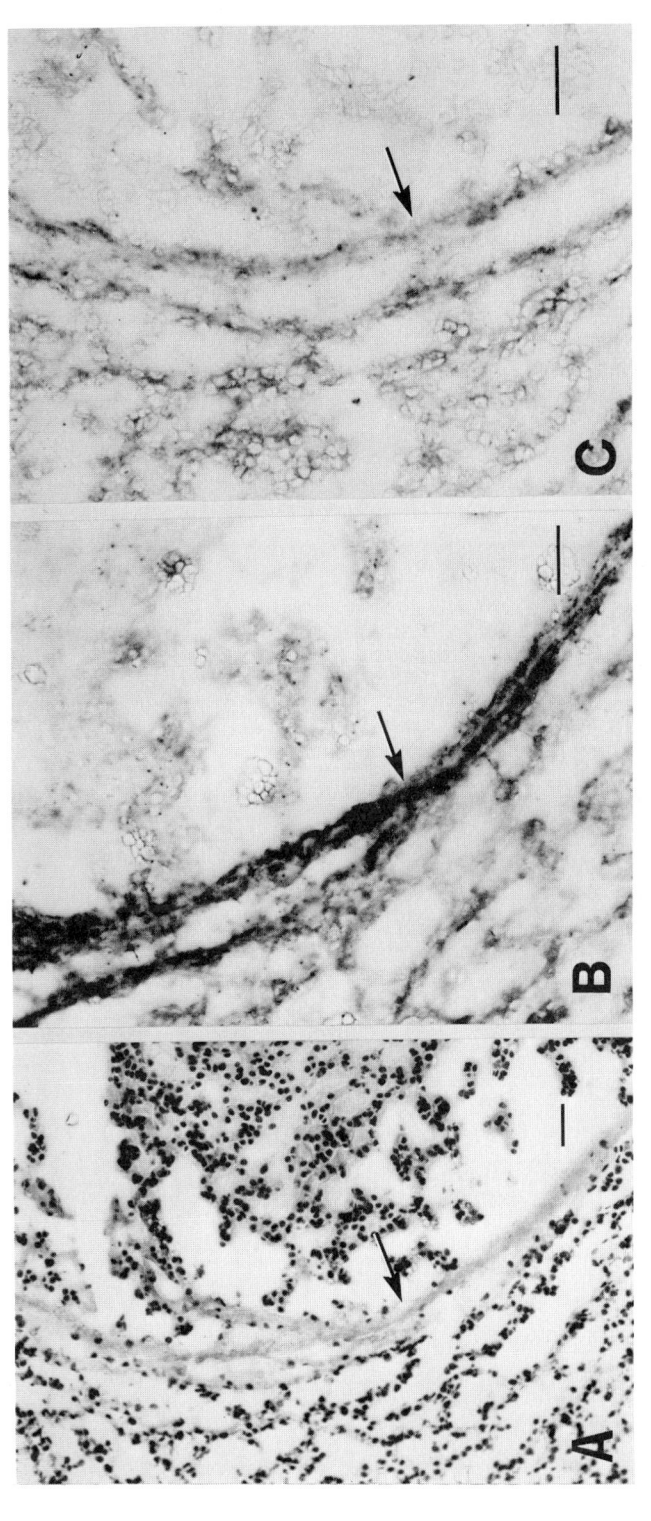

Fig. 15. Immunohistological studies of AAV-5005-induced angiosarcoma. (A) Frozen section stained with hematoxylin and eosin showing a blood-filled space lined with endothelial cells (arrow). (B) Frozen section stained with antifactor VIII showing the localization of factor VIII to the lining cells (arrow). (C) Frozen section stained with a control antibody, antihuman placental lactogen. Note the lack of staining of the endothelial lining cells (arrow). Bar, 20 μm.

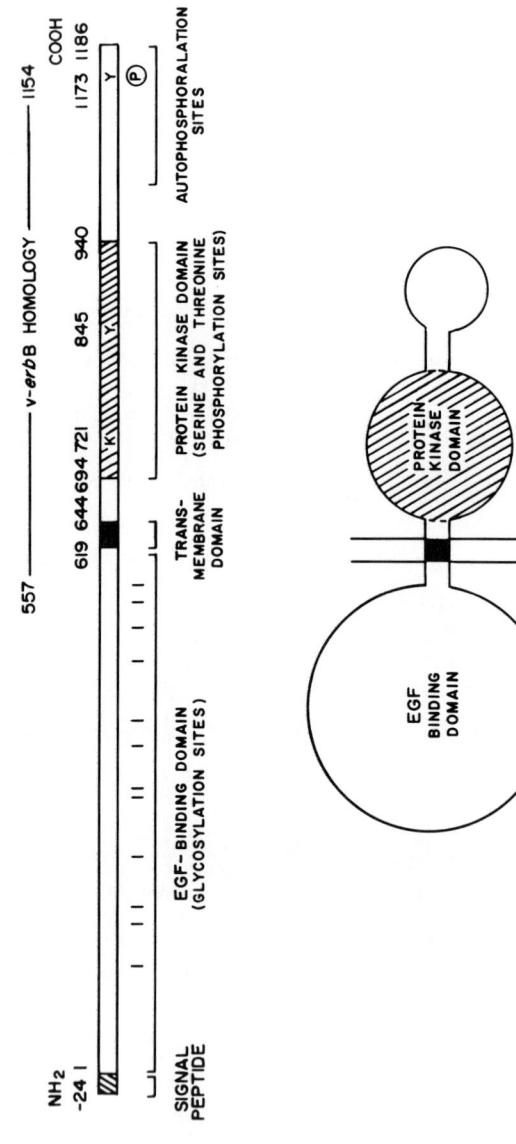

From: Tony Hunter, *Nature* *311*: 414 (1984)

Fig. 16. Schematic depicting the functional domains of the EGF receptor.

in proteins provided by RAV-I. RAV-I infects many tissue types.
Presumably, the transduced c-erbB sequences also gain entry to
many cell types. Yet, the viruses cause disease only in the lineages that encompass erythroblasts and angioblasts. Furthermore,
highly related viruses, such as the erythroblastosis- and angiosarcoma-inducing transductions of c-erbB that originated in
chicken 5005 (Figs. 10 and 11), appear to cause erythroblastosis
or angiosarcoma but not both diseases. These fascinating observations suggest that cell lineages that arise from the primitive
blood islands are 1) unusually susceptible to transformation by
the c-erbB domains of the EGF receptor and 2) are undergoing
differentiation with respect to how they respond to signals
initiated by c-erbB-encoded proteins.

Figure 16 shows a schematic of the EGF receptor gene product
which I have copied from a recent article by Tony Hunter. The
c-erbB protein product includes a transmembrane domain, an src-
related kinase domain and a COOH-terminal domain with the
tyrosine that is the major site of autophosphorylation. Erythroblastosis-inducing proviral insertions result in the expression
of a protein that is the EGF receptor minus its EGF-binding
domain. Interestingly, viruses that transduce c-erbB sequences
cause erythroblastosis, angiosarcomas or fibrosarcoma. However,
neither fibrosarcomas nor angiosarcomas appear to be induced by
proviral insertions in c-erb. We therefore think that the induction of these diseases may require truncation of the COOH-
terminal as well as the NH_2-terminal domains of the EGF receptor
(Figs. 8 and 16). One of the present goals of our research is to
use the new c-erbB transducing viruses to define sequences in
c-erbB that determine differences in disease potential.

ACKNOWLEDGMENT

   I would like to thank Dr. B. A. Woda of the University of
Massachusetts Medical School for helping with the diagnosis of
the angiosarcomas.

SELECTED REFERENCES

1. Miles, B.D. and Robinson, H.L. (1985). J. Virol. 54, 295.
2. Tracy, S.E., Woda, B.A. and Robinson, H.L. (1985). J. Virol.
   54, 304.

PATHOGENESIS OF MURINE RETROVIRAL INFECTIONS

Robert A. Yetter
Janet W. Hartley
Torgny N. Fredrickson
Herbert C. Morse III

Laboratory of Immunopathology
National Institute of Allergy and Infectious Diseases
National Institutes of Health
Bethesda, Maryland

Abnormalities in mice induced by murine leukemia viruses (MuLV) are the result of integrations of those viruses into the genomes of mice (Table I). These integrations may take place either in the germ cell or the somatic cell. Germ cell integrations are rare events. In strains of mice that produce high levels of ectropic virus from early enough in life to allow transplacental infection, they may occur every seven to 20 generations. Compatibility at $\underline{Fv-1}$ is required for these integrations. That is, n-tropic integrations occur in $\underline{Fv-1}^n$ mice and b-tropic integrations in $\underline{Fv-1}^b$ mice. Most of these integrations are silent. There are occasional phenotypic alterations which include coat color mutations, such as dilute, as seen in DBA, and the lethal yellow mutation.

More common is the integration in the somatic cell. These occur in high frequency in all strains of mice that produce high levels of ectropic virus. As with the germ cell integration, $\underline{Fv-1}$ compatibility is required. Again, most of these integrations are silent. Phenotypic alterations due to somatic cell integrations may be oncogenic or nononcogenic. Nononcogenic alterations

TABLE I. Effects of Integration of MuLV

Germ cell	Somatic cell

1. Rare event
 	
  High ecotropic MuLV
  expression early
  n-Tropic integrations
  in $\underline{Fv-1}^n$
  b-Tropic integrations
  in $\underline{Fv-1}^b$
 	
2. Most are silent
 	
3. Phenotypic alterations
  include d, A^y
	1. High frequency in high
	  ecotropic virus strains
	
	2. Most are silent
	
	3. Phenotypic alterations include
	
	  a. Deformed vibrissae
	  b. Greying with age
	  c. Neurological disease
	
	4. Oncogenic sequellae
	
	  a. Short latent period
	
	    1) Recombination with
	       cellular genes--MSV
	    2) Recombination with non-
	       ecotropic viral genes--
	       SFFV
	
	  b. Long latent period, pro-
	     moter, enhancer insertion
	
	    1) Ecotropic viruses
	    2) MCF viruses

may be either pathogenic or nonpathogenic. Deformed vibrissae is the result of injection of neonatal mice with such ecotropic viruses as Friend or Moloney. Greying with age is a phenomenon seen in certain black strains of mice that produce high levels of ecotropic virus from early in life. As the mice get older they turn grey, sometimes starting as early as 1 month of age. One of the pathogenic results of somatic cell integrations is neurologic disease. Inoculation of neonatal mice with ecotropic viruses isolated from certain strains of California wild mice or with Moloney variants induces a disease which resembles amyotrophic lateral sclerosis.

Oncogenic sequellae cover a wide range of diseases, including erythroleukemias, myelogenous leukemias, lymphomas of T and B cells and sarcomas. They can, however, be separated into two major groups: the short latent period diseases and the long latent period diseases. Short latent period diseases tend to be the result of insertion of replication defective viruses. These viruses become replication defective during recombination. In some cases, murine sarcoma virus (MSV) for example, the recombination is with cellular sequences, the proto-oncogenes. Another possibility is recombination with nonecotropic viral sequences, as is the case with Friend spleen focus-forming virus (SFFV). Long latent period diseases are thought to be due to insertion of promoter and enhancer sequences into the genome in such a place that they can affect viral or cellular genes. Viruses associated with long latent period disease are ecotropic viruses, such as Gross passage A and SL3, and the recombinant mink cell focus-forming (MCF) viruses.

Leukemogenesis is the result of a continuous interplay between the virus and host genes. From the time that ecotropic viruses are produced they can be limited in their spread by certain host genes. Fv-1 and Fv-4 may restrict the replication of ecotropic viruses. Antibody, a result of immune responses controlled by H-2-linked genes, such as Rgv-1 and Rfv-1, may neutralize the virus. It should be pointed out, however, that an immune response at this point may be a two-edged sword. The same immune response that produces antibody may produce lymphokines such as IL-3 and CSF-2 that could maintain a potential target cell type for leukemogenesis. If the viruses spread and recombine they are still subject to control by host genes. Ecotropic type viruses are restricted by Fv-1, Fv-4 and the immune response. Oncogene transducing type viruses come under the control of other genes: Fv-2 which restricts Friend SFFV and Ab-1 and Ab-2 which affect Abelson virus. Viruses that recombine to form MCF viruses

may be restricted by <u>Rmcf</u>. If the viruses are not restricted and
spread to new cell types, transformation can occur; but a cellular immune response may still prevent clonal outgrowth of the
tumor.

Having given this rather brief overview of pathogenic mechanisms in MuLV systems, I would like to turn to a system that we
have been working with in our laboratory. This virus is of particular interest since it induces a polyclonal lymphoproliferative disease that is associated with hypergammaglobulinemia and
profound immunosuppression. The virus that we have been working
with is a variant of the Duplan-Laterjet radiation leukemia
virus. The Duplan-Laterjet virus differs from most other radiation leukemia viruses in that they require neonatal inoculation
and result in thymic lymphomas. The Duplan-Laterjet virus, from
its initial isolation, could be transmitted by inoculation of
both neonates and adults, and has been associated with what were
described as non-T cell lymphomas in C57BL/6 mice. After several
passages of these tumors through B6 mice by inoculation with
cell-free filtrate, Haas derived a bone marrow stromal cell line
which he called RCN-BM5. Filtered culture supernatants of this
line, when injected into either neonatal or adult B6 mice, produced a disease that was at first termed a reticulum cell sarcoma
type B. The more modern classification of this, after Pattengale,
was an immunoblastic B cell lymphoma. Studies showed, however,
that cells from this tumor could not be transplanted into nonimmunosuppressed hosts, could not be readily grown in culture
and remained diploid throughout the course of the disease. Consequently, the disease was reclassified as a non-neoplastic
proliferation of B immunoblasts.

The lymphoproliferative disease is induced by injection of
filtered culture supernatants of the RCN-BM5 cell line, which
contains a mixture of b-tropic viruses, MCF virus, ecotropic
virus and pseudotypes of both virions. Pseudotyped MCF virus, an

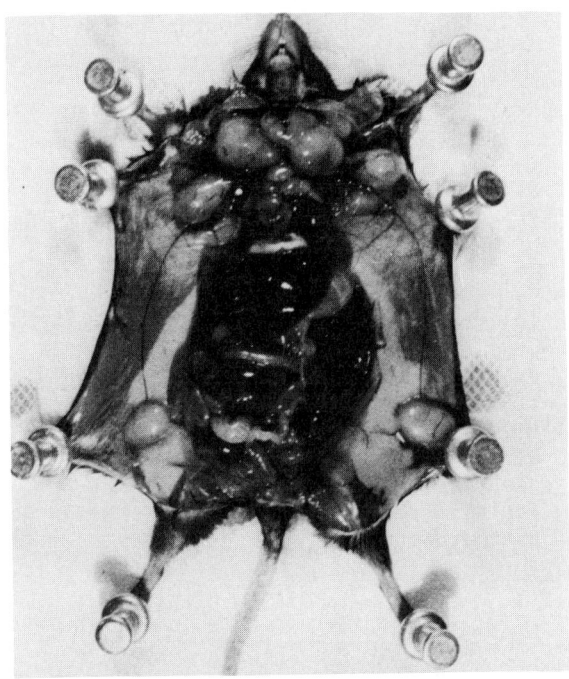

Fig. 1.   B6 mouse with lymphadenopathy and splenomegaly.

MCF genome inside an ecotropic coat, will produce disease. However, cloned ecotropic virus or cloned MCF virus, when injected
into either neonatal or adult mice, will not cause disease.

Classically the disease in the susceptible B6 mouse presents
as massive lymphadenopathy and splenomegaly (Fig. 1). Both
peripheral and mesenteric nodes are enlarged as is the spleen.
The thymus is usually not involved; what you see in Figure 1 are
parathymic lymph nodes. On the occasions that the thymus is
enlarged it is due to infiltration rather than proliferation of
thymocytes. Enlargement of nonlymphoid organs such as the liver
is occasionally seen. Again this is due to infiltration.

Microscopically, early in the course of disease, we see
proliferation of lymphocytes in the periarteriolar lymphocytic
sheath. Large numbers of immunoblasts are present. There is

Table II. Strain Distribution of Sensitivity
to Disease Induced by BM5 Virus

Sensi-tivity	Disease	Mor-tality	$Fv-1^{b/b}$	$Fv-1^{n/n}$ or $^{n/b}$
High	Progressive lymphadenopathy, splenomegaly	+	C57BL/6, C57BL/10, I/St, B10.F	(C57BL/6 × CBA/N)F_1
Moderate	Early lymphadeno-pathy, regression, residual histo-pathology	-	BDP	
Resistant	No adenopathy or splenomegaly, little if any histopathology	-	BALB/c, A, AL, AU, LG, RIIIS, SEC/1	NFS, CBA/N

hyperplasia of the germinal centers, and breakdown of the margin
of the periarteriolar lymphocytic sheath. As the disease progresses there is continued proliferation in the periarteriolar
lymphocytic sheath, with an increased number of immunoblasts.
Eventually the normal architecture of the organ is obliterated.
At this point we begin to see perivascular infiltrations of nonlymphoid organs, for example the liver, kidney, lungs and heart.
These infiltrations contribute to the neoplastic appearance of
the disease but it should be pointed out that even at this stage
lymphocytes from spleen or lymph node cannot be transplanted to
nonimmunosuppressed hosts and cannot be grown in culture.

Table II shows a strain distribution of sensitivity to
disease induced by BM5 virus. Mice fall into one of three groups.
The highly sensitive group is characterized by progressive
lymphadenopathy, splenomegaly and ultimately death. It includes
the $Fv-1^b$ strains, C57BL/6, C57BL/10, I/St and B10.F. The moderately sensitive group which shows early lymphadenopathy, and

residual histopathology with no mortality, includes only the $Fv-1^b$ strain, BDP. The resistant group shows no adenopathy or splenomegaly, little, if any, histopathology and no mortality. This group includes the $Fv-1^b$ strains, BALB/c, A, AL, AU, LG, RIIIS and SEC. Since the viruses that induce this disease are b-tropic, it is not surprising that the $Fv-1^n$ strains NFS and CBA/N are resistant to the disease. We would expect an $Fv-1^{n/b}F_1$ to be resistant since such mice are resistant to both n- and b-tropic viruses. However, the $Fv-1^{n/b}F_1$ B6 × CBA/N is highly sensitive, indicating that $Fv-1$ is not playing its usual role in modification of this disease. Another interesting point is that CBA/N carries the resistance allele at $Rmcf$. Resistance determined by $Rmcf$ is dominant. Again we would expect this gene to contribute to resistance in the F_1 yet it does not. Thus there are two genes that we know to affect the replication of virus which do not seem to be having the expected effect on the course of disease. All $Fv-1^b$ strains are not uniformly sensitive; hence there must be some other host gene affecting the outcome of infection. One gene that was studied was the major histocompatibility complex, in order to determine whether the unusual $H-2^p$ haplotype of BDP was responsible for moderate sensitivity to the disease. We found that B10.F, which is also $H-2^p$, is highly sensitive; thus its $H-2$ haplotype is unlikely to be the reason for BDP being only moderately sensitive.

Figure 2 shows a time course of the disease in three strains of mice: B6, BDP and BALB/c. All of these mice were injected with a filtered culture supernatant at 1 month of age. By 1 week after injection in the B6 mouse there are increased levels of serum immunoglobulin. By 3 weeks after infection high levels of ecotropic and moderate levels of MCF virus can be found in the spleen. We also begin to see splenomegaly and the early histological changes that I referred to previously. By 4 weeks after infection we start to see changes in cell surface antigens of

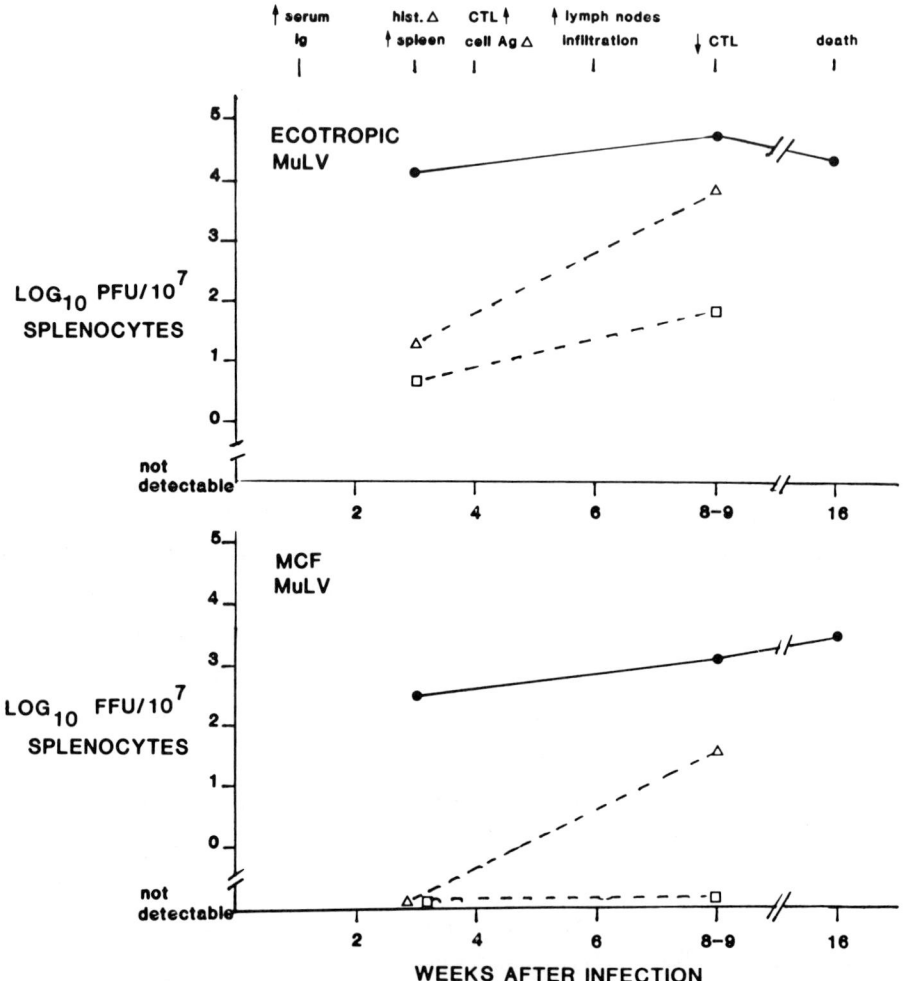

Fig. 2. Strain distribution of sensitivity to disease induced by BM5 virus. ●——●, C57BL/6; △---△, BDP; □---□, BALB/c. The notations at the top refer only to the disease in B6 mice.

lymphocytes. These include decreased amounts of surface immuno-globulin per B cell and an increased percentage of IgG2-positive cells. It is interesting that there are normal percentages of both T and B cells. This in a spleen that is five to seven times normal size, which would indicate that we have both T and B cell proliferation at this stage of the disease. Also at this time we

see an enhanced cytotoxic T lymphocyte response to alloantigens.
By 6 weeks into the disease, there are readily palpable lymph
nodes and we see the first signs of infiltration into nonlymphoid
organs. By 8 to 9 weeks, virus levels are at about the same level
as at the outset of disease. The cytotoxic T lymphocyte response
is suppressed. By 15 weeks the immunosuppression in these animals
has become clinically relevant. Normally B6 mice are resistant to
ectromelia. Fifteen weeks after infection with BM5 virus, ectromelia kills B6 mice. Sixteen weeks after infection virus levels
again are approximately the same as at the outset. This is also
the time when the first deaths due to the disease occur. No B6
mice survive to 6 months after infection.

The course in the BDP mouse is somewhat different. Three
weeks after infection we see low levels of ecotropic virus in the
spleen. MCF virus is not readily detectable in the spleen. Histologically the spleens look reactive. At this time there is a
slight increase in serum immunoglobulin levels. By 8 to 9 weeks
after infection ecotropic virus levels approximate those that we
would see in the B6 mouse. Low levels of MCF virus can be found
in the spleen. Histologically the animals show a picture of early
disease. Lymph nodes are palpable, and serum immunoglobulin
levels are eight times normal. Hypergammaglobulinemia is developing in the BDP. By 6 months after infection the lymphadenopathy
has regressed and histopathologically we see a picture of early
disease.

In BALB/c, the resistant strain, 3 weeks after infection low
levels of ecotropic virus could be found, but MCF virus was not
detectable. Histopathologically the animals were unremarkable.
Eight to 9 weeks after infection there was a slight increase in
ecotropic virus, MCF virus was still not detectable and the
animals were still histopathologically unremarkable. There was
no sign of hypergammaglobulinemia. By 6 months after infection

the BALB/c mice showed no sign of disease, either grossly or on histopathological examination.

What we are dealing with then is a non-neoplastic polyclonal proliferation of B immunoblasts. This is associated with a profound immunosuppression. It is induced by a mixed population of b-tropic, ecotropic and MCF MuLV. The susceptibility of various mouse strains to this disease indicate that Fv-1 and Rmcf are not playing the roles that we would expect them to play in modification of this disease. Further, there is some other gene or genes that affects the outcome of infection. Finally, this disease can be induced in both neonates and adults of susceptible strains, which makes this system amenable to studies of vaccine intervention in lymphoproliferative and immunosuppressive disease.

ACKNOWLEDGMENT

R. A. Yetter is a special fellow of the Leukemia Society of America. The authors would like to thank Mrs. Joan Austin for excellent technical assistance.

EQUINE RETROVIRUS INFECTION

Leroy Coggins

North Carolina State University
School of Veterinary Medicine
Raleigh, North Carolina

Interest in equine infectious anemia (EIA), though longstand-
ing, has varied over the years with the number of horses. In the
early 1930s and 1940s, there were many horses and much disease;
but in the 1960s, the horse population increased with the growing
number of pleasure horses and race horses, and a significant
amount of the disease developed, especially among racing horses.
In New York State, EIA became a problem in the 1960s and threatened to close some of the race tracks. Consequently, New York
State, beginning in the mid-1960s, has spent several million
dollars in the development of diagnostic tests and ways of controlling the infection. In the mid-1960s, the only ways available
to diagnose the disease involved the observation of clinical
signs or the inoculation of animals (injection of blood from a
horse suspected of having the disease into a susceptible horse).
Veterinarians were able to diagnose the disease only if the
clinical signs were severe and typical.

The clinical signs include a very high fever (up to 107°F
or 108°F), a rapid decrease in blood packed cell volume, anemia
(which can be very severe in the chronic, recurring disease), a
rapid loss in weight, edema of the lower parts of the body and
the legs and an enlarged spleen, which can be palpated through

the rectum. Many animals with these signs will die. If blood is
taken from a sick animal and inoculated into a susceptible horse,
it is possible to produce clinical disease. The pathology that
is seen in animals that die or are sacrificed includes lymphadenopathy, hemorrhages, edema, thrombosis of some of the vessels
(including mesenteric vessels and those in the testes), lymphocytic infiltrates in the liver and hemosiderin in the liver and
circulating leukocytes. Whole red blood cells are often seen in
Kupfer cells, usually with hemosiderin.

In the late 1960s, there was no virus assay and no accurate
or dependable serological assay. Using my experience with African
swine fever, a disease producing both acute and chronic states
and involving macrophages and the lymphoid system, I tried to
develop techniques for a serologic test or a test for viral antigens. In very acutely infected animals, about 10 days after initial infection with a virulent strain of the virus, such as the
Wyoming strain, engorgement of the spleen and hyperemia of the
lymph nodes associated with the spleen occur. When material is
taken from the spleen at this stage of infection and put into a
gel immunodiffusion test with serum from a survivor animal, an
immunoprecipitin line forms. The antigen from the spleen had to
be taken before precipitating antibody developed in the animal.
Such antibody usually appears at about 2 weeks after infection.
Not all animals produce enough antigen in the spleen to give this
reaction. This finding did, however, provide us with a reliable
serological test that could be used for screening horses for EIA
infection. This test detected variable levels of antibody. The
spleen sample is placed in the inner well, survivor serum is
placed in the three outside wells and, if antibody is present, it
deflects the control line (Fig. 1). After tissue culture-adapted
virus became available, it was used as the antigen source and is
currently used throughout the country in the official tests. If
there is a surplus of antibody in the test reaction, there is

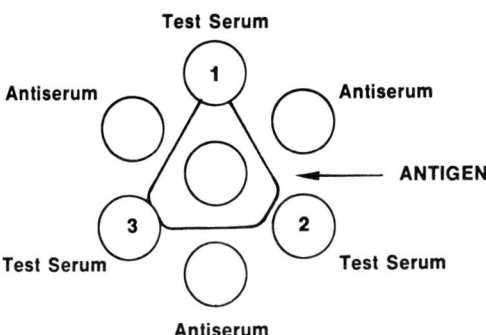

Fig. 1.   Immunodiffusion test for diagnosis of EIA. Test serum in well no. 1 is negative. Test sera in wells no. 2 and 3 are positive and contain specific antibody against EIA virus.

some dissolution of the precipitin line. A majority of infected animals give lines in this range. Using the immunodiffusion test, primarily with ponies inoculated intravenously, we measured the time from experimental inoculation to detection of precipitating antibody. Between 2 and 3 weeks after inoculation, 65% of the animals became positive on immunodiffusion test. By 4 weeks, 88% were positive and, by 45 days, all of the animals produced pre- cipitating antibody (Table I). From observations in the field and the laboratory we knew that variable incubation periods existed with this disease. In some instances it took as long as 3 months after inoculation before clinical disease appeared, and the literature reports studies in which incubation periods were as short as 5 to 6 days. Therefore, we were concerned about how long it might take for antibody to be produced. However, by using the virulent Wyoming strain, incubation periods were consistently 5 to 7 days. When material was from horses in the field, incuba- tion periods as long as 3 months before clinical signs appeared were seen. These animals developed antibody by 45 days after inoculation even though clinical disease was not evident until 1 to 2 months later. Thus antibody can develop several months before the clinical signs are seen. From the literature and from

TABLE I. Appearance of EIA Antibody,
Detected by Immunodiffusion Test,
in 57 Experimentally Inoculated Ponies

Post inocu- lation week	Number of ponies	
	Test positive for first time	Cumulative data (%)
2nd	1	1 (2)
3rd	36	37 (65)
4th	13	50 (88)
5th	3	53 (93)
Later than 5th	4[a]	57 (100)

[a]The longest time before antibody was detected was 45 days
in one pony.

our previous experience, we believed that, once a horse is
infected, it remains infected for life. Blood was taken from
horses positive in the immunodiffusion test and from horses that
were negative in the immunodiffusion test and inoculated into
experimental ponies. Initially, small amounts of blood, 25 ml,
were used; but in some cases, this amount did not seem to be
enough blood. It was later found to be important that the blood
be kept refrigerated or fresh. It probably had to contain viable
leukocytes. Eventually, 250 ml of blood was taken from positive
animals under field conditions for transfusion. Eighty-five EIA
test-negative ponies were inoculated with whole blood from
antibody-positive horses. Eighty-three of the experimental animals developed febrile reactions, 80 of them showed anemia and
64 showed decreases in platelet counts. Lower platelet counts
occurred at about the same time as the febrile reaction or
slightly earlier. Eighty-four developed EIA precipitating antibody and 78 had mononuclear infiltrations of the liver and
spleen.

Blood samples from 78 antibody-negative horses were inoculated into experimental animals. The donors were animals that
were in some cases from the same farm where there were outbreaks
of EIA disease. Two animals developed febrile reactions,
decreases in platelet counts and lowered blood packed cell
volume. One pony developed EIA precipitating antibody, and both
ponies had mononuclear infiltrates of the liver and spleen. We
later found that the donor resulting in the antibody-positive
recipient was in the incubation stage of EIA infection and
developed clinical EIA.

From these data (Table II) it was concluded that the immunodiffusion test was at least 95% accurate as an indicator of
infection in the horse. The test was developed in 1970, it became
official in 1973 and since that time between 200,000 and 700,000
horses have been tested annually. Most of those horses have been
moving, going to race tracks, horse shows and so forth. The incidence of positive tests was initially about 6%. During the past
year, 700,000 horses were tested in this country and less than
0.1% were positive.

There are three major possible means for transmission of the
virus. The first is through contaminated needles or other instruments used by horsemen and veterinarians. It was common at race
tracks for the same needle to be used for multiple inoculations;
but, even after that practice was discontinued in the 1950s and
1960s, we still had problems with outbreaks of EIA infection on
breeding farms. Of course, blood transfusion is an effective way
of transmitting this infection. Second, transmission can occur
from the mare to her offspring either in utero or through colostrum. Finally, blood-sucking insects, primarily the horsefly, can
transmit the infection.

The transmission from infected horses seems to be related to
the clinical condition of the infected animal. Data were collected on seven mares and their offspring. When the mares showed

TABLE II. Correlation of immunodiffusion test and pony infectivity test

Donor horses EIA anti-body status	No.	Experimental ponies with positive results in infectivity test					
		Rectal temp. increased	Decreased packed cell volume	Smaller platelet count	Microscopic lesions	EIA anti-body	No. affected with EIA/no. in study
Test positive	85	83	80	64	78[a]	84	85/85[b]
Test negative	78	2	2	2	2	1	1/78[c]

[a] Only 78 ponies were examined histologically.

[b] The one horse in which infective EIA virus was not demonstrated was destroyed before it could be retested, and it is assumed that the EIA virus was inactivated in transit to the laboratory.

[c] This single failure was due to a horse in the incubation stage of EIA infection.

clinical signs during gestation or at the time of foaling, all
seven foals became infected. Of 45 mares which were positive on
immunodiffusion tests, but showed no clinical signs of disease,
only five had infected foals. In a study at Louisiana State, 20
positive mares had foals; two of the 20 foals became infected.
These studies did not establish whether transmission occurred in
utero or by way of colostrum. Also in some of these cases, there
were possibilities for insect transmission. They all had clinical
signs. We have not noticed any tolerance to infection by this
virus. All the foals with demonstrated viremia maintained precipitating antibody in their blood. The difficulty in determining if
transmission occurs in a foal is that if they receive colostrum,
then they will have passive antibody for up to 6 months and react
positively in the immunodiffusion test.

Both virus and antibody can be found in the fetus. One mare
which was in isolation aborted a fetus. The immunodiffusion test
for antibody had been positive, she developed clinical signs, was
kept in isolation and aborted her fetus at 6 months of gestation.
The foal was infected with the virus which was recovered by animal inoculation and the fetal serum was positive on the antibody
test.

The virus is in the blood indefinitely in an infected horse
but is not necessarily in the plasma or in the serum. A research
group in Japan looked at virus titers in the serum of an infected
horse and the associated febrile responses. Each time a febrile
response occurred, free virus appeared in the serum and a different antigenic type appeared. However, if whole blood was
examined, virus could be recovered throughout.

We have also looked at in vivo neutralization potential of
serum antibody. Pony 163 was a long-term carrier that had been
experimentally inoculated and had been kept in isolation. Blood
was collected 5 years after the original infection. The plasma
was mixed with 3 logs of virus. Plasma given by itself did not

cause infection, showing that plasma alone did not have virus. When either 99 ml of plasma or 9 ml was used with homologous Wyoming strain of virus, no infection resulted. When normal plasma was mixed with 3 logs of this virus, there was an incubation period of 7 days. This incubation period has been a consistent finding with the Wyoming virus. Using plasma and virus from different locations, or using blood taken at different times during disease, will cause infection with a little bit longer incubation period. Using less than about 3 logs of virus, the incubation period with Wyoming strain is about 2 weeks.

The clinical disease can be recrudesced in an inapparent carrier by using corticosteroids. This was originally described by the Japanese and confirmed by us in a few field cases given corticosteriods for 5 days.

Two long-term carriers, pony 163 and pony 7, maintained in isolation, were followed over 10 to 12 years. Pony 163 received the Wyoming strain initially in 1971. Whole blood was infectious for some time. Then there was a period when whole blood was not infectious and only blood cells or washed leukocytes were infectious. It is not known how common this type of animal is. There are, however, some animals that, although they cannot transmit the infection routinely with whole blood, their leukocytes are infectious.

In acute cases, neutralizing antibody generally is not detectable in in vitro tests. It does not appear until after about 45 days. It is present in pony 163. The serum of acute cases is infectious; but, in ponies 7 and 163, serum was not infectious, whereas whole blood was infectious. In acute cases there are about 7 or 8 logs of virus in whole blood. One milliliter of blood from pony 7 has routinely been infectious over a period of 10 years; whereas as much as 250 ml of blood from pony 163 has not been infectious in the last 7 or 8 years. The leukocyte portion of whole blood is infectious from acute cases.

Leukocytes from pony 163 have been infectious unless they are washed or if repeated inoculations are made. We have not seen clinical disease in these two ponies since the first year after inoculation. In addition, it has not been possible to demonstrate transmission by interrupted feeding of horseflies on these two ponies. In contrast, transmission can be demonstrated with a single horsefly from an acute case. Stable flies and mosquitoes will also transmit infection from acute cases.

I think our model is of most value in the area of diagnosis. Diagnosis is important because, once a horse becomes infected, it remains infected for life and precipitating antibody remains there for life. The transmission of EIA infection can be controlled by controlling the infected horse.

PATHOGENESIS OF BOVINE RETROVIRUS INFECTION

Martin J. Van Der Maaten

National Animal Disease Center
U.S. Department of Agriculture
Ames, Iowa

Due to the fact that there is very little information available regarding the pathogenesis of bovine leukemia virus (BLV)
infections and bovine lymphosarcoma, much of this chapter will
deal with related, but somewhat peripheral, subjects.

VIRUS TRANSMISSION

As we consider the possible means by which BLV may escape
from the persistently infected host we should review a few important basic facts regarding BLV infections: 1) BLV infections,
once established, persist for the life of the host; 2) there is
a concommitant and persistent antibody response to viral proteins; and 3) virus is associated with lymphoid cells where
expression is stringently controlled at the transcriptional
level; thus there is virtually no free virus present in, or shed
from infected animals. Given these facts, one would expect that
BLV would be transmitted with considerable difficulty, requiring
prolonged and close contact. This is, in fact, the situation. It
is also apparent that the escape of virus from the persistently
infected host would be cell-associated and that the infectivity
present in various secretions or excretions would depend on the

normal cellular content of these substances. Any factor, physio-
logic, inflammatory or traumatic, which would increase the cellular content (particularly the lymphocytic component) of secretions would, of course, favor virus transmission. Experimental
studies have provided substantial support for these predictions.
BLV infectivity, in general, has not been identified in saliva,
nasal secretions, urine or feces. Exceptions to this are a study
in which the collection of large quantities of saliva resulted
in the identification of infectivity, a study which reported the
presence of BLV antigen (but not infectivity) in urine, and the
identification of BLV infectivity associated with the cellular
component of bronchoalveolar washings. Studies of colostrum and
milk from infected cows have revealed the presence of BLV infectivity, presumably due to the cellular content of these secretions. Tests of bovine semen and calves sired by BLV-infected
sires have, with one exception, failed to incriminate semen as
a vehicle for the transmission of BLV. The exception involved
tests of semen from one bull, the semen having been collected
as a result of the manipulation and massage of the urethra and
accessory glands per-rectum. This method of semen collection is
known to result in the presence of blood in the semen and it is
presumed that the contaminating blood cells were the source of
the infectivity found in the study. Tests of the fluids used to
flush embryos from the female reproductive tract for embryo
transfer procedures have identified BLV infectivity but this is
not unexpected because these fluids are routinely contaminated
with blood. BLV has never been identified in the embryos themselves. The transmission of BLV from an infected dam to her fetus
during gestation has been adequately documented. The estimates of
the frequency with which this occurs range from 3 to 20% with the
variations possibly being influenced by the genetic constitution
of the animals involved. Other studies, in which infected cows
were followed through several pregnancies, indicated that the

TABLE I.   Identification of BLV Infectivity
in Bovine Tissues, Secretions or Excretions

Material tested	Result	Reference
Saliva	-	(1)
	+	(2)
Nasal secretions	-	(1,3)
Bronchoalveolar washings	+	(3)
Urine	-	(1,2)
	(+)?	(4)
Feces	-	(2)
Colostrum and milk	+	(1,5-7)
Blood	+	(7-11); many others
Semen	-	(1,12,13)
	(+)?	(14)
Uterine flush fluids	+	(15)
Embryos	-	(15,16)

in utero transmission of BLV seemed to be rather random in that
cows which had, or had not, given birth to infected calves in one
pregnancy did not seem to repeatedly produce similar infected, or
uninfected, calves in subsequent pregnancies. A summarization of
potential sources of infectious BLV is presented in Table I.

ROUTES OF SUSCEPTIBILITY

A second approach to the study of transmission of BLV infections among cattle involved the identification of routes by which
cattle were susceptible to infection with BLV. These studies

included inocula consisting of either infectious cell culture
fluid containing free virus or, more commonly, peripheral blood
lymphocytes from persistently infected cattle. In several experiments, the inocula used represented doses of infectious material
which would greatly exceed any that one would expect animals to
encounter under natural conditions but the results establish at
least a base line from which to estimate relative susceptibility.
Tests of oral infectivity in newborn calves revealed that they
were susceptible to infection using large numbers of lymphocytes
but similar tests of 3-day-old and 3-week-old calves indicated a
rather rapidly rising resistance to infection by this route.
Intranasal instillation of free virus revealed that cattle were
susceptible to exposure by this route if cell-free virus was
present but, as discussed previously, there is little evidence
that significant quantities of free virus are ever present in the
environment. Similarly, the intrauterine instillation of large
quantities of lymphocytes infected some, but not all, of the
recipient cows thus indicating that this is not a route of high
susceptibility. It was only by the intradermal or intracutaneous
inoculation of lymphocytes or free virus that infections were
routinely established with small doses of virus or small numbers
of lymphocytes. In one study it was, in fact, established that
the intradermal inoculation of as little as 0.025 cubic milli-
meters of whole blood from an infected donor could result in
transmission of the virus to susceptible calves. A summary of
studies designed to determine routes of susceptibility to BLV
infection, along with an arbitrary scoring indicating the
probable importance of these routes, is presented in Table II.

The evidence that most BLV transmissions are effected by
blood cells and the demonstration that the skin is very susceptible to infection leaves little doubt that the intervention of
man and management or veterinary practices may greatly influence
the transmission of BLV. It is obvious that blood transfusions

TABLE II.   Routes of Susceptibility to Infection with BLV

Route of exposure	Inoculum	Susceptibility to infection	Reference
Intravenous	BLV-infected cells	+++	(10,11); many others
Intraperitoneal	Virus	+++	(17)
Intranasal	BLV-infected cells	(+)?	(5,18)
Intratracheal	BLV-infected cells	++	(19)
Aerosol	Virus	++	(18)
Oral	BLV-infected cells	(+)?	(8,18,19)
Intrauterine	BLV-infected cells	(+)?	(18,19)
Intradermal	BLV-infected cells	+++	(18,19)
	Virus	+++	(18)

from persistently infected cattle would readily transmit infections as would the use of "vaccine" preparations consisting of whole blood products similar to those sometimes used for the immunization of cattle against blood parasites. Studies of infected herds where blood samples had been collected with a common needle suggest that this practice can transmit infection and it is likely that many routine minor surgical procedures such as castration, dehorning and ear tagging provide considerable potential for the transfer of blood cells between animals. Vaccination with a common needle might also be suspected although a study conducted in England involving the intradermal tuberculin

test indicated that transmission occurred only when the needle
was intentionally contaminated with blood; in routine use there
was apparently insufficient transfer of blood cells to cause BLV
transmission. The demonstrated dermal susceptibility to infection
also indicates that there is a potential for insect transmission
of BLV, a subject that will be presented in more detail in this
volume (Miller, J.M. "Bovine Leukemia Virus Vaccines").

There is little data available concerning the pathogenesis of
BLV infections. In an initial study conducted in our laboratory
we thought we found evidence that the intradermal inoculation of
BLV-infected lymphocytes resulted in the initial appearance of
virus in the spleen, thus bypassing the regional lymph nodes and
indicating that the spleen was a primary or requisite site for
BLV replication. Additional studies failed to support this initial observation however, and we subsequently found that the
removal of the spleen prior to inoculation had no apparent effect
on the initiation of BLV infections. Similarly, splenectomy of
animals with established persistent BLV infections had no apparent effect on the persistence of infection and we thus concluded
that the spleen plays no special role in BLV infections.

The very initial stage of BLV infection may include a transient true viremia with the appearance of free virus in the plasma
but this soon diasappears, probably due to the developing immune
response. An additional detectable response to infection is the
appearance and persistence of a population of lymphocytes which,
when examined by electron microscopy, have alterations of the
nuclear membrane which have been referred to as nuclear pockets
or nuclear projections. The significance of these structures has
not been fully determined.

If the long-term or ultimate results of BLV infection are
considered, cattle seem to fall into three groups. The first, and
largest of these groups, consists of those animals that develop a
persistent infection and immune response but remain normal in all

other respects. The second group, representing perhaps 30 to 35%
of all BLV-infected cattle, develops a persistent lymphocytosis.
The lymphocytosis is due to an expansion of the B lymphocyte
population. Some of these B cells carry the BLV information but
others do not and it has been suggested that they are a population that is expanded because it is responding to the infection.
It has frequently been surmised that persistent lymphocytosis
is an initial or prodromal stage in tumor development but this
is probably not true. Studies at the University of Pennsylvania
have, in fact, indicated that hereditary factors may control or
influence both the development of persistent lymphocytosis and
tumor development but that these seem to be separate and distinct
entities. They conclude that persistent lymphocytosis is a benign
response to infection with BLV and not an initial stage in the
development of lymphosarcoma. Persistent lymphocytosis is, however, sufficiently marked and frequent that it served as a useful
diagnostic tool for identification of herds at risk of developing
lymphosarcoma in the years before BLV was identified and the more
specific serological tests were devised for diagnostic purposes.

A third, and much smaller, group consists of those animals
that develop lymphosarcoma. Attempts to obtain broadly based
estimates of the prevalence of tumor development among BLV-
infected cattle have met with serious problems. Condemnations at
abattoirs in this country have been in the range of 10 to 20 per
100,000 cattle slaughtered for the past several years; but with
no accurate information regarding deaths from lymphosarcoma on
farms, and in the absence of any statistically based estimates of
the prevalence of BLV infection in our cattle herds, any attempt
to establish a tumor incidence is merely a guess. This situation
is further compounded by the fact that the average age of the
United States cattle population is declining and thus an ever
increasing number of animals are being culled from herds before
they reach the 4 to 8 year age range when maximum tumor incidence

might be expected. In Europe, where some control programs are in
progress, better information regarding prevalence of infection
is available; but, once infected animals are identified, they are
sent to slaughter, probably long before tumors would develop. The
best estimates of tumor incidence can be gained from a limited
study in an area of southern France in which it was found that
about 0.09% per year of the total cattle population or 0.31% of
the BLV-infected cattle developed tumors each year.

In conclusion I would like to note a few factors which may be
important in influencing the course of BLV infections. The fact
that the infection persists in the presence of antibody provides
abundant proof that immune responses cannot repress established
infections. We did find, however, that we could not infect newborn calves if BLV-infected blood cells were fed alone with
colostrum containing high levels of BLV antibody. In a subsequent
study we fed BLV antibody-positive colostrum to newborn calves
and then inoculated the animals intradermally with BLV-infected
lymphocytes. There was still evidence of protection but, in one
animal, when the colostral antibody disappeared at 4 months of
age, an active BLV infection emerged. Thus there is evidence that
passive antibody can effect a prolonged suppression of infection
without entirely eliminating the virus.

Studies at the University of Pennsylvania have shown that the
plasma, but not the serum, of infected cattle contains a factor
that suppresses BLV replication at the transcriptional level.
Preliminary characterization studies indicate that the activity
is associated with a substance having a molecular weight of about
150,000; it is susceptible to destruction by proteases but not by
nucleases, lipase or amylase. The factor does not seem to be
antibody or interferon and it is not effective in blocking the
replication of murine (Rauscher) or feline leukemia virus. We
obviously look forward to learning more about this substance from
future research.

It is also possible that other viral infections may influence the course of BLV infection. A number of years ago we isolated a virus from cattle that is structurally similar, but antigentically distint, from maedi-visna virus of sheep. Inoculation of this virus into calves resulted in a transient viremia and lymphocytosis of several weeks to a few months duration. During this time the hemolymph nodes in these animals enlarged, and remained so, due to a proliferative response but there was no evidence of prolonged or progressive illness in these cattle. A year later these animals were inoculated with BLV and they subsequently developed a lymphocytosis in the range of 30,000 to 100,000 lymphocytes per cubic millimeter of blood. This response was far in excess of what we usually encountered following BLV inoculation and causes us to speculate that the prior infection with the maedi-visna-like virus may have, in some way, prepared or predisposed these cattle to mount an excessive lymphocytic response to the BLV infection.

REFERENCES

1. Miller, J.M. and Van Der Maaten, M.J. (1979). J. Natl. Cancer Inst. 62, 425.
2. Ressang, A. et al. (1982). Zentrabl. Veterinarmed. [B] 29, 137.
3. Roberts, D.H. and Bushnell, S. (1982). Vet. Rec. 111, 501.
4. Gupta, P. and Ferrer, J.F. (1980). Int. J. Cancer 25, 663.
5. Straub, O.C. (1982). In "4th Int. Symp. Bovine Leukosis," p. 299.
6. Ferrer, J.F. and Piper, C.F. (1981). Cancer Res. 41, 4906.
7. Romero, C.H. et al. (1982). Pesq. Vet. Bras. 2, 9.
8. Mammerickx, M., Portetelle, D., Burny, A. et al. (1981). Zentrabl. Veterinarmed. [B] 28, 69.
9. Roberts, D.H., Lucas, M.H., Wibberley, G. et al. (1981). J. Biol. Stand. 9, 469.
10. Van Der Maaten, M.J., Miller, J.M., Schmerr, M.J. et al. (1981). Am. J. Vet. Res. 42, 1498.
11. Van Der Maaten, M.J. et al. (1982). In "4th Int. Symp. Bovine Leukosis," p. 225.
12. Kaja, R.W. and Olson, C. (1982). Theriogenology 18, 107.

13. Baumgartener, L.E., Crowley, J., Entine, S. et al. (1978).
    Zentrabl. Veterinarmed. [B] 25, 202.
14. Lucas, M.H., Dawson, M., Chasey, D. et al. (1980). Vet. Rec.
    106, 128.
15. Bouillant, A.M.P. et al. (1981). Ann. Rech. Vet. 12, 531.
16. Eaglesome, M.D., Mitchell, D., Betteridge, K.J. et al.
    (1982). Vet. Rec. 111, 122.
17. Van Der Maaten, M.J. and Miller, J.M. (1976). Bibl.
    Haematologica 43, 377.
18. Van Der Maaten, M.J. and Miller, J.M. (1977). Adv. Comp.
    Leuk. Res, p. 29.
19. Roberts, D.H., Lucan, M.H. and Wibberley, G. (1982). Vet.
    Rec. 110, 222.

THE PATHOBIOLOGY OF MACAQUE RETROVIRUSES
CLOSELY RELATED TO HUMAN T CELL LYMPHOTROPIC VIRUSES

P. J. Kanki,[1/2] R. D. Hunt[2]
and M. E. Essex[1]

[1]Department of Cancer Biology
Harvard School of Public Health
Boston, Massachusetts

[2]New England Regional Primate Research Center
Southborough, Massachusetts

Years of research on exogenous retroviruses in various inbred and outbred animal systems have provided the basis for comparative studies in human oncogenesis and the pathogenesis of immunosuppressive disease. There is now strong evidence that human T cell lymphotropic virus type I (HTLV-I) is the etiologic agent of a unique T cell malignancy, adult T cell leukemia/lymphoma (1,2). Gallo and coworkers first described this human retrovirus in 1980, isolated from a patient with aggressive T cell lymphoma (3-8). There are presently over 100 isolates of HTLV-I. Most are from Japan, the Caribbean Basin, Central Africa, South America and the United States; such endemic loci are additionally identified by the increased prevalence of healthy HTLV carriers as determined serologically, and the elevated presence of tumor cases. All of the isolates are similar by nucleic acid homology and serologic comparisons of their proteins; these have been collectively termed HTLV-I (9,10). A second member of the HTLV family, HTLV-II, was isolated from cultured spleen cells of a patient with a variant form of hairy cell leukemia (11,12).

Antigenic comparisons between HTLV-I and HTLV-II gag-encoded
proteins show these viruses share group-specific but not type-
specific determinants (11,13,14). Lee and colleagues have shown
that despite approximately 90% nucleic acid divergence between
these two HTLV types, considerable serologic crossreactivity
can be demonstrated resulting from conservation in the deduced
amino acid sequence of the major env gene products (15). The
relationship of HTLV-II to human disease is yet unknown.

A third member of the HTLV family was recently described by
Gallo and coworkers (16-18). This is the prototype virus isolated from patients with the acquired immune deficiency syndrome
(AIDS), also known as lymphadenopathy-associated virus (LAV) or
AIDS-related virus (ARV). Similar to HTLV-I and II, the AIDS
virus is T4 cell tropic, and epidemiologic studies indicate that
these viruses are most readily transmitted via sexual contact,
blood or blood product transmission. Recent data on the incidence
of AIDS cases and the prevalence of HTLV-III antibody-positive
individuals indicate that this disease is of worldwide public
health significance.

The HTLV family of viruses therefore represents a new and
important group of human pathogens. The need for animal model
systems in which one can study these viruses and the pathogenesis
of their associated diseases is obvious. It is now known that the
macaque monkey is naturally infected with two T lymphotropic
retroviruses, one closely related to HTLV-I and the second more
closely related to HTLV-III; these have been designated STLV-I
and STLV-III, respectively. Studies of these primate viruses
indicate numerous parallels to the human systems and no doubt
will provide a relevant model system for the understanding of
HTLV viruses and the pathogenesis of their associated diseases.

STLV-I

Miyoshi and coworkers first reported on the presence of antibodies to HTLV-I in Japanese macaques, Macaca fuscata (19). Phytohemagglutinin-stimulated lymphocytes from seropositive macaques showed type C virus particles identical to HTLV-I after 6 days in short-term culture. In cocultivation procedures the macaque virus was capable of transforming seronegative macaque and human lymphocytes (20,21). These HTLV-I transformed cells exhibited the adult T cell leukemia antigen when tested with the appropriate antisera in a fixed immunofluorescence assay (19-21). Subsequent serologic surveys by numerous investigators have shown the presence of antibodies to HTLV-I in numerous Old World primates, ranging from 0-44% (22-27). These include species of the genus Macaca, African green monkeys (Cercopithecus aethiops), baboons (Papio sp) and chimpanzees (Pan troglodytes); whereas New World primates and Prosimians have been uniformly seronegative. Familial clustering and an age dependence of STLV-I antibodies have been demonstrated (25,26). Horizontal transmission as judged by seroconversion has been observed from mother to infant and male to female in Japanese macaque studies (25,26,28). Studies in Indonesia and Japan with wild-caught Macaca fascicularis and M. fuscata, respectively, showed geographic clustering of seropositive macaques, similar but not coincident with the clustering of seropositive human populations.

In vivo transmission of lymphomatous tissue from a Papio hamadryas (originally from the Sukhumi, USSR colony) to naive baboons, macaques and owl monkeys resulted in seroconversion to HTLV-I detected by indirect enzyme-linked immunosorbent assay (ELISA) (27). A virus-producing cell line (designated 991-1) was established from fresh peripheral blood lymphocytes of an antibody-positive Papio cynocephalus recipient in the presence of interleukin-2. The cell line released typical type C virus particles with extracellular reverse transcriptase and reacted positively with monoclonal antibody against p19 of HTLV-I and antisera to p24 of HTLV-I. Proviral sequence analysis demonstrated that the baboon virus was more related to HTLV-I than to HTLV-II, yet distinct from both (29).

We have recently reported the first eivdence for the association of STLV-I to the development of spontaneous lymphoma in three species of macaque. A seroepidemiologic survey was conducted in which sera from Macaca cyclopis, M. fascicularis and Macaca mulatta were examined for the presence of antibodies to HTLV-I. For each species, serum samples from healthy macaques and macaques with the histopathologic diagnosis of malignant lymphoma or lymphoproliferative disorder were included (30). Among healthy M. cyclopis, the Taiwanese Rock macaque, were 20 serum samples from macaques captured and housed in their native country, Taiwan; all other macaques were from the New England Regional Primate Research Center colony (NERPRC).

Malignant lymphoma is not a common spontaneous neoplasm of macaques (31,32). The NERPRC has observed relatively high prevalence of this tumor over the past 12 years (33). All cases were diagnosed lymphoma of the non-Hodgkin's type with considerable variability in histopathologic appearance and distribution. Lymphoproliferative sizes of 24,000 daltons (p24), 45,000 daltons (gp45) and 61,000 daltons (gp61) as has been previously described. These proteins were not immunoprecipitated by human serum negative for HTLV-membrane antigen (HTLV-MA). HTLV-MA-positive serum from macaques with malignant lymphoma, lymphoproliferative disorder or healthy seropositives recognized the same viral-encoded proteins as human reference positive sera. These were not recognized by seronegative macaque serum samples.

The polymorphic nature of various HTLV-I glycoproteins has been described (34). HTLV-MA-positive serum samples from macaques were also capable of recognizing the major antigens in other

HTLV-I isolates such as MT-2, C5-MJ, MJ and C91PL (unpublished data). Thus it appears that the STLV-I virus is very closely related to HTLV-I by major antigen crossreactivity. It also appears that STLV-I, like its human counterpart, may be associated with a spontaneous lymphoid abnormality. The study of this virus and its disease association may provide valuable insight into the mechanism of HTLV-I-induced oncogenesis.

STLV-III

There is now strong evidence for an etiologic relationship of HTLV-III and AIDS. This member of the HTLV family is characerized by its cytopathic effect and T4 tropism; however, there are many features of this virus such as its unique genetic structure and its apparent rapid mutation rate that are distinct. To our knowledge, there have been no previous reports of a similar agent found naturally in animals. The isolation and preliminary characterization of a cytopathic T cell tropic retrovirus from three immunodeficient macaques and one macaque with malignant lymphoma have recently been described (35,36). Investigators at the NERPRC successfully isolated this virus by cocultivation of peripheral blood lymphocytes, splenic lymphocytes or cell-free serum samples on Hut-78, a well-characterized mature human T cell line. Analysis of cell-free supernatants for reverse transcriptase yielded positive results for Mg^{++}-dependent activity 12 to 18 days after initiation or cocultivation. Maximum reverse transcriptase levels were detected approximately 10 days later, and have been maintained for over 4 months in culture. Hut-78 cells infected with the macaque retrovirus demonstrated a characteristic cytopathic effect with the formation of pleomorphic, multinucleated giant cells.

Filtered cell-free supernatants from cells infected with the macaque virus isolates could efficiently infect fresh human

T lymphocytes grown in the presence of T cell growth factor.
Studies by N. Letvin and colleagues demonstrated the T4 tropism
of this virus. Peripheral blood lymphocytes prepared from heparinized human blood were treated with monoclonal antibody + complement and T4- and T8-enriched cell populations were isolated.

All four macaque retrovirus isolates demonstrated similar
ultrastructural morphology in studies conducted by N. King and
coworkers. Type C retroviral particles were observed in infected
cells, where nucleoids were seen only in particles in the process of budding. Mature, extracellular viral particles had a
cylindrical-shaped nucleoid, also a feature of HTLV-III. Two of
the macaques from which virus was isolated also demonstrated
similar type C retrovirus particles in lymph node biopsy
specimens.

We have serologically identified and characterized the
macaque retrovirus by radioimmunoprecipitation techniques. Virus-
specific proteins of 160 kilodaltons (kd), 120 kd, 55 kd and
24 kd were identified; all similar in size to the major gag- and
env-encoded proteins of HTLV-III (17,18,37,38). These protein
species were similarly recognized by macaque serum samples and
human reference serum samples from AIDS-related complex (ARC) and
AIDS patients, positive for HTLV-III antibodies. Monoclonal disorder (LPD) is a unique lymphoid abnormality characterized by
nodular aggregates of mature lymphocytes in nonlymphoid organs.
LPD has been linked with Macaque immunodeficiency syndrome
observed at the NERPRC (39,40).

Serum samples were tested with a membrane immunofluorescence
assay for evidence of antibody directed to HTLV-MA as previously
described (41,42). The assay detects two glycoproteins (gp61 and
gp45) expressed on HTLV-I-infected cells that are in part encoded
by the env gene of HTLV-I (34,43). These two glycoproteins are
the most immunogenic species recognized in people exposed to this
virus in contrast to the viral core proteins (i.e., p24 and p19)

which are the antigen targets used in most other assays for the detection of HTLV antibodies. Immunofluorescence was conducted on two reference HTLV-I-infected cell lines, Hut-102 and MT-2. All positive sera were tested on uninfected T (8402) and B (NC 37) lymphoid cell lines to rule out nonspecificity.

The rate of seropositivity to HTLV-MA in M. cyclopis from Taiwan and M. cyclopis raised in captivity at the NERPRC are similar (10% and 14%, respectively). Notably, three of four M. cyclopis with LPD were positive for antibodies to HTLV-MA. One of 31 healthy M. mulatta from the NERPRC were seropositive for HTLV-MA. In contrast five of six M. mulatta with lymphoma or LPD were seropositive. Two of 30 healthy M. fascicularis had antibodies to HTLV-MA while all three macaques with lymphoma were seropositive. In total, 11 of 13 (84.6%) macaques with lymphoma or LPD had antibodies to HTLV-MA, whereas seven of 95 healthy macaques were seropositive. The association of lymphoid abnormalities or malignancies with evidence of exposure to HTLV is statistically significant at a p value $<6.27 \times 10^{-9}$, the Fisher exact statistic.

Macaque sera were also used for radioimmunoprecipitation and sodium dodecyl sulfate-polyacrylamide gel electrophoresis (SDS-PAGE). When Hut-102 (a reference HTLV-I-infected cell line) whole cell lysate was used as the antigenic source, human reference serum positive for antibodies to HTLV-MA immunoprecipitated proteins with antibodies directed to the major core protein of HTLV-III, p24, also immunoprecipitated a 24 kd species in the macaque virus-infected cell lysate. Macaque sera with antibodies to the macaque virus were also capable of immunoprecipitating the major gag-encoded proteins of HTLV-III, p55 and p24. The env-related glycoproteins of HTLV-III are the most immunogenic antigens in exposed people (37); however, macaque antibody-positive sera showed minimal crossreactivity with the gp120 and gp160 of HTLV-III. Therefore demonstrating the apparent type immunoreactivity of the env-coded glycoproteins, consistent with observations in other retrovirus systems.

An immunodeficiency syndrome of macaque monkeys has been described at the NERPRC characterized by infection with a variety of opportunistic infections, impaired T cell function and lympho-proliferative disorders (39,40). Type D retroviruses have been isolated at the NERPRC and at least two other primate colonies where a similar immunodeficiency syndrome has been described, however most of the macaques in this study were apparently free of type D retrovirus based on repeated unsuccessful isolation attempts and negative serology (44-47). We would therefore hypothesize that the macaque T lymphotropic retroviruses may be etiologically linked to an immunodeficiency syndrome, thus pro-viding an excellent animal model for the study of HTLV-III and the pathogenesis of AIDS. The close relationship of STLV-III to HTLV-III at an antigenic level may provide valuable insight into the development of an AIDS vaccine.

REFERENCES

1. Takatsuki, K., Uchiyama, T., Ueshima, Y. et al. (1979). Jpn. J. Clin. Oncol. 9, 317.
2. Takatsuki, K., Uchiyama, T., Sagawa, K. et al. (1976). Top. Hematol. 415, 73.
3. Poiesz, B., Ruscetti, F.W., Gazdar, A.F. et al. (1980). Proc. Natl. Acad. Sci. 77, 7415.
4. Reitz, M.S., Jr., Poiesz, B.J., Ruscetti, F.W. et al. (1981). Proc. Natl. Acad. Sci. 78, 1887.
5. Rho, H.M., Poiesz, B., Ruscetti, F.W. et al. (1981). Virology 112, 335.
6. Kalyanaraman, V.S., Sarngadharan, M.G., Poiesz, B. et al. (1981). J. Virol. 38, 906.
7. Poiesz, B.J., Ruscetti, F.W., Reitz, M.S. et al. (1981). Nature 294, 268.
8. Kalyanaraman, V.S., Sarngardharan, M.G., Bunn, P.A. et al. (1981). Nature 294, 271.
9. Popovic, M., Reitz, M.S., Sarngadharan, M.G. (1982). Nature 300, 63.
10. Popovic, M., Sarin, P.S., Robert-Guroff, M. et al. (1983). Science 219, 856.

11. Kalyanaraman, V.S., Sarngadharan, M.G., Robert-Guroff, M. et al. (1982). Science 218, 571.
12. Saxon, A., Stevens, R.H. and Golde, D.W. (1978). Ann. Intern. Med. 88, 323.
13. Kalyanaraman, V.S., Sarngadharan, M.G., Poiesz, B. et al. (1981). J. Virol. 38, 906.
14. Robert-Guroff, M., Ruscetti, F.W., Posner, L.E. et al. (1981). J. Exp. Med. 154, 1957.
15. Lee, T.H., Coligan, J.E., McLane, M.F. et al. (1984). Proc. Natl. Acad. Sci. 81, 7579.
16. Popovic, M., Sarngadharan, M.O., Read, E. et al. (1984). Science 224, 497.
17. Schupbach, J., Popovic, M., Gilden, R.V. et al. (1984). Science 224, 503.
18. Sarngadharan, M.G., Popovic, M., Bruch, L. et al. (1984). Science 224, 506.
19. Miyoshi, I., Ohtsuki, Y., Fujishita, M. et al. (1982). Gann 73, 848.
20. Miyoshi, I., Tagushi, H., Fujishita, M. et al. (1981). Lancet 1, 1016.
21. Miyoshi, I., Tagushi, H., Fujishita, M. et al. (1981). Lancet 2, 166.
22. Hayami, M., Ishikawa, K., Komuro, A. et al. (1983). Lancet 2, 620.
23. Hunsmann, G., Schneider, J., Schmitt, J. et al. (1983). Int. J. Cancer 32, 329.
24. Ishida, T., Yamamoto, K., Kaneko, R. et al. (1983). Microbiol. Immunol. 27, 297.
25. Miyoshi, I., Fujishita, M., Taguchi, H. et al. (1983). Int. J. Cancer 32, 333.
26. Hayami, M., Komuro, A. and Nozawa, K. (1984). Int. J. Cancer 33, 179.
27. Saxinger, W.C., Lange-Wantzin, G., Thomsen. K. et al. (1984). In "Human T-cell Leukemia Viruses" (R.C. Gallo, M. Essex and L. Gross, eds.), p. 323. Cold Spring Harbor Press, New York.
28. Miyoshi, I., Fujishita, M., Taguchi, H. et al. (1983). Lancet 1, 241.
29. Guo, H.-G., Wong-Staal, F. and Gallo, R.C. (1984). Science 223, 1195.
30. Homma, T., Kanki, P.J., King, N.W., Jr. et al. (1984). Science 225, 716.
31. O'Gara, R.W. and Adamson, R.H. (1972). In "Pathology of Simian Primates" (R.N.T.W. Fiennes, ed.), p. 190. Karger, Basel, Switzerland.
32. Manning, J.R.S. and Griesemer, R.A. (1974). Lab. Anim. Sci. 24, 204.
33. Hunt, R.D., Blake, B.J., Chalifoux, L.V. et al. (1983). Proc. Natl. Acad. Sci. 80, 5085.

34. Lee, T.H., Homma, T., Schultz, K.T. et al. (1984). In "Human T-cell Leukemia Viruses" (R.C. Gallo, M. Essex and L. Gross, eds.), p. 111. Cold Spring Harbor Press, New York.
35. Daniel, M.D., Letvin, N.L., King, N.W. et al. (1985). Science 228, 1201.
36. Kanki, P.J., McLane, M.F., King, N.W. et al. (1985). Science 228, 1199.
37. Barin, F., McLane, M.F., Allan, J.S. et al. (1985). Science 228, 1094.
38. Allan, J.S., Coligan, J.E., Barin, F. et al. (1985). Science 228, 1091.
39. Letvin, N., Eaton, K.A., Aldrich, W.R. et al. (1983). Proc. Natl. Acad. Sci. 80, 2718.
40. King, N.W., Hunt, R.D. and Letvin, N. (1983). North Am. J. Pathol. 113, 382.
41. Essex, M., McLane, M.F., Lee, T.H. et al. (1983). Science 220, 859.
42. Essex, M., McLane, M.F., Lee, T.H. et al. (1983). Science 221, 1061.
43. Lee, T.H., Coligan, J.E., Homma, T. et al. (1984). Proc. Natl. Acad. Sci. 81, 3856.
44. Daniel, M.D., King, N.W., Letvin, N.L. et al. (1984). Science 223, 602.
45. Stromberg, K., Benveniste, R.E., Arthur, L.O. et al. (1984). Science 224, 289.
46. Marx, P.A., Maul, D.H., Osborn, K.G. et al. (1984). Science 223, 1083.
47. Letvin, N., Daniel, M.D., Sehgal, P. et al. (1984). J. Virol. 52, 683.

STUDIES IN NONHUMAN PRIMATES ON RETROVIRUSES
ASSOCIATED WITH AN ACQUIRED IMMUNE DEFICIENCY SYNDROME

A. A. van Es
W. van Vreeswijk

Primate Center TNO
Rijswijk, The Netherlands

L. J. Lowenstine

California Primate Research Center
Davis, California

P. Bentvelzen

Radiobiological Institute TNO
Rijswijk, The Netherlands

Considerable evidence accumulates for the etiological role of a novel retrovirus in the recent epidemic of the acquired immune deficiency syndrome (AIDS) in man (1-3). Many nonhuman primates have been inoculated with samples, like blood, from AIDS patients or with virus preparations named either lymphadenopathy-associated virus (LAV), human T cell lymphotropic virus type III (HTLV-III) or AIDS-related retrovirus (ARV).

In the Dutch Primate Center chimpanzees and rhesus monkeys were inoculated in 1982 with blood from one of the first AIDS patients in the Netherlands. Only the chimpanzees proved to replicate the retrovirus as demonstrated by the presence of antiviral antibodies, detected by means of a solid phase

radioimmunoassay, and by the presence of a provirus in some
leukocytes as revealed by spot blot hybridization.

A collaborative program was started with L. Montagnier
(Institut Pasteur, Paris). Lymphocytes of chimpanzees and rhesus
monkeys were infected in vitro with so-called LAV. The cells of
all the tested chimpanzees proved to replicate LAV at a high
rate, as determined by a reverse transcriptase assay of the culture supernatants. Cells of only three of 10 tested rhesus monkeys proved to be positive in this test. Virus production proved
to be approximately 10 times lower than in cultures of infected
chimpanzee lymphocytes. The infected cells were injected back
into the donors. The animals were thereafter inoculated five
times with purified LAV. Within a month the chimpanzees proved
to be infected, whereas the rhesus monkeys remained negative in
various tests during an observation period of 1 year. No morbid-
ity has been noted in the animals, although the chimpanzees
showed a transient lymphopenia.

A serological survey of 100 chimpanzees kept in the Dutch
Primate Center revealed four additional positives for antibodies
to LAV/HTLV-III. It is unlikely that this seropositivity is due
to (sexual) contact with the intentionally infected chimpanzees.
These animals have been used for studies on human hepatitis
viruses. An investigation is presently being conducted as to
whether the human samples used in these studies were contaminated
with the AIDS retrovirus.

Since 1969 four outbreaks of the so-called simian acquired
immune deficiency syndrome (SAIDS) have occurred in rhesus monkeys and stump-tail macaques at the California Primate Research
Center. This syndrome results in rare opportunistic infections
and malignancies (4,5). Inoculation of materials from diseased
animals into healthy animals led to the development of lymphadenopathy, splenomegaly, neutropenia, polymyositis and skin
lesions resembling human Kaposi sarcoma, in a proportion of the

animals. A type D retrovirus seems to be involved (6-8) which is related to the Mason-Pfizer monkey virus (MPMV), isolated from a rhesus monkey sebaceous gland tumor. The MPMV when inoculated into newborn rhesus monkeys induces lymphoid cell depletion and thymic atrophy followed by opportunistic infections (9).

We have looked for a relationship between susceptibility to the pathogenic action of the SAIDS agent and the RhLA system. This system is the major histocompatibility complex of the rhesus monkey and is comparable to the human HLA and murine H-2 systems. This gene complex has been extensively studied in the Dutch Primate Center (10,11). It comprises A and B regions coding for classical, serologically defined antigens present on B and T cells and various other tissues. The D/DR gene codes for antigens involved in mixed lymphocyte culture stimulation.

This study on the RhLA-SAIDS association was initiated in view of the association between H-2 and susceptibility to the pathogenic effect of some retroviruses in mice (12,13). Fifteen unrelated rhesus monkeys were typed for the DR locus in addition to the other RhLA loci and then inoculated with homogenized tissues from monkeys with SAIDS. The animals were checked daily for signs of disease. The diagnosis of SAIDS was only made if the animals, in addition to lymphadenopathy, fulfilled at least four of the following criteria: splenomegaly, weight loss ($\leq$10%), anemia (packed cell volume $\leq$30%), lymphoid depletion, persistent untreatable diarrhea and chronic or opportunistic infections.

As can be concluded from Table I seven of the 15 tested animals carried the DR-1-RhLA antigen. Six of these animals developed SAIDS. Two diseased animals carried the DR-2 antigen. Only one of the seven resistant monkeys carried DR-1. The excess of DR-1 in the group of affected animals suggests strongly that this allele causes susceptibility to the SAIDS virus. This hypothesis is presently tested in genetically well-defined monkey

TABLE I.   RhLA-DR Phenotype Distribution
in Relationship to Susceptibility to SAIDS

	Sex	DR locus
Susceptible		
1	F	2
2	M	2
3	M	1
4	M	1
5	F	1
6	M	1
7	M	1
8	M	1
Resistant		
1	F	1
2	F	2
3	F	2
4	F	3
5	M	3
6	M	4
7	M	4

groups in the Dutch Primate Center in which segregation of susceptibility to AIDS, possibly in association with RhLA-DR, can be investigated.

REFERENCES

1. Barré-Sinoussi, F., Chermann, J.C., Rey, F. et al. (1983). Science 220, 868.
2. Gallo, R.C., Salahuddin, S.Z., Popovic, M. et al. (1984). Science 224, 500.
3. Levy, J.A., Hoffman, A.D., Kramer, S.M. et al. (1984). Science 225, 840.
4. London, W.T., Madden, D.L., Gravell, M. et al. (1983). Lancet 2, 869.
5. Henrickson, R.V., Maul, P.H., Lerche, N.W. et al. (1984). Lab. Animal Sci. 34, 140.
6. Daniel, M.O., Norval, W.K., Letvin, N.L. et al. (1984). Science 223, 602.

7. Marx, S.A., Maul, D.H., Osborn, K.G. et al. (1984). Science 223, 1083.
8. Stromberg, K., Benveniste, R.E., Arthur, L.O. et al. (1984). Science 224, 289.
9. Fine, D.L., Landon, J.C., Pienta, R.J. et al. (1975). J. Natl. Cancer Inst. 54, 651.
10. Balner, H. (1981). In "Ia Antigens and Their Analogs in Man and Other Animals" (S. Ferrone and C.D. David, eds.), vol. 2. Boca Raton, Florida.
11. Van Es, A.A. and Balner, H. (1978). Tissue Antigens 12, 275.
12. Lilly, F. (1966). Genetics 53, 525.
13. Mühlbock, 0. and Dux, A. (1974). J. Natl. Cancer Inst. 53, 993.

HOST IMMUNITY
AND RETROVIRUS DISEASE

PROSPECTS FOR CHEMOTHERAPEUTIC OR CHEMOPROPHYLACTIC INTERVENTION IN AIDS-RELATED RETROVIRUS INFECTION

William M. Shannon

Kettering-Meyer Laboratory
Southern Research Institute
Birmingham, Alabama

In terms of the potential control measures that might be employed in combating AIDS, this volume has thus far discussed only the potential development of vaccines and possible immuno-therapy for use in the prevention and treatment ot AIDS-related retrovirus infections. At this point, it might be appropriate to examine the prospects for chemotherapeutic intervention and possibly even chemoprophylaxis in the control of AIDS virus infection.

Obviously, until there is an effective and useful immuniza-tion for the prevention of human AIDS-related retrovirus infec-tion, there will be many new individuals who will develop the disease and there will be large numbers of deaths due to this devastating illness. I think, therefore, that a concerted effort should be made to find selective antiviral drugs that are effec-tive against retrovirus infections. Such drugs might be extremely useful in the control of AIDS infection and for prophylactic treatment of those who are at the highest risk of developing AIDS.

Most of the research efforts in antiviral chemotherapy in recent years have been directed primarily toward the herpes viruses (1). There are a number of reasons for this focus on the herpes viruses. First of all, most of our success has been in this particular area of antiviral research and it has been like the fellow who lost his wallet one evening and was later seen at the street corner searching for it under the street lamp, simply because the light was better there. A second factor, of course, has been the large-scale epidemic of genital herpes virus infections. This has focused the attention of the pharmaceutical industry and others so that there has been a resurgence of interest in the development of antiviral drugs for use in the treatment of herpes virus infections. Additional funding has therefore been funneled into the effort to develop more potent and more effective antiviral compounds.

Shown in Figure 1 are the chemical structures of selected purine and pyrimidine nucleoside analogues which have demonstated significant activity against the herpes viruses. We are indeed fortunate to have a number of clinically effective agents, some of which have received FDA approval and are licensed for general use in this country. All of these drugs could be very useful in controlling the opportunistic infections with various herpes viruses that one sees in immunocompromised patients, such as in the AIDS patients. The halogenated pyrimidine nucleoside analogues, 5-iodo-2'-deoxyuridine (IdUrd) and trifluorothymidine (F_3dThd), are both licensed for use in the topical treatment of herpetic eye infections (1-5). Other compounds have been synthesized that have greater selectivity in their activity against herpes group viruses: 5'-amino-5-iodo-2',5'-dideoxyuridine (AIddUrd) (4), the fluorinated pyrimidine nucleoside analogues represented by 2'-fluoro-5-iodo-arabinosylcytosine (FIAC) (6) and, of course, acyclovir (1,7-9). These compounds are activated in the infected cell by the herpes virus-induced deoxypyrimidine kinase and this, therefore, results in an order of magnitude greater specificity for inhibition of the virus. Of these compounds, acyclovir has recently been licensed by the FDA for use

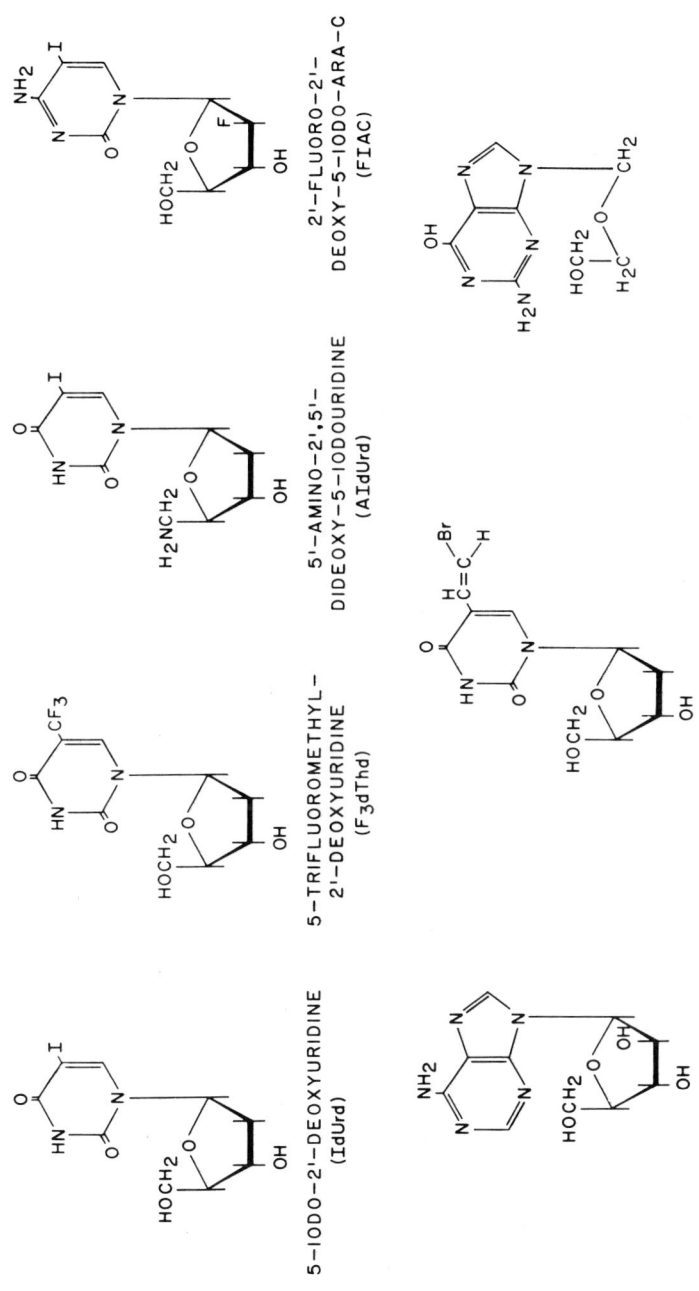

Fig. 1. Selected nucleoside analogues with significant antiviral activity against herpes viruses.

in primary genital herpes and mucocutaneous herpes in the immunosuppressed host. 9-β-D-Arabinofuranosyladenine (araA) has, of
course, been licensed for many years for ophthalmic use against
herpes virus-induced eye infections (1,10). It was also the first
antiviral drug found effective against generalized herpes virus
infections and which was licensed for systemic use in man (1,10).
It has been the drug of choice for the treatment of life-
threatening or severe herpes virus infections such as herpes
encephalitis (11), neonatal herpes (12) and generalized herpes
virus infections in immunosuppressed patients (13).

Southern Research Institute, in collaboration with the Parke-
Davis Company, was involved in much of the early preclinical work
on araA conducted back in the late 1960s and early 1970s. At that
time, we reported the activity of araA against the retroviruses,
both avian and murine retroviruses in vitro (14,15) and murine
retroviruses in vivo (16). Subsequently, it was found that araA
triphosphate (araATP) inhibits reverse transcriptase (17). Looking at the metabolism of araA (Fig. 2), one sees that it is
deaminated in mammalian cells to ara-hypoxanthine (araH) by the
action of the ubiquitous enzyme adenosine deaminase. It is
phosphorylated by several kinases to the mono-, di- and triphosphates and it is the triphosphate that is responsible for the
inhibition of the RNA-dependent DNA polymerase of retroviruses.
This compound, araATP, is a competitive inhibitor of both the
herpes virus-induced DNA polymerase and the retrovirus reverse
transcriptase with respect to the normal substrate, dATP. This
is not the only mechanism of action of araA however; there are
others. We note, for example, that it inhibits ribonucleotide
reductase in herpes virus-infected cells and it appears to do
this preferentially. One can therefore discern two steps in the
DNA synthetic pathway that are blocked by this drug (Fig. 2),
and there may be other sites of action as well (18).

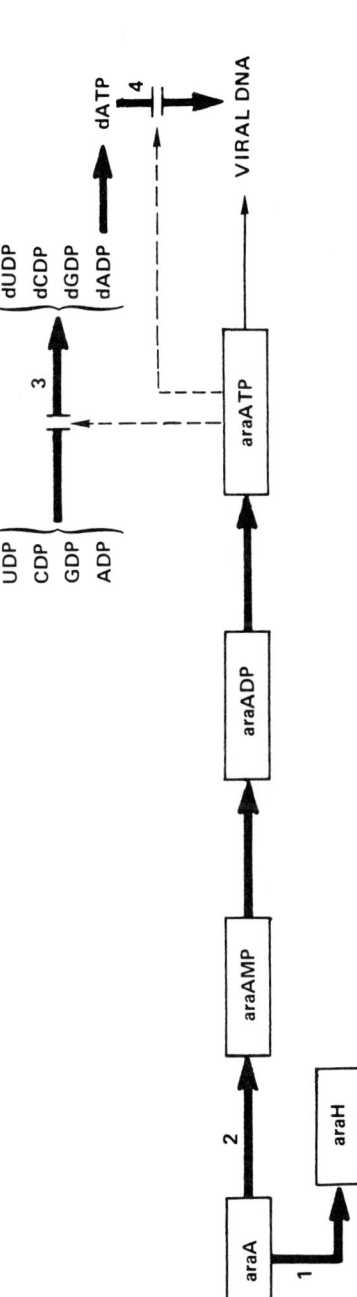

Fig. 2. Metabolism and possible biochemical targets for the antiviral action of araA. The large arrows indicate the metabolic pathways; the smaller broken arrows indicate the known effects of araATP on specific enzyme systems. 1) adenosine deaminase, 2) cellular adenosine kinase and cellular deoxycytidine kinase, 3) virus-induced ribonucleotide reductase and 4) virus-induced DNA polymerase.

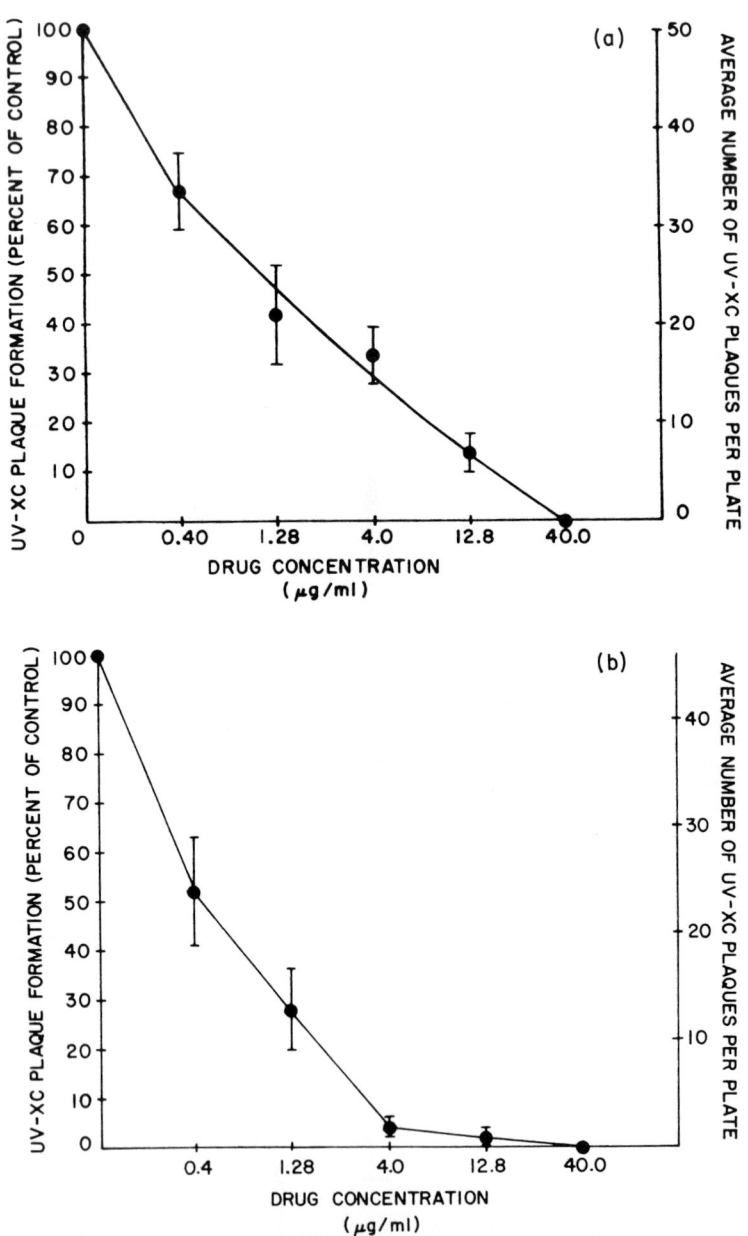

Fig. 3.   Inhibition of (a) Gross and (b) Rauscher MLV replication in Swiss mouse embryo cells by araA.

Some of the early data that we obtained with araA as an inhibitor of retrovirus replication are shown in Figure 3. Using the extremely reproducible UV-XC plaque assay technique for murine leukemia viruses that was developed by Rowe, Pugh and Hartley some years ago (19), we examined araA for antiviral activity in a plaque reduction test. Gross or Rauscher murine leukemia virus (MLV) replication in mouse embryo cells was inhibited in a dose-dependent manner by nontoxic concentrations of araA. We followed this observation up in vivo by testing araA against Rauscher MLV in mice and we found significant inhibition of Rauscher virus-induced tumorigenesis (Table I). Indicator mice that received spleen homogenates from virus-infected animals developed significant splenomegaly, whereas mice that received spleen homogenates from virus-infected animals treated with 240 or 360 mg/kg/day had spleen weights that were similar to that of the uninfected controls.

Another compound that should be given some attention is cyclaradine, the carbocyclic analogue of araA (Fig. 4), synthesized by Dr. Robert Vince of the University of Minnesota (20).

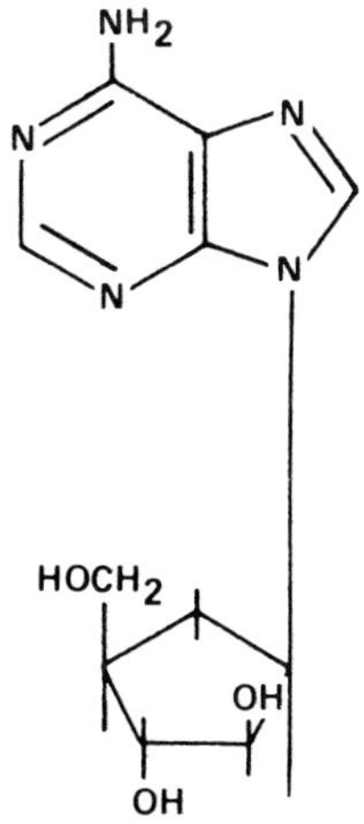

Fig. 4. Chemical structure of cyclaradine, the carbocyclic analogue of araA.

Table I. Reduction in Rauscher MLV Titers in the Plasma and Spleens of araA (NSC 404241)-Treated Mice as Determined by Splenomegaly Bioassay in Indicator Mice[a]

Drug dosage[b]	Average spleen weight of indicator mice on day 21 (g)	% Inhibition[c]	Significance (P)[d]
Plasma			
0 (uninfected controls)	0.132	—	
0 (virus-infected controls)	0.426	—	
araA, 240 mg/kg/day	ND[e]	—	
araA, 360 mg/kg/day	0.167	88.1	<0.05
Spleen			
0 (uninfected controls)	0.131	—	
0 (virus-infected controls)	1.090	—	
araA, 240 mg/kg/day	0.154	97.6	<0.0025
araA, 360 mg/kg/day	0.139	99.2	<0.0005

(continued)

248

Table I (continued)

---

[a]Indicator mice were inoculated i.p. with serial 10-fold dilutions of 10% plasma or spleen homogenates from surviving mice.

[b]Drug was administered i.p., every 3 hours × 8, on days 1, 5 and 9.

[c]The percentage of inhibition of splenomegaly was calculated as follows:

$$1 - \frac{\text{Net spleen weight increase in the presence of drug}}{\text{Net spleen weight increase in the absence of drug}} \times 100$$

[d]P = probability ($\underline{t}$ test) that reduction in splenomegaly was due to chance.

[e]Not done.

TABLE II. Evaluation of Carbocyclic Analogues of 5-Substituted Uracil Nucleosides Against Herpes Simplex Virus[a]

Compound no.	X	Type 1, strain 377		Type 2, strain MS	
		VR	MIC$_{50}$ mcg/ml	VR	MIC$_{50}$ mcg/ml
2a	H	0			
2b	CH$_3$	5.4	0.8	3.2	7.0
2c	F	0		0	
2d	Br	6.2	0.3	1.5	32
2e	I	6.5	0.4	2.9	32
		7.1	0.3	3.4	20
		7.9	0.1		
		7.4	0.4		
2f	NH$_2$	0.1			
2g	NHCH$_3$	4.2	10	1.2	229
		3.9	15		
		4.5	25		
2h	NHC$_4$H$_9$	2.0	290	0.7	1000
2i	N(CH$_3$)$_2$	0			
3a	H	0			
3b	CH$_3$	0.4		0	
3c-3g	F,Br,I,NH$_2$	0			
4a-4g	F,Br,I,NH$_2$	0			
4h	CH$_2$OH	0.3		0	
6a	Br	1.3	92		
		0.9	100		
6b	Br	0			
6d	I	2.4	10		
		1.6	25		
IdUrd		7.4	0.3	5.0	1.0
AraA		2.7	9.8	2.3	20.1

[a]Antiviral assays were performed with HSV-1 and HSV-2 replicating in primary rabbit kidney cell cultures.

This compound has a methylene group instead of an oxygen in the carbohydrate moiety so that, instead of a tetrahydrofuranose ring, it has a cyclopentane ring. This endows the compound with stability against cleavage by phosphorylases and hydrolases. It also makes it a deaminase-resistant molecule. The compound is quite effective against herpes virus infections and we reported earlier that it is as effective as acyclovir in the treatment of genital herpes virus infections in the guinea pig model (21). Schering Corporation is currently performing safety and toxicology studies with this drug. Cyclaradine is also active against retroviruses in vitro (17) and is therefore a candidate antiviral for evaluation in AIDS.

In our laboratories at Southern Research Institute, Dr. Y. Fulmer Shealy has made a number of carbocyclic analogues of both purine and pyrimidine nucleosides (Table II). Among a series of these carbocyclic nucleoside analogues, some have been found with high virus ratings (VRs) (22). The carbocyclic analogue of 5-iodo-2'-deoxyuridine (C-IdUrd) possessed significant and potent antiviral activity with a low MIC_{50}. This compound is much more potent than the true nucleoside analogue against herpes viruses. It passes the blood-brain-barrier and it is significantly effective against herpes encephalitis in mice (Shannon, W.M., L. Westbrook, Y.F. Shealy et al., unpublished data). C-IdUrd is also active against Gross MLV in cell culture (Fig. 5), with significant inhibition of virus replication observed at noncytotoxic concentrations.

Another promising compound that has been shown to have activity against MLV is ribavirin (Fig. 6). Dr. Robert Sidwell initially reported this compound to possess activity against Friend leukemia virus (23). Subsequently, the activity of ribavirin against Gross and Rauscher leukemia viruses both in vitro and in vivo was demonstrated in our laboratories (Fig. 7 and Table III) (16). One has to administer a relatively high dose level of drug

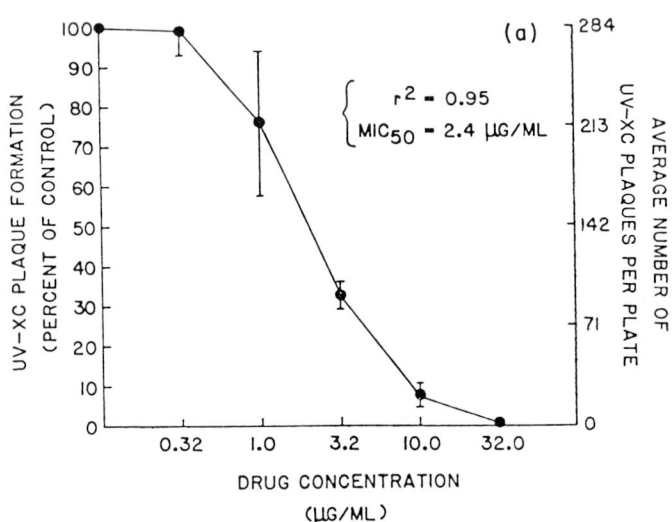

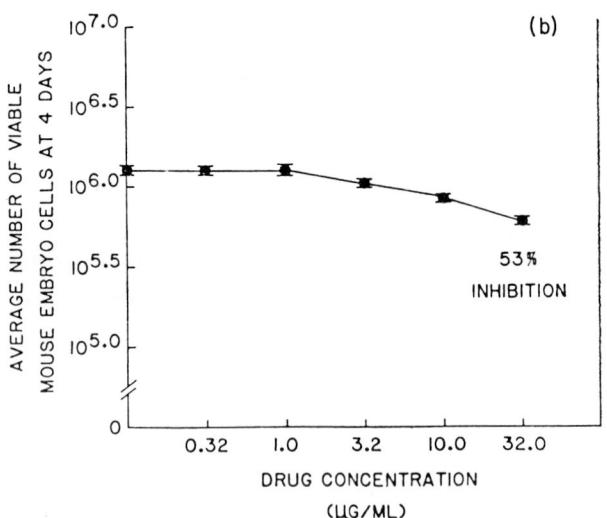

Fig. 5.   (a) Inhibition of Gross MLV replication in mouse
embryo cells by the carbocyclic analogue of IdUrd. (b) Effect of
carbocyclic IdUrd on host cell multiplication.

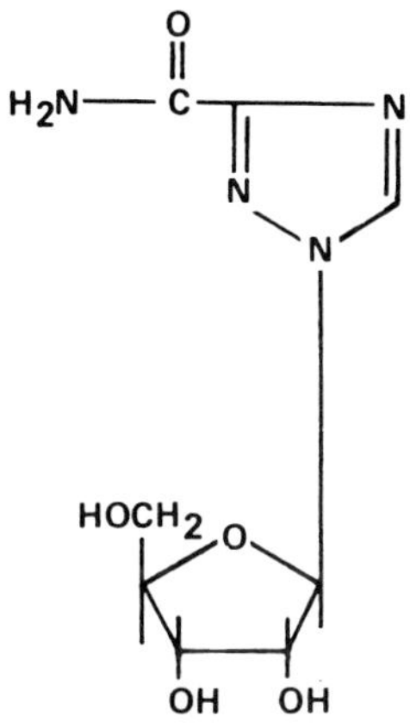

1-β-D-Ribofuranosyl-1,2,4-triazole-3-carboxamide
(Ribavirin)

Fig. 6.   Chemical structure of ribavirin.

(75 mg/kg; i.e., a dose level which is approaching the LD_{20})
before significant antiviral efficacy is observed with ribavirin.
Nevertheless, this drug should be examined for activity against
AIDS-related retroviruses.

Phosphonoacetic acid (PAA), a DNA polymerase inhibitor which
inhibits herpes virus replication, has also been found to significantly inhibit MLV replication in cell culture (Fig. 8) (16)
and to inhibit MLV reverse transcriptase in a dose-dependent
manner (17). PAA acts as a noncompetitive inhibitor of the DNA
polymerase by interacting with the enzyme at the pyrophosphate
binding site, so it is different from some of the nucleoside
triphosphates, such as araATP, which are competitive inhibitors
of the enzyme (Fig. 9). Therefore, if one puts araA and PAA
together in combination, one gets a synergistic response and
better inhibition ot MLV replication than one can obtain with
either compound alone (17). If one plots the fraction of the

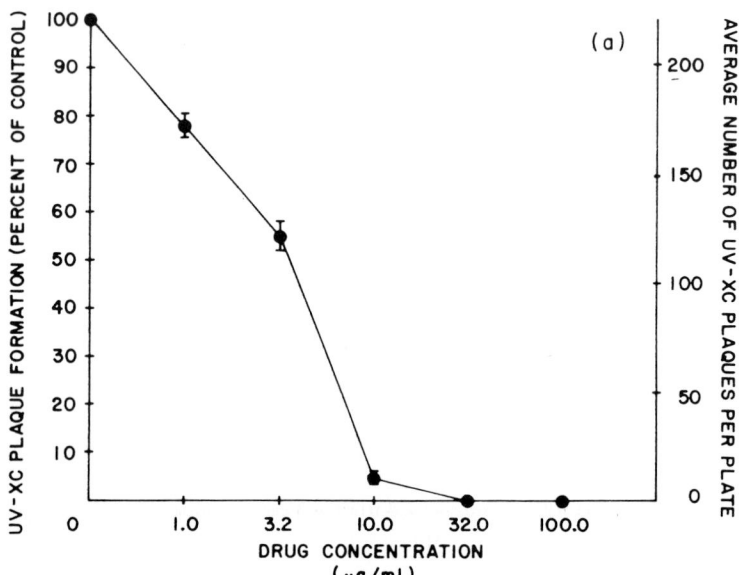

Fig. 7. (a) Effect of 1-β-D-ribofuranosyl-1,2,4-triazole-3-carboxamide (virazole; ribavirin; NSC 163039) on Gross MLV replication in Swiss mouse embryo cells. (b) Effect of virazole (ribavirin) treatment on host cell multicplication.

PAA concentration versus the fraction of the araA concentration that gives ≧90% inhibition of MLV replication in vitro, one obtains an isobologram which clearly indicates a synergistic effect with these two compounds (Fig. 10). Many antiviral chemotherapists have become quite aware of the possibilities of putting drugs together in combination. I think that the great progress that has been made in anticancer chemotherapy, using combinations of drugs, could also be achieved in the antiviral chemotherapy area through combination drug treatment.

Besides araA, cyclaradine and ribavirin, a number of other classes of compounds have been examined for antiretrovirus activity. A large number of rifamycin SV compounds were looked at in the early 1970s. Hundreds of these were examined for activity in

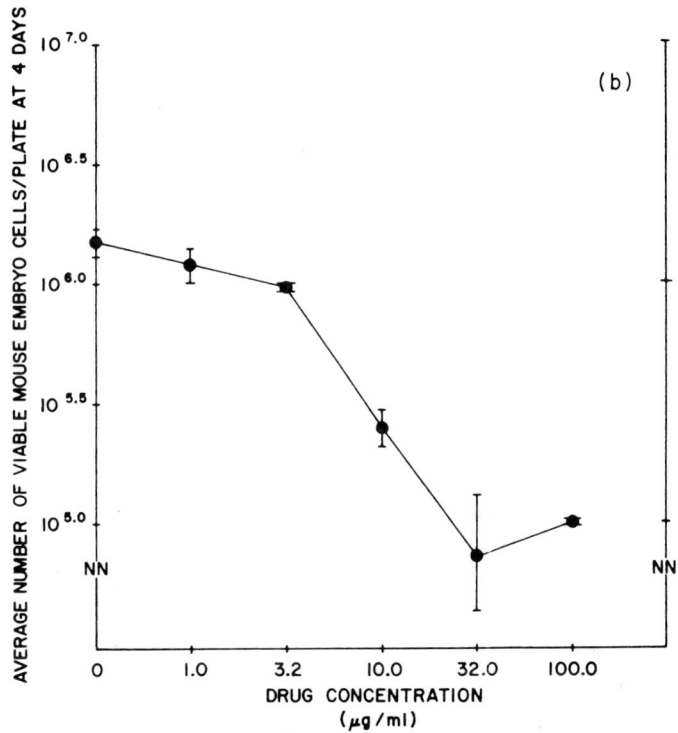

Fig. 7b.

vitro, but none of them really showed much activity in infected
animals. Many of them were potent inhibitors of reverse transcriptase in cell-free enzyme systems, but most of these compounds
had difficulty penetrating cells. Those that did show activity
in intact cells in vitro were too toxic for possible use (16,17).
The same situation held with 3-deazauridine. This was an active
compound in vitro, but had no useful activity in vivo (16,17).
The other candidate antiviral compound which was of interest in
those years was pyrazofurin, previously named pyrazomycin (Fig.
11). This is a C-nucleoside antibiotic which was produced at Eli
Lilly Company and which was examined as an anticancer agent for
awhile in multiple-drug regimens. This compound, which has

TABLE III. Effect of Virazole (Ribavirin; NSC 163039) on Rauscher MLV-Induced Splenomegaly in Swiss Mice

Drug dose[a] (mg/kg/day)	Toxicity control mortality (dead/total)	Average spleen weight on day 21 (g)	Inhibition of splenomegaly[b] (%)	Significance (P)[c]
0 (uninfected controls)	0/10	0.163	—	—
0 (virus-infected controls)	0/20	0.746	—	—
9.4	0/10	0.573	30	>0.05
18.8	0/10	0.661	15	>0.05
37.5	0/10	0.515	40	>0.05
75.0	2/10	0.427	55	<0.05

[a] Drug was administered i.p. once daily for 14 days beginning 4 hours after virus inoculation.

[b] The percentage of inhibition of splenomegaly was calculated as follows:

$$1 - \frac{\text{Net spleen weight increase in the presence of drug}}{\text{Net spleen weight increase in the absence of drug}} \times 100$$

[c] P = probability (t test) that reduction in splenomegaly was due to chance.

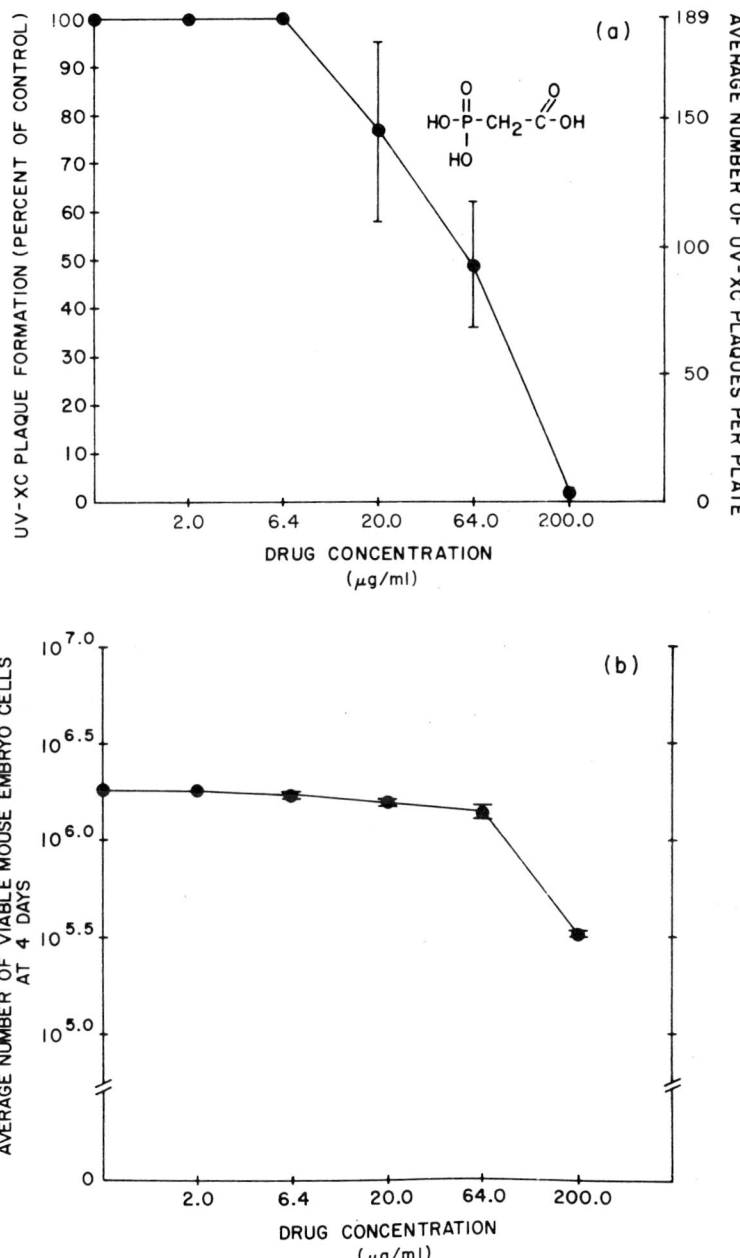

Fig. 8.   Effect of PAA (a) on the replication of Gross MLV
in Swiss mouse embryo cells and (b) on host cell multiplication.

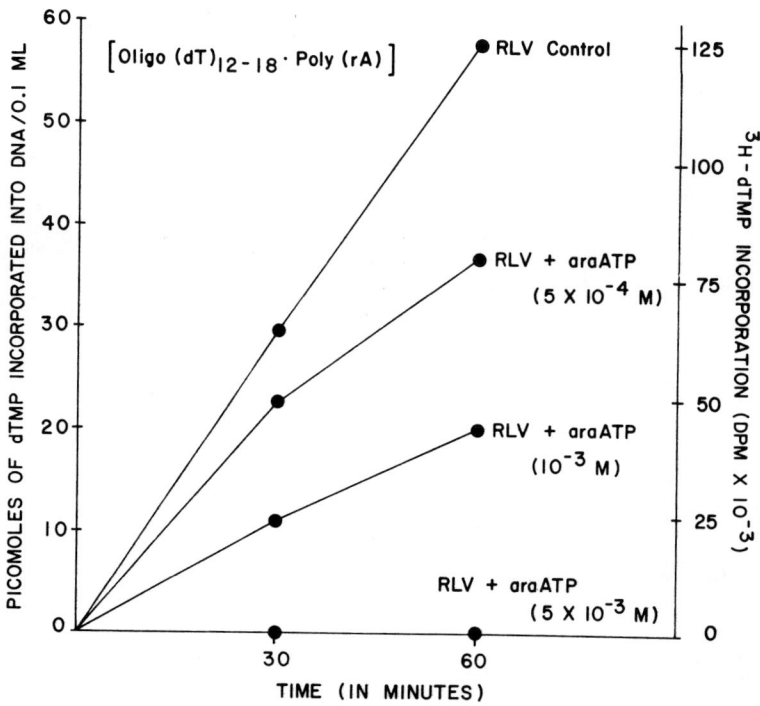

Fig. 9.   Inhibition of Rauscher MLV reverse transcriptase activity by araATP.

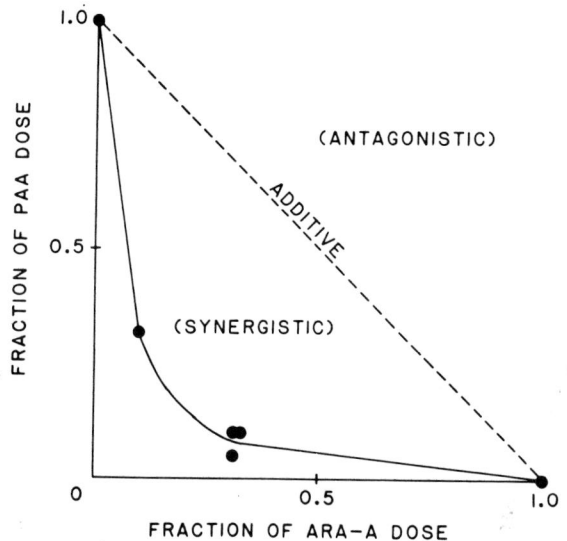

Fig. 10. Isobologram for ≥90% inhibition of Gross MLV replication in Swiss mouse embryo cells by araA, PAA and the combination of araA + PAA.

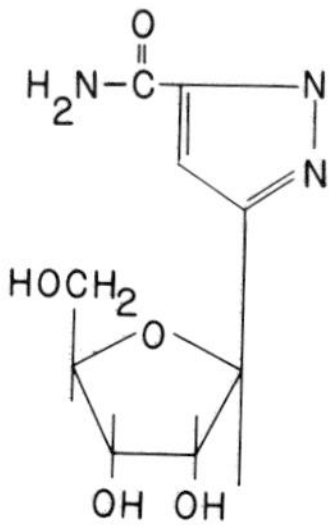

Fig. 11. Chemical structure of pyrazofurin (pyrazomycin).

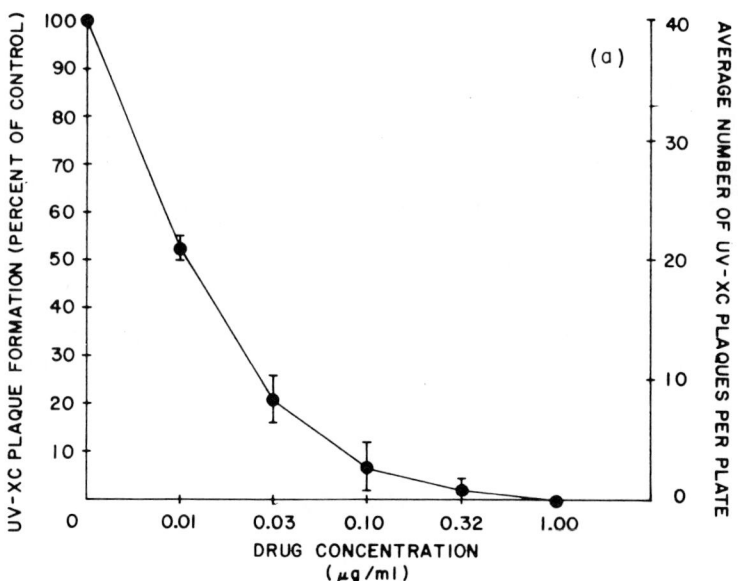

Fig. 12.   (a) Inhibition of Gross MLV replication in Swiss
mouse embryo cells by pyrazofurin (pyrazomycin; NSC 143095).
(b) Effect of pyrazofurin (pyrazomycin) treatment on host cell
multiplication.

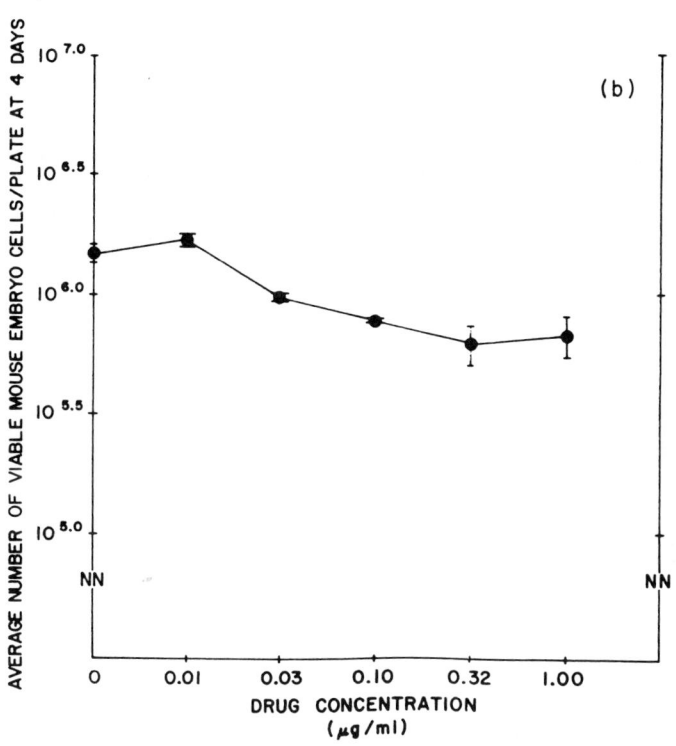

Fig. 12b.

TABLE IV. Inhibitory Effect of Pyrazofurin (Pyrazomycin; NSC 143095) on Rauscher MLV-Induced Splenomegaly in Swiss Mice

Drug dose[a] (mg/kg/day)	Toxicity control mortality (dead/total)	Average spleen weight on day 21 (g)	Inhibition of splenomegaly[b] (%)	Significance (P)[c]
0 (uninfected controls)	1/10	0.173	—	—
0 (virus-infected controls)	0/20	0.799	—	—
1.25	1/10	0.507	46.6	<0.01
2.5	1/10	0.221	92.3	<0.001
5.0	5/10	0.119	100.0	<0.001

[a] Drug was administered to mice i.p., on an every 3 day × 7 schedule, beginning 4 hours after virus inoculation.

[b] The percentage of inhibition of splenomegaly was calculated as follows:

$$1 - \frac{\text{Net spleen weight increase in the presence of drug}}{\text{Net spleen weight increase in the absence of drug}} \times 100$$

[c] P = probability (t test) that reduction in splenomegaly was due to chance.

broad-spectrum antiviral activity (17), is also significantly active against Gross MLV replication in cell culture at noncytotoxic concentrations (Fig. 12) (16). One should note the very low MIC_{50} of 0.01 µg/ml which indicates that pyrazofurin is an extremely potent inhibitor of MLV replication. Treatment of Rauscher virus-infected mice with pyrazofurin at dose levels as low as 2.5 mg/kg/day, on a q3d $\times$ 7 schedule for 21 days, resulted in significant inhibition of splenomegaly in these animals (16) (Table IV). This compound should also be tested for activity against AIDS-related retroviruses.

The "take-home message" here really is that there are a number of candidate antiviral compounds that have shown significant activity against other retroviruses and that could be evaluated in the various animal models as described above. Some of these compounds could have clinically useful activity against human AIDS-related retroviruses and I think this possibility certainly demands further investigation.

REFERENCES

1. Galasso, G.J., Merigan, T.C. and Buchanan, R.A. (1984). "Antiviral Agents and Viral Diseases of Man," 2nd ed. Raven Press, New York.
2. Bauer, D.J. (1977). "The Specific Treatment of Virus Diseases." University Park Press, Baltimore.
3. Coster, D.J., Jones, B.R. and McGill, J.I. (1979). Br. J. Ophthalmol. 63, 418.
4. Prusoff, W.H., Chen, M.S., Fischer, P.H. et al. (1979). Pharmacol. Ther. 7, 1.
5. Heidelberger, C. and King, D. (1979). Pharmacol. Ther. 6, 427.
6. Fox, J.J., Lopez, C. and Watanabe, K.A. (1981). In "Medicinal Chemistry Advances" (F.G. De Las Heras and S. Vega, eds.), p. 27. Pergamon Press, Oxford.
7. Elion, G.B. (1982). In "Acyclovir Symposium" (D.H. King and G.J. Galasso, eds.). Am. J. Med. 71(1A), 7.
8. Meyers, J.D., Wade, J.C., Mitchell, C.D. et al. (1982). In "Acyclovir Symposium" (D.H. King and G.J. Galasso, eds.). Am. J. Med. 73(1A), 229.

9. Bryson, Y.J., Dillon, M., Lovett, M. et al. (1983). N. Engl. J. Med. 308, 916.
10. Pavan-Langston, D., Buchanan, R.A. and Alford, C.A., Jr. (1975). "Adenine Arabinoside: An Antiviral Agent." Raven Press, New York.
11. Whitley, R.J., Soong, S.-J., Dolin, R. et al. (1977). N. Engl. J. Med. 297, 289.
12. Whitley, R.J., Nahmias, A.J., Soong, S.-J. et al. (1980). Pediatrics 66, 495.
13. Whitley, R.J., Soong, S.-J., Dolin, R. et al. (1982). N. Engl. J. Med. 307, 971.
14. Sohabel, F.M., Jr. (1968). Chemotherapy 13, 321.
15. Shannon, W.M., Westbrook, L. and Schabel, F.M., Jr. (1974). Proc. Soc. Exp. Biol. Med. 145, 542.
16. Shannon, W.M. (1977). Ann. NY Acad. Sci. 284, 472.
17. Shannon, W.M. and Schabel, F.M., Jr. (1980). Pharmacol. Ther. 11, 263.
18. Shannon, W.M. (1984). In "Antiviral Agents and Viral Diseases of Man" (G.J. Galasso, T.C. Merigan and R.A. Buchanan, eds.), 2nd ed. Raven Press, New York.
19. Rowe, W.P., Pugh, W.E. and Hartley, J. (1970). Virology 42, 1136.
20. Vince, R. and Daluge, S. (1977). J. Med. Chem. 20, 612.
21. Vince, R., Daluge, S., Lee, H. et al. (1983). Science 221, 1405.
22. Shealy, Y.F., O'Dell, C.A., Shannon, W.M. et al. (1983). J. Med. Chem. 26, 156.
23. Sidwell, R.W., Robins, R.K. and Hillyard, I.W. (1979). Pharmacol. Ther. 6, 123.

THE SEROEPIDEMIOLOGY OF HUMAN AIDS

Luc Montagnier

Viral Oncology Unit
Institut Pasteur
Paris, France

The discovery of the retrovirus considered as the causative agent of AIDS has made it possible to detect specific humoral responses against viral antigens and therefore to begin the seroepidemiology of viral infection.

The virus was first named by us lymphadenopathy-associated virus (LAV), since it was isolated from a patient with lymphadenopathy and is known also as T leukemia or lymphotropic virus) type III (HTLV-III) or AIDS-related virus (ARV) (review 1 and 2).

VIRAL ANTIGENS

The main structural proteins of LAV are all antigenic. Upon metabolic labeling of the virus with $[^{35}S]$cysteine, three main proteins can be detected upon sodium dodecyl sulfate-polyacrylamide gel electrophoresis (SDS-PAGE) with respective molecular weights (MW) of 25,000, 18,000 and 13,000. These proteins are associated with the core (nucleoid) of the virus.

In the higher molecular weight zone, it was more difficult to detect viral proteins, including the hypothetic viral glycoproteins, since some cellular proteins such as actins seem to be tightly associated with purified viruses.

The viral glycoprotein could be clearly detected only after immunoprecipitation with patients' sera of [^{35}S]cysteine-labeled virus: its MW is around 110,000 daltons. Its glycosylation was shown by labeling with [^{14}C]glucosamine, binding to lectins (concanavalin A, lentyl-lectin) and reduction of its apparent MW to 80,000 after endoglycosydase H treatment.

Its viral nature was demonstrated by its association with purified virions banded in sucrose gradients. This protein is highly antigenic and is precipitated by most, if not all, AIDS and "pre-AIDS" patients' sera. When the immunoblotting (Western) technique is used, besides the 110 Kgp, three lower MW proteins are recognized by patients' sera, with MW of 68, 41 and 34 Kd, respectively. They are presumably fragments of the gp110 (3).

We have analyzed viral proteins labeled with [^{35}S]methionine by two-dimensional gel analysis. The typical p25 protein gives two spots recognized by the antibodies from the patients. There is also a protein in the range of 43 K. This protein comigrates with actin.

WHAT IS THE RELATIONSHIP OF LAV TO OTHER RETROVIRUSES?

Proteins of LAV and HTLV-III were compared. Three proteins, p13, p18 and p25, have the same size. Also, by immunoprecipitation, HTLV-III was found to have the gp110 protein. Using uninfected T cells, these proteins are not found, although there are a number of cellular proteins in the range 40 to 50 Kd. In two-dimensional gel electrophoresis, p25 proteins of LAV and HTLV-III migrate at the same isoelectric point. Their antigenicities are the same as determined by immunoprecipitation with a panel of patient sera.

We have recently cloned LAV1 virus proviral DNA. The viral DNA is about 9.2 Kb. The restriction map analysis shows some microheterogeneity; from this particular viral isolate, two clones were obtained, differing by one HindIII restriction site, which was missing in one clone. This clone, J19, has a map which is similar to the map obtained from HTLV-III (4).

Clearly, the two viruses are nearly identical if not exactly the same. All of the other isolates are related to the first isolate. We have now made more than 31 isolates at the Pasteur Institut from AIDS and pre-AIDS patients. There were also two isolates made from two healthy carriers.

All of the isolates are identical in proteins, antigenicity and morphology in electron microscopy; they may differ in more subtle ways which might appear when they will be cloned.

We have also compared LAV with other animal retroviruses. By immunoprecipitation, some crossreactivity was seen with the equine infectious anemia virus (EIAV). Sera from horses infected with EIAV could immunoprecipitate the p25 protein of LAV. However, the reverse is not true; serum from patients do not immuno-precipitate the p26 protein of EIAV (5). In order to explain this difference, we assume that there is only one or a few common epitopes shared by the two viruses and that the horse sera but none of the human sera recognize these epitopes. Using molecular probes, we could not find hybridization with the RNA of EIAV. The homology is probably small between LAV and EIAV. However, they are similar in two aspects, morphology and antigenic sites.

We also compared LAV with the two other known human retro-viruses, HTLV-I and HTLV-II. This work was done in collaboration with V.S. Kalyanaraman and D. Francis at the Centers for Disease Control (CDC). p24 from HTLV-I or HTLV-II was labeled with I^{125} and used in competition immunoprecipitation studies. There was no competition between LAV, EIAV and other virus core proteins using these labeled probes. Conversely, several LAV isolates could all immune compete with LAV1 p25 protein (6). In summary, there is no detectable crossreactivity between LAV and either HTLV-I or

HTLV-II core major proteins. This also holds true for other viral proteins, such as p18 and gp110.

Two-dimensional gel electrophoresis comparisons of the p25 protein of LAV and the p24 protein of HTLV-I show very different isoelectric points. The pI for LAV p25 is in the range of 6.5 to 6.7. HTLV-I p24 gives several spots around pH 7 (Krust, B., personal communication).

All of the human retroviruses have a Mg^{++}-dependent reverse transcriptase, but this is also found in a number of animal retroviruses. The tropism of the human retroviruses is mostly directed at T4 cells, but the molecular bases for these tropisms may not be the same in each case. The tropism of HTLV-I and HTLV-II seems to be based on some regulatory sequences of the long terminal repeat or in the PX protein region. In the case of LAV, the tropism seems to be controlled, at least partly, by the binding of the viral glycoprotein to the T4 molecule itself. Recently we have shown in collaboration with D. Klatzmann and J.C. Gluckman that, using monoclonal antibodies to the T4 molecule, virus infection could be prevented. Other monoclonal antibodies directed to other surface markers on T cells cannot prevent infection. These results suggest that the T4 molecule is at least a part of the receptor for LAV on the surface of T4 cells (7).

We were able to show the strict tropism of LAV to T4 cells by using cells from the healthy brother of an AIDS patient, both of whom were hemophiliacs. LAV could be released only from the T4 fraction of cells and not from the T8 fraction. The T4 marker on these cells was less exposed during virus production (8). Perhaps the binding of LAV glycoprotein to the T4 molecule impairs binding of the monoclonal antibodies to the latter.

The tropism is not very strict in that the virus could also be adapted to growth on B cell lines transformed by Epstein-Barr virus (9). These lines may also express transiently the T4 receptor, thus accounting for the growth on such lines.

The virus is cytopathic for lymphocytes. Electron microscope studies show a number of particles produced by dying cells or giant cells. This is not observed in HTLV-I and HTLV-II cell lines.

Thus there are a number of differences between the two groups of human retroviruses. In morphology, the core is very small and concentric in LAV (or HTLV-III), but very large and similar to C type murine viruses in HTLV-I and HTLV-II. There is either no or unsignificant crossreactivity between the major core proteins. No homology among the nucleic acid components using cloned DNA probes could be detected.

The classification of the human retroviruses in the retroviridae family is still uncertain. There are clearly two groups so far. In the family of retroviridae, LAV may be placed as the EIAV, in the lentiviridae subfamily. More definite evidence for this will come from the sequences of structural proteins and from the sequence of DNAs.

The last part of this chapter will deal with serological studies in several high risk groups. Because AIDS is a life-threatening disease, it is important that the tests give no false positive or false negative results. Since viral antigens are always contaminated with cellular proteins, we must have two types of controls, sera of noninfected individuals and cells not infected by the virus which may be producing cellular proteins recognizable by the patients' sera. We have studied sera from AIDS and pre-AIDS patients and from blood donors. It is known in the case of the AIDS patients that their sera are by no means normal. Such sera are hypergammaglobulinemic (IgG). They contain immune complexes and often have antibody against cellular proteins from T lymphocytes. Of course, the situation in healthy blood donors is not as complex.

TABLE I. Tests for Detection of Anti-LAV Antibodies

Principle	Protein denaturation	Antigens recognized
ELISA	Yes or no	gp110, p25, p18
RIPA	No	gp110, p25, p18, p68, p34 (p55, p40)
IFA	No	gp110
Immunoblotting (Western)	Yes	p25, p18, p68, p34 (gp110), gp41 (p55, p40)

In Table I is a list of the main tests which can be used to detect LAV antibodies. There are two types of tests, those which use native proteins and those which use denatured proteins. Whatever the technique used, purification of the virus is critical and should respect the integrity of the glycoprotein, which can be easily detached from the virion. He can also use acetone-fixed cells infected with LAV and detect viral antigens by immunofluorescence. This test shows a good correlation with the other tests and seems to detect mostly the glycoprotein. Radioimmunoprecipitation detects the p25 protein when labeling is done with [35S]methionine. Using [35S]cysteine, all four of the major proteins are detected. This is the most sensitive and specific test available so far. The Western blot technique is also highly sensitive, recognizing the major core proteins. Often, it does not measure the intact gp because this glycoprotein is not transferred well onto the papers. Three proteins of 34, 41 and 68 Kd can be detected well by this technique. They probably represent fragments of the glycoprotein.

Some of these tests are only laboratory tests while others can be used on a large scale. We have been using an enzyme-

linked immunosorbent assay (ELISA) test in studies done in collaboration with Drs. F. Brun-Vézinet and C. Rouzioux (10,11). The
control for nonspecific binding consists of wells coated with a
crude cytoplasmic lysate from uninfected lymphocytes of the same
donor. Sera are considered as positive when binding to viral
antigens over that to cellular antigens leads to a difference in
optical density higher than 0.3.

RESULTS

We first studied a group of French AIDS and pre-AIDS patients
from whom we have isolated virus similar to LAV. They all had
antibodies against the p25 viral protein and were positive by
ELISA except one case, in which the results were negative. In
this case, it was found that this patient's serum was positive
against the p18 protein and the glycoprotein. In no case were
antibodies against HTLV-I p24. In France, HTLV infection is very
rare, so we could not easily be confused by the HTLV problem.

An interesting observation was made of the two hemophiliac
brothers. One developed AIDS in the beginning of 1983. His
brother is still completely healthy. We could isolate the virus
from their lymphocytes. The healthy carrier did not have any
immune depression and had a higher titer of antibody. A drop of
antibody titer was noted at the onset of AIDS in his brother. We
could find antibodies against the p25 protein in 50 to 94% of the
AIDS patients depending on their groups. For instance, we found
a very high incidence in the African patients from Zaire and a
lower incidence in French patients. The American patients are
between these two groups. In 75% of the pre-AIDS (lymphadenopathy) patients, we could also find antibodies against p25. By
using the cysteine-labeled virus, we could find antibodies in
nearly 100% of the cases. Only a very young infant which could

not mount an immune response was found to be negative by this test.

The situation for the AIDS virus is not very different from what is seen in animal retroviral infections, where antibodies against the envelope protein are generally present. LAV anti-gp antibodies probably reflect recent expression of virus, with or without lysis of the infected cells. If there is cell and virus lysis, then the host can mount an immune response against the internal core proteins.

Results obtained in France and in the New York area show a high incidence of seropositivity in AIDS and pre-AIDS patients. A lower, but still high, percentage were positive in the asymptomatic homosexual groups.

We have conducted similar studies in Zaire in collaboration with our colleagues of CDC, NIH and members of the Institute for Tropical Diseases in Antwerp in groups of hospitalized patients diagnosed with AIDS in October, 1983 (11). By two tests, these patients showed a high incidence of antibodies: 94% by radioimmunoprecipitation assay (RIPA), 89% by ELISA. This study also gave us some information about the distribution of the virus in the general population. Our first control group included patients in the same two hospitals of Kinshasa having infectious or noninfectious diseases, different from AIDS. Surprisingly, 23% were positive in this control group. Analyzed in more detail, this group showed an interesting correlation between seropositivity and low T4:T8 ratios. Sixty-two percent of the group (5/8) with a T4:T8 ratio less than 0.7 were positive. Fifty percent had less than 400 T4 cells/mm3. Only 1/18 (5%) was positive in a group in which the ratio was higher than 0.7. Thus, perhaps in relation to LAV infection, this group had some immunodepression and diseases other than those fitting the CDC criteria for AIDS.

In a group of noninfectious patients of another Kinshasa hospital, 7% were positive. In a group of young healthy mothers,

whose serum was collected in 1980, 5% were positive. So the background incidence of seropositivity against LAV is higher in Zaire
than in the United States or in France. In France, out of 330
blood donors and laboratory workers, only one was found to be
positive for LAV antibodies by the ELISA test.

Blood taken in 1977 from a Zairian woman was also positive.
She died in 1978 from what was considered retrospectively to be
AIDS. These results suggest that the virus was present in Africa
at that time and that the epidemic may have begun earlier in
Zaire than in the United States or in France.

We have also looked for antibodies in sera of patients with
classical Kaposi's sarcoma (KS). This study was done in collaboration with Dr. Papaevangelo in Greece (12). Of 10 cases, not one
was positive for LAV antibodies. This suggested that classical
KS, which is a slowly developing disease, is not related to LAV
infection.

Another high risk group is that of hemophiliacs. We asked
whether LAV positivity correlated with the way in which they
were treated for hemophilia. Three groups were studied. One was
a group of French hemophiliacs heavily treated with commercial
factor VIII and IX preparations. Fifty percent of this group were
positive for LAV antibodies by ELISA analysis. The second group
included French patients treated occasionally with factor VIII or
IX. Only 10% were positive. The third group were Belgian hemophiliacs treated with local preparations of cryoprecipitates of
factor VIII. Only 3.4% were positive (13). These results show
that the antigens came from commercial preparations made from a
pool of plasma prepared from sera contributed by donors including
high risk donors.

These results do not tell whether positive individuals had
been infected with the virus. One could assume as well that they
had mounted immune responses against inactivated viral proteins.
This is, however, unlikely. Active infection of chimpanzees with

LAV results in a rapid seroconversion. In rhesus monkeys, which
appear to be nonpermissive to the virus, there was no antibody
response after inoculation of the virus. So it is possible that
all of the seropositive individuals have had live virus infections, an unknown fraction of which will come down later with
AIDS.

We have followed up the antibody response in some patients.
In the case of the two hemophiliac brothers, the brother with
AIDS was already seropositive by June, 1981, or perhaps even
before. As previously mentioned, his antibody titer dropped at
the time of onset of the disease. We have seen this phenomenon
in several other patients. Now this patient is completely seronegative by ELISA but is positive by the glycoprotein test. His
healthy brother still has a high titer of antibodies. There may,
therefore, be a drop in antibodies with disease onset, although
this is not a general phenomenon since some AIDS patients continue to show a high titer of antibodies. The parents were seronegative, suggesting that transmission had not occurred in this
family from the parents to the children, but probably by the
preparations of factor IX.

Figure 1 shows the SDS-PAGE of immunoprecipitation from
patients' sera using [^{35}S]cysteine-labeled virus. Serum from a
young woman with Pneumocystis carinii (PCP) infection in 1984
taken 8 days before she died showed only weak antibodies to the
glycoprotein and the p25 protein. This case is interesting
because we had serum from this patient taken the previous year.
At that time the serum was highly positive for p25 antibodies.
This suggests that not only the titer but also the specificity of
the antibodies may vary as disease develops. Virus could not be
isolated from her blood. Her husband's serum was completely negative. One healthy homosexual had antibodies against all of the
viral proteins. Virus could be isolated from his blood. There may
be some correlation between the type of antibody produced and

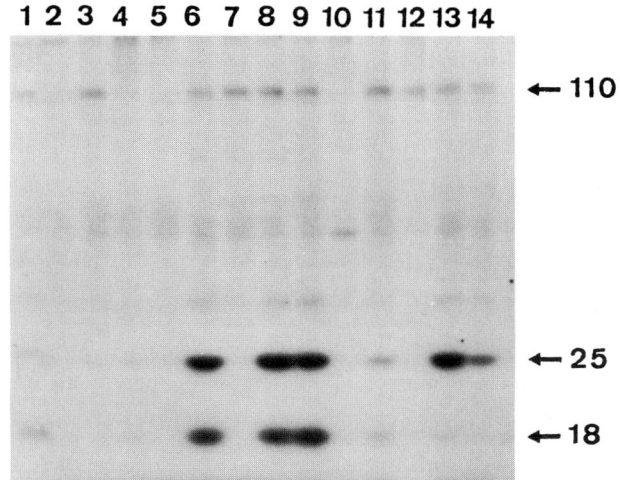

Fig. 1. SDS-PAGE of immunoprecipitates of [^{35}S]cysteine-labeled viral lysate immunoprecipitated with different sera. Lanes 1 and 3: adult AIDS patients. Lane 6: 18-month-old-girl, AIDS. Lane 7: father. Lane 8: mother of patient in lane 6, both healthy. Lane 9: lymphadenopathy syndrome. Lanes 2, 4 and 5: healthy donors. Lanes 10 to 14: AIDS patient, bone marrow grafted. Lane 10: 7 days before graft. Lane 11: 15 days after graft. Lane 13: 7 months later. Lane 14: 24 months later (onset of AIDS). (Reproduced from Montagnier et al. (1985). Virology 144, 283, by permission of Academic Press.)

viremia. An 18-month-old girl with AIDS is highly positive for all types of antibodies. Her mother is also highly positive for all antibodies, whereas her father is positive only for the glycoprotein. A virus could be isolated from the girl and is under characterization. Lanes 10 to 14 analyze sera from a patient who received a bone marrow graft in 1982. Serum taken before grafting was negative but serum taken 5 days after the graft was positive. Probably the patient received the virus from the graft donor or from the accompanying transfusions. Two months later the patient became negative again. Seven months later he showed an immune response against p25. Now he is negative against the p25 protein but still retains the antibodies to the glycoprotein. This study shows again some fluctuation of the antibody response. The finding of seropositive individuals in France who do not belong to the classical high risk groups can mean one of two things. It may indicate that the virus is now spreading in the general population as we have seen in Zaire. It is also possible that in these groups the virus was present before the AIDS epidemic and that there are two phases in the AIDS virus history. First, there were sporadic cases of LAV-induced AIDS. Then, when the virus entered the susceptible homosexual population, it changed its mode of transmission and its pathogenicity. We are investigating the possibility that the virus was associated with other types of diseases that have existed before AIDS.

From our data, four situations are found in which antibodies can be detected against this virus. The first is that of healthy, asymptomatic carriers. These constitute a problem because such individuals can donate blood and propagate the virus by sexual contacts. The second is that of individuals in whom immune depression can be measured but in whom there are no clinical signs of disease. The third is found in patients diagnosed with lymphadenopathy syndrome or AIDS-related complex. A minor proportion (10%?), however, can later develop full-blown AIDS. The fourth is that of patients with full-blown AIDS, having KS, opportunistic infections or both.

It is unknown why some individuals develop disease while others have only the benign form. This is a general problem in viral diseases. It is of prime importance to understand why some develop AIDS and how to prevent it.

ACKNOWLEDGMENTS

The author wishes to thank his colleagues of the Pasteur Institute who have participated in the described work and also Drs. Brun-Vézinet, Rouzioux, Gluckman, Klatzmann, Rozenbaum and

Brunet, whose collaboration was also essential in the discovery and characterization of LAV.

REFERENCES

1. Montagnier, L. et al. (1984). In "Human T Cell Leukemia Lymphoma Viruses" (R C. Gallo, M.E. Essex and L. Gross, eds.), p. 363, vol. 1. Cold Spring Harbor Laboratory, Cold Spring Harbor, New York.
2. Montagnier, L. et al. (1985). In "Retroviruses in Human Lymphoma/leukemia" (M. Miwa et al., eds.). Sci. Soc. Press, Tokyo/VNU Science Press, Utrecht, Japan. In press.
3. Montagnier, L. et al. (1985). Virology 144, 283.
4. Alizon, M., Sonigo, P., Barré-Sinoussi, F. et al. (1984). Nature (London) 312, 757.
5. Montagnier, L. et al. (1984). Ann. Virol. (Inst. Pasteur) 135E, 119.
6. Kalyanaraman, V.S., Cabradille, C.D., Getchell, J.P. et al. (1984). Science 225, 321.
7. Klatzmann, D., Champagne, E., Chamaret, S. et al. (1984). Nature (London) 312, 763.
8. Klatzmann, D., Barré-Sinoussi, F., Nugeyre, M.T. et al. (1984). Science 225, 59.
9. Montagnier, L., Gruest, J., Chamaret, S. et al. (1984). Science 225, 63.
10. Brun-Vézinet, F., Rouzioux, C., Barré-Sinoussi, F. et al. (1984). Lancet 1, 1253.
11. Brun-Vézinet, F. et al. (1984). Science 220, 859.
12. Papaevangelou, G., Economidou, J., Kallinikos, J. et al. (1984). Lancet 2, 642.
13. Rouzioux, C., Brun-Vézinet, F., Courouce, A.M. et al. (1985). Ann. Intern. Med. 102, 476.

IMMUNOSUPPRESSION INDUCED BY THE FRIEND MURINE LEUKEMIA VIRUS COMPLEX IN MICE WITH THE Rfv-3$^{r/s}$ GENOTYPE

Richard P. Morrison
Jane Nishio
Bruce Chesebro

Laboratory of Persistent Viral Diseases
Rocky Mountain Laboratories
National Institute of Allergy and Infectious Diseases
National Institutes of Health
Hamilton, Montana

Infection by oncogenic retroviruses is frequently associated with immunosuppression (1). In the case of the erytholeukemia-inducing Friend murine leukemia virus complex (FV), suppression of functions of B lymphocytes, T lymphocytes and macrophages have been observed in infected and leukemia mice (2-5). However, some mouse strains develop a strong anti-FV humoral immune response during the course of active FV infection (6). This response is controlled in part by a single non-H-2 gene, designated Rfv-3. Anti-FV antibody made in mice with the Rfv-3$^{r/s}$ genotype, such as (B10.A × A)F$_1$, was found to eliminate established viremia and to reduce levels of virus-releasing cells in the spleen by 10,000-fold, in spite of the continued presence of leukemic splenomegaly (7). Because of the unusual coexistence of a significant antiviral immune response and progressive leukemia in (B10.A × A)F$_1$ mice, we decided to test these mice for their ability to respond immunologically to nonviral antigens during the course of FV leukemia. BALB/c mice were used as controls because of their known susceptibility to FV-induced

immunosuppression (2) and their lack of a humoral immune response
to FV during active infection (7).

Mice were inoculated with sheep red blood cells (SRBC) 18 or
21 days after FV infection. Spleens were analyzed for plaque-
forming cells (PFC) 7 or 4 days later, respectively, so that all
mice were tested 25 days after inoculation. Control groups were
given SRBC but were not infected with FV. The results indicated
that splenic anti-SRBC PFC responses were suppressed during FV
infection in both Rfv-3$^{r/s}$ and Rfv-3$^{s/s}$ mouse strains (Table I).
The suppression of IgG PFC at day 7 was more extensive (3.95-
4.28 $\log_{10}$) than suppression of IgM PFC at day 4 (2.4 $\log_{10}$) or
at day 7 (1.2-1.6 $\log_{10}$). The IgM PFC response in infected
(B10.A × A)F$_1$ mice was actually higher on day 7 than on day 4; in
contrast the IgM PFC in uninfected mice always decreased significantly between days 4 and 7. This suggested that in FV-infected
(B10.A × A)F$_1$ mice the IgM anti-SRBC response might have been
delayed kinetically, rather than simply suppressed in magnitude.

Since infection with FV induced rapid splenomegaly, it was
possible that the decreases in spleen PFC responses observed
were the result of some local splenic alterations, rather than
systemic immunosuppression. Therefore, plasma from mice infected
and immunized as before was tested for anti-SRBC antibodies. The
data indicated that both 4 and 7 days after SRBC immunization
agglutination titers were decreased in FV-infected mice of both
Rfv-3 genotypes (Table II). Additional experiments using plasma
treated with 2-mercaptoethanol indicated that in infected mice
most antibodies at both 4 and 7 days were of the IgM class,
whereas uninfected mice had mostly IgG by day 7 (data not shown).
Thus the plasma data agreed entirely with data from splenic PFC
and indicated that the suppression observed was indeed systemic
rather than local.

From the above results it was not possible to conclude which
cells in the immune system were affected by FC infection. Both

TABLE I. Suppression of Direct and Indirect Anti-SRBC PFC Response 25 days after FV Inoculation in Mice with the $Rfv\text{-}3^{r/s}$ or $Rfv\text{-}3^{s/s}$ Genotype

Mouse strain	Rfv-3 genotype	FV infected	$\log_{10}$ PFC/spleen		
			4 Days	7 Days	
			Direct	Direct	Indirect-direct
(B10.A × A)F$_1$	r/s	−	4.94 ± 0.04	4.01 ± 0.13	4.87 ± 0.08
(B10.A × A)F$_1$	r/s	+	2.48 ± 0.07	2.84 ± 0.14	0.92 ± 0.45
BALB/c	s/s	−	5.04 ± 0.03	4.31 ± 0.06	4.51 ± 0.11
BALB/c	s/s	+	2.68 ± 0.10	2.71 ± 0.14	0.23 ± 0.23

Mice were infected by inoculation intravenously with 1000 spleen focus-forming units of FV complex on day 0. All mice were immunized on either day 18 or 21 by intraperitoneal inoculation of 0.25 ml of a 10% suspension of washed sheep erythrocytes, and spleens were removed 4 or 7 days later (25 days after FV inoculation) for titration of PFC responses. P values for t test comparison of infected vs. uninfected mice were <0.001 in all cases. There were nine or 10 mice in each experimental group.

TABLE II. Suppression of Plasma Anti-SRBC Titer
25 days After FV Inoculation in Mice
with the Rfv-3$^{r/s}$ or Rfv-3$^{s/s}$ Genotypes

Mouse strain	Rfv-3 genotype	FV infected	Log$_{10}$ anti-SRBC titer	
			4 Days	7 Days
(B10.A × A)F$_1$	r/s	−	9.40 ± 0.16	13.8 ± 0.13
(B10.A × A)F$_1$	r/s	+	6.40 ± 0.37	9.0 ± 0.38
BALB/c	s/s	−	10.9 ± 0.23	14.6 ± 0.31
BALB/c	s/s	+	6.63 ± 0.18	10.5 ± 0.75

Mice were infected with FV complex and immunized with sheep erythrocytes as in Table I. There were eight to 10 mice per group. Mice were bled 4 or 7 days after SRBC immunization (25 days after FV inoculation). Plasma was tested for hemagglutination of SRBC by mixing 50 μl of two-fold serial plasma dilutions with 25 μl of a 1% SRBC suspension; after 45 minute incubation cells were washed three times and 50 μl of a 1/100 dilution of rabbit antimouse immunoglobulin was added. Agglutination titer was read after 4 hours at 4°C as the reciprocal of the highest dilution giving distinct agglutination.

the IgM and IgG responses to SRBC are T lymphocyte-dependent. Suppressed B lymphocyte, T lymphocyte or accessory cell function could have produced the observed results. Therefore, to test B lymphocytes directly we immunized one group of (B10.A × A)F$_1$ mice with a T lymphocyte-independent antigen, TNP-Ficoll (Biosearch, San Rafael, California). The response to this antigen was reduced but not eliminated during FV infection, similar to the situation with IgM anti-SRBC PFC (Table III). Thus, immunosuppression induced by FV appeared to act at least in part at the level of B lymphocytes. However, the total absence of the SRBC-specific IgG response, compared to the reduced but still present SRBC-specific IgM response, suggested that during FV infection perhaps there was also an alteration in helper T cell function needed for the maturation of the IgG response.

TABLE III. Suppression of PFC Response to TNP-Ficoll
in (B10.A × A)F$_1$ Mice 25 Days After FV Inoculation

Mouse strain	FV infected	Log$_{10}$ PFC/spleen
(B10.A × A)F$_1$	-	4.72 ± 0.12
(B10.A × A)F$_1$	+	2.65 ± 0.18

Mice were FV infected by intravenous inoculation with FV
complex (1000 spleen focus-forming units). Twenty-one days
later mice were immunized intraperitoneally with 10 μg TNP-
Ficoll, and 4 days later spleens were tested for TNP-specific
PFC using TNP-conjugated sheep erythrocytes. There were five
mice in each group.

The mechanism of immunosuppression by FV is unclear. The
Friend helper virus component (F-MuLV) of the FV complex is known
to be capable of infecting and/or inducing leukemias of a variety
of hemopoietic cell types (8). It seems likely that infection of
B or T lymphocytes or macrophages might have diverse immunosuppressive effects. Thus suppression might occur simultaneously at
many levels of the immune system.

It was surprising to discover that Rfv-3$^{r/s}$ and Rfv-3$^{s/s}$ mice
were equally immunosuppressed to SRBC, whereas only Rfv-3$^{r/s}$ mice
could make a significant humoral immune response to FV itself.
The anti-FV response in Rfv-3$^{r/s}$ mice might have been partially
suppressed similar to the IgM anti-SRBC response; however, this
seemed unlikely because the anti-FV titers in these mice were
equal to titers seen in other strains of mice who were not
immunosuppressed to SRBC (data not shown). At present we have no
explanation for these differences in immune response. However,
one possibility might be the fact that the immune response to FV
is initiated early after infection, perhaps before the overwhelming immunosuppression has taken place. It is also possible that
chronic FV infection provides a continuous stimulus to the immune

system which leads to a detectable antibody response in (B10.A ×
A)F$_1$ mice. In contrast, the response to a single immunization
with SRBC may be more sensitive to suppression.

There are several interesting similarities between the status
of FV-infected (B10.A × A)F$_1$ mice and AIDS virus-infected human
patients. In both cases individuals are immunosuppressed, and
surprisingly both have detectable antiviral antibodies. Furthermore, expression of infectious virus is limited, making virus
isolation difficult to achieve. The reason for the coexistence
of immunosuppression and a positive antiviral immune response in
AIDS is paradoxical. Understanding of the mechanisms involved may
be extremely important in attempts to develop effective vaccines
and manipulate parameters of immune protection in these retroviral diseases. FV infection in (B10.A × A)F$_1$ mice appears to be
a useful model for further study of these phenomena.

REFERENCES

1. Dent, P.B. (1972). Prog. Med. Virol. 14, 1.
2. Ceglowski, W.S. and Friedman, H. (1968). J. Immunol. 101,
   594.
3. Ceglowski, W.S. and Friedman, H. (1970). J. Immunol. 105,
   1406.
4. Friedman, H. and Ceglowski, W.S. (1971). J. Immunol. 107,
   1673.
5. Mortensen, R.F., Ceglowski, W.S. and Friedman, H. (1974).
   J. Immunol. 112, 2077.
6. Doig, D. and Chesebro, B. (1979). J. Exp. Med. 150, 10.
7. Chesebro, B., Wehrly, K., Doig, D. et al. (1979). Proc. Natl.
   Acad. Sci. 76, 5784.
8. Chesebro, B., Portis, J., Wehrly, K. et al. (1983). Virology
   128, 221.

RETROVIRUS INDUCTION OF IMMUNODEFICIENCY AND LYMPHOPROLIFERATIVE DISEASE IN MICE

Donald E. Mosier[1]

Institute for Cancer Research
Philadelphia, Pennsylvania

Robert A. Yetter
Herbert C. Morse III

Laboratory of Immunopathology
National Institute of Allergy
and Infectious Diseases
National Institutes of Health
Bethesda, Maryland

This chapter deals with the profound immunosuppressive effects of a complex mouse retrovirus that has been described in this volume by Morse et al. ("Biology of Murine Leukemia Viruses") and Yetter et al. ("Pathogenesis of Murine Retroviral Infections"). The virus mixture is the Dupan-Laterjet isolate of radiation leukemia virus that causes non-T cell lymphomas in adult mice (1). The particular viral isolates that we have been using were made by Martin Haas and are passaged in vitro culture (2). The question I will focus on in this chapter is why this virus mixture is so acutely immunosuppressive in adult mice. I will first describe this disease in more detail and convince you that immunosuppression is involved.

---

[1]Present address: Medical Biology Institute, LaJolla, California.

285

The major feature of the disease in C57BL/6 mice caused
by this mixture of ecotropic and mink cell focus-forming (MCF)
viruses is a rapid, profound lymphoproliferation of T lymphocytes, B lymphocytes and some non-T and non-B lymphoid cells. The
proliferating cell populations are complex. There is rapid polyclonal activation of B cells with enormous increases in secreted
immunoglobulins. There is also rapid induction of immunosuppression, and this affects every possible immune response that the
mouse could make. Dr. Yetter presented the evidence that viral
replication continues, uncontrolled by host immune responses or
by viral immune response genes that might, in theory, control
replication of the virus mixture. Finally, mice die some 4 to
6 months after virus inoculation. In our colony, which is a
specific pathogen-free colony, death is usually caused by massive
lymphadenopathy compromising the upper airways. We have observed
intercurrent infections in the mice, including recurring infections with mouse hepatitis virus. Two mice appeared to die of
Pneumocystis carinii pneumonia.

When adult C57BL/6 mice are inoculated with this virus intraperitoneally, a substantial increase in the size of the spleen
occurs within 1 week. (The observations described here are those
found in spleen but hold as well for lymph node and peripheral
blood.) There is an increase in the total number of B cells during the first 4 weeks and continuing throughout the course of the
disease. The percentage of T cells drops, but the absolute number
of T cells is slightly increased. A lot of these T cells are
blasts, and there is a significant increase in the total number
of both T and B blast cells in the spleen (Table I).

One change observed in the spleens is a large increase in
surface IgM^+ cells. Virus-infected mice have cells bearing the
normal amount of surface IgM, cells which have low intensity IgM
and very few cells with no surface markers. When Patengale et al.
(3) originally described this disease, they claimed that up to

TABLE I. Changes in C57BL/6 Splenic Lymphocyte Populations Induced by LP-BM5 Murine Leukemia Virus

Time post-infection (wk)	Blast cells[a] (× 10^-6)	Proportion of blast cells (%)	Median cell size[b]	T cells (× 10^-6)	Thy-1+ cells (%)	B cells (× 10^-6)	sIg+ cells (%)
1	59 ± 5[c]	29 ± 3	332 ± 7	47 ± 4	23 ± 3	120 ± 10	59 ± 2
2	96 ± 16	36 ± 3	343 ± 9	59 ± 10	22 ± 7	165 ± 28	62 ± 1
3	105 ± 7	39 ± 4	353 ± 12	35 ± 3	13 ± 4	153 ± 11	57 ± 3
4	136 ± 26	41 ± 4	396 ± 6	43 ± 8	13 ± 4	176 ± 34	53 ± 5
Control values	34 ± 3	29 ± 3	325 ± 13	40 ± 4	34 ± 2	62 ± 6	53 ± 5

[a]Blast cell number measured by increase in light-scatter signal on FACS.

[b]Median channel number of light-scatter signal on FACS. Increasing numbers indicate increasing volume of blast cells.

[c]Underlined values are significantly different from controls at p <0.05.

[Reproduced from Mosier, D.E., Yetter, R.A. and Morse, H.C. (1985). J. Exp. Med. 161, 766, by copyright permission of The Rockefeller University Press.]

90% of B cells were involved in the lymphoproliferative process. We find that most of the low density IgM is cytophylic IgM binding to the cells from the serum. The number of B cells found in the lymphoid organs is accordingly less.

There is a rapid increase in serum immunoglobulin levels following the injection of virus into adult mice. At 1 week, levels of IgM, IgG3 and IgG1 are increased. No increase was found in IgA.

One of the advantages of working in the mouse system is that in vitro studies, in vitro reconstitution studies and in vivo studies can be done. We (4) have recently reported such a series of experiments, and they are summarized in Table II. In one in vivo experiment, mice were injected with virus and found to be profoundly immunosuppressed 4 weeks later. The sheep red blood cell (SRBC) response, a T-dependent antibody response, was suppressed. If the spleens from these mice were put into tissue culture, they did not make a response to SRBC. If normal and infected spleen cells were mixed, an intermediate response was obtained, suggesting that there was not an active mechanism of immunosuppression operating in the 4 day culture system.

A number of proliferative responses were measured following virus infection using two mitogens, phytohemagglutinin (PHA) and concanavalin A (con A), which primarily activate T cells, and two others, lipopolysaccharide (LPS) and anti-μ antibodies, which in the mouse activate B cell proliferation (Fig. 1). There was rapid loss of proliferative responsiveness to T cell mitogens, a somewhat slower loss of the proliferative response to LPS and a transient elevation of the response to anti-μ antibodies which then rapidly falls at later points after infection. The phenomenon of transient immunoenhancement is more pronounced in lymph node B cells than in spleen. It lasts for 2 weeks after infection but, thereafter, the response falls off dramatically. Not only are the T cell blastogenic responses to mitogens depressed, T cell

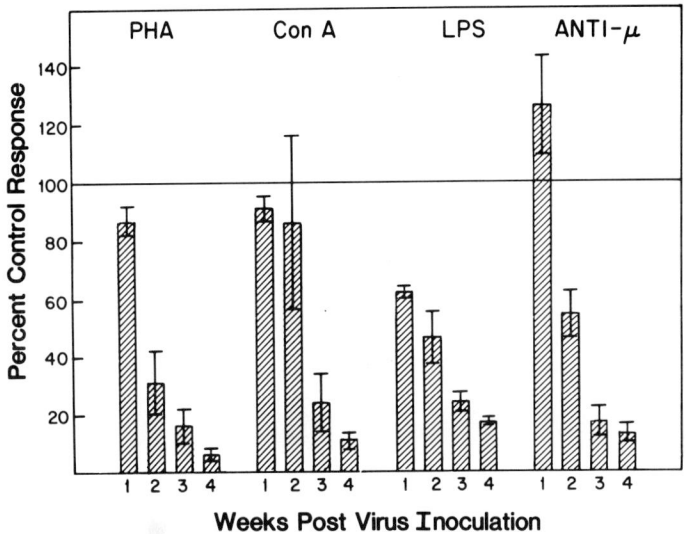

Fig. 1. Proliferative responses of spleen cells from LP-BM5 murine leukemia virus-infected C57BL/6 mice were compared to responses of age- and sex-matched controls at weekly intervals following virus injection. Cells were stimulated with PHA, con A, LPS or goat anti-μ and uptake of [^{3}H]thymidine was determined after 3 days of culture. Data were normalized to the control response for each mitogen for the duration of the experiment. Vertical bars represent the standard error of the mean. [Reproduced from Mosier, D.E., Yetter, R.A. and Morse, H.C. (1985). J. Exp. Med. 161, 766, by copyright permission of The Rockefeller University Press.]

responses to alloantigens in mixed lymphocyte reactions are also depressed. These responses are profoundly and rapidly suppressed with 3 weeks of infection.

Using an in vitro culture system, we examined whether the defect in the antibody response to SRBC is at the level of the T helper cell or the responding B cell. B cells were separated from both virus-infected mice and normal mice. Through mix and match experiments, defects in both T and B cells were found following virus infection. There is a decrease in T helper cells, and a decrease in the ability of B cells from normal mice to

TABLE II. Infection of C57BL/6 Mice with LP-BM5 Murine Leukemia Virus (MuLV) Depresses In Vivo and In Vitro Antibody Responses to SRBC

Mouse cells used	PFC/10^6 cells[a]		PFC/spleen	
	SRBC	IgM	SRBC	IgM
In vivo				
LP-BM5 MuLV-infected C57BL/6 (SRBC-immunized)	<1	672 ± 13	220 ± 49	355,000 ± 21,850
LP-BM5 MuLV-infected C57BL/6 (unimmunized)	<1	795 ± 51	227 ± 58	419,000 ± 10,030
Normal C57BL/6 (SRBC-immunized)	184 ± 35	413 ± 23	35,117 ± 4,606	81,500 ± 9,262

(continued)

TABLE II (continued)

Mouse cells used	SRBC PFC/culture[b]
In vitro	
LP-BM5 MuLV-infected C57BL/6 (5×10^6)	0
Normal C57BL/6 (5×10^6)	$440 \overset{\times}{\div} 1.03$
LP-BM5 MuLV-infected and normal spleen cells, 1:1 mixture (5×10^6 total)	$247 \overset{\times}{\div} 1.02$

[a]Numbers are the mean ± SEM of PFC determined using three mice per group.

[b]Numbers are the mean $\overset{\times}{\div}$ SE factor of five replicate cultures containing 5×10^6 cells each.

[Reproduced from Mosier, D.E., Yetter, R.A. and Morse, H.C. (1985). J. Exp. Med. 161, 766, by copyright permission of The Rockefeller University Press.]

TABLE III. LP-BM5 Murine Leukemia Virus Infection
Makes B Cells Unresponsive to Normal T Cell Help

Source of B cells and macrophages	PFC[b] against	Source of T cells[a]	
		Normal mice	LP-BM5-infected mice
Normal mice	SRBC	78	12
	IgM	690	1407[c]
LP-BM5 infected	SRBC	0	0
	IgM	40	25

[a]Numbers are PFC/10^6 B cells and macrophages, and represent the geometric mean of five replicate cultures per group.

[b]2×10^6 nylon wool-passed T cells were added to 5×10^6 T-depleted spleen cells (B cells plus macrophages) and SRBC- and IgM-specific PFC determined after 4 days of culture.

[c]Mean is significantly higher than corresponding group with normal T cells (p <0.01).

[Reproduced from Mosier, D.E., Yetter, R.A. and Morse, H.C. (1985). J. Exp. Med. 161, 766, by copyright permission of The Rockefeller University Press.]

respond to SRBC (Table III). When T helper cells from the virus-infected mice were added to normal B cells, an insignificant SRBC response was obtained. There was elevated polyclonal IgM synthesis suggesting that T cells from infected mice are making something that can stimulate IgM production by normal B cells.

In very recent experiments, the course of this disease in C57BL/6 nude mice was followed. These mice lack functional T cells. The disease was different in nude mice. It was much slower in onset, the extent of lymphoproliferation was much reduced, it was not a fatal disease and the onset of B cell immunosuppression in spleen was delayed. Some B cells in lymph node had normal function throughout the course of the disease in the nude mice.

Therefore, some of the immunosuppression seen in C57BL/6 mice may be dependent on normal T:B collaboration.

Is this virus directly immunosuppressive when added to normal cells in vitro? It is not. A variety of responses have been measured after adding the virus directly to culture and there is no immunosuppressive or immunostimulatory effect. Could the immunosuppression be reversed using exogenous interleukin 2? The proliferative responses of cells from virus-infected mice could not be restored by adding interleukin 2 to cultures. The severe immunosuppression was irreversible.

This lymphoproliferative disease eventually kills the mice. The injection of virus results in profound immunosuppression, detectable literally within days of viral injection. There is an early polyclonal activation of B cells which continues. There is some augmentation of early responses within a week of virus injection; thereafter, all the immune responses we could measure rapidly decline. There is no evidence that addition of virus to cultures is immunosuppressive. The working hypothesis is that the immunosuppression results from the total polyclonal activation of T and B cells, preempting them from responding to any specific antigen. We do not know whether they are responding to the viral antigens or not. The mouse model has some unique advantages for studying retroviral immunosuppression. Much is known about the genes that control viral resistance and viral replication in mice and a great deal is known about the immune system. This would seem to be an ideal system in which to study the rapid onset of virus-induced immunosuppression.

REFERENCES

1. Laterjet, R. and Duplan, J.F. (1962). Int. J. Radiat. Biol. 5, 339.
2. Haas, M. and Meshorer, A. (1979). J. Natl. Cancer Inst. 63, 427.

3. Patengale, P.K., Taylor, C.R., Twomey, T. et al. (1982). Am.
   J. Pathol. 107, 362.
4. Mosier, D.E., Yetter, R.A. and Morse, H.C. (1985). J. Exp.
   Med. 161, 766.

PATHOGENESIS OF EQUINE INFECTIOUS ANEMIA

Travis C. McGuire

Department of Veterinary Microbiology and Pathology
Washington State University
Pullman, Washington

The most characteristic feature of equine infectious anemia
(EIA) virus infection is recurrent episodes of clinical disease,
predominantly fever and anemia. The clinical episodes last only
a few days with the horses appearing relatively normal during
the intervening periods. In recently infected horses the clinical
episodes can occur as often as 2 weeks apart; as the infection
progresses the time between clinical episodes increases to a
few months and eventually no clinical episodes occur. Viremia
correlates directly with the clinical episodes suggesting that
increased virus replication results in clinical signs and
lesions.

Persistence of EIA virus can be explained by proviral integration with latency. The recurrent virus expression correlates
with the presence of new antigenic variants of the virus as
defined by neutralization. Variation seems to be caused by amino
acid changes in neutralization-sensitive epitopes on the surface
glycoproteins. Data indicate that a new variant appears, replicates, causes disease and is removed by newly formed neutralizing
antibody. New variants likely arise from persistently infected
cells.

The virus replicates in monocytes and macrophages and during
acute phases of the diseases, infected cells are present in a
variety of organs. Virus-infected cells are most prominent in the
spleen, lymph nodes and liver. However, most organs have infected
cells during the peak viremia. After about 3 months of infection,
infected cells are rare when tissue sections are examined by
immunofluorescence.

The most characteristic morphologic lesion caused by EIA
virus infection occurs in the liver. Lymphocytes and macrophages
accumulate in the periportal areas and in severe cases comprise
approximately one-fourth the area of a section. In the central
part of the lobule, the hepatocytes have anoxic degeneration
caused in part by the anemia. Kupffer cells are swollen and many
contain stainable iron. When frozen sections are reacted with
fluorescent-labeled antibodies to EIA virus, viral antigens are
easily demonstrated in the cytoplasm of Kupffer cells and in an
occasional macrophage in the cellular accumulations in the periportal areas. It is assumed that the lymphocytes are responding
to viral antigens although this assumption has not been proven.
Interestingly, the severity of the liver lesions as measured by
the amount of mononuclear cell accumulation correlates positively
with the number and intensity of the recurring febrile episodes.
Infected horses which have been clinically normal for several
months have a normal appearing liver when examined histologically. Accumulations of lymphocytes and macrophages can occur in
several other organs including interstitial areas of the kidney,
adrenal, meninges and lung.

Glomeruli in the kidneys of infected horses have accumulations of neutrophils and mononuclear cells and a marked thicken-
ing of the basement membrane. Electron microscopy reveals dense
granular deposits in the basement membrane. Deposits of immunoglobulin and C3 are present when examined with fluorescent-
labeled antibodies to these substances. When isolated glomeruli

are eluted with a low pH buffer, antibodies to EIA virus are
recovered. Identification of the viral proteins involved in the
immune complex-mediated glomerulitis have not been made. The
glomerular lesion does not progress to the point of causing
proteinuria.

The anemia is caused by both increased erythrocyte destruction and decreased erythropoiesis. There is a marked decrease in
the erythrocyte life span during active disease. Erythrocytes are
osmotically fragile and some lyse in the circulation as evidenced
by hemoglobin in the plasma in very acute cases and by decreased
or absent serum haptoglobin in other cases. Intravascular hemoly-
sis only rarely progresses to hemoglobinuria. Indirect bilirubin
increases and erythrophagocytosis by macrophages is common. In
active cases of EIA virus infection erythrocytes have C3 on their
surface as revealed by Coombs' testing with a specific antibody
to equine C3. However, Coombs' testing fails to detect IgG,
IgG(T), IgM or immunoglobulin light chain. The cause of the C3
on the erythrocyte surface cannot readily be explained by cold
hemagglutinins. A current hypothesis is based on the fact that
EIA virus causes hemagglutination and it is assumed that viral
subunits bind to erythrocytes, antiviral antibody binds and complement is activated. Antibody amounts could be below the detectable threshold while a small number of C1q molecules bound could
lead to the activation of hundreds more C3b molecules which could
bind to the erythrocytes. Complement activation by antigen-
antibody complexes leads to decreased circulating C3 amounts in
active infection (Table I).

The decreased erythropoiesis can be demonstrated during
active disease by an increased myeloid-erythroid ratio in the
bone marrow and by ferrokinetics. Studies with ^{59}Fe reveal a
decrease in the plasma iron turnover rate and in the percentage
iron utilization. One cause of the erythroid suppression seems to
be a temporary iron deficiency. During febrile periods there is a

TABLE I.   Complement Activation in Horses with EIA

C3 deposits in glomeruli

C3-coated erythrocytes

Decreased plasma C3 amounts

---

marked decrease in serum iron and a decresse in the percentage
saturation of transferrin as measured by the iron binding capacity. At the same time there is an increase in stainable iron in
the macrophages. Whether other virus-induced effects contribute
to the erythroid suppression is not known.

There is no increase in susceptibility to other infections
in EIA virus-infected horses. B lymphocytes are present in normal
numbers and T lymphocytes respond to phytolectins with a normal
response. The only evidence of an altered lymphoid immune
response is the specific suppression of an IgG subclass, IgG(T)
(Table II). IgG(T) differs from IgG in that it does not fix complement, does not bind to monocytes and neutrophils, does not
precipitate antigens with repeating determinants and floculates
instead of precipitating with other antigens. In EIA virus infection, specific IgG(T) antibodies to EIA virus block complement
fixation by IgG when IgG(T) predominates. However, total amounts
of serum IgG(T) decrease at 2 months post infection, and are
still decreased 1 year after infection. In contrast, IgG amounts
were significantly increased at both times after infection.
Immunoglobulin metabolism studies demonstrated a decrease in
synthesis of IgG(T) in EIA virus-infected horses when compared
to normal horses. No difference was noted in the amounts of IgG
synthesis in EIA virus-infected and normal horses. In addition,
EIA virus-infected horses produced less IgG(T) antibody to DNP
immunization than did normal horses. The significance of the
IgG(T) subclass specific suppression in EIA virus-infected horses
is unknown as is the mechanism of suppression.

TABLE II. Evaluation of Immunosuppression in Horses with EIA

Evaluation susceptibility to infection	Result
B lymphocyte numbers	Normal
Lymphocyte response to lectins	Normal
Serum IgG	Increased
Serum IgM	Increased (early)
Serum IgG(T)	Decreased
IgG(T) synthesis	Decreased

Even though neutralizing antibody can be demonstrated against the virus used for infection or in other homologous reactions, all virus present in the serum of infected horses is not neutralized. Most of the infectious EIA virus in the serum of infected horses 22 to 27 days after infection can be removed by treatment with rabbit anti-equine gamma globulin but not by rabbit antiserum to equine albumin or normal rabbit serum. These results demonstrate infectious EIA virus-antibody complexes in the serum and provide a source of virus for infection of susceptible cells.

Attempts to study infected cell surface antigens as targets of the immune system have demonstrated small amounts of direct lymphocyte cytotoxicity. Antibodies from infected horse sera bind to the surface of EIA virus-infected dermal cells; however, no antibody-dependent cellular cytotoxicity is demonstrated. Results with viral-induced cell surface antigens need to be extended to include virus-infected macrophages.

With regard to the potential of EIA virus as a model of human retrovirus infection, there are at least two important areas for contribution.

1. Since EIA virus infects and grows primarily in macrophages, there is an opportunity to study a nononcogenic

retrovirus which has a restricted nonlymphoid host cell range. Since the primary target for virus replication is the monocyte/macrophage system, important areas of study are mechanisms of virus persistence, subsequent virus expression and resulting disease.

2. Rapid antigenic variation of the envelope glycoproteins in the same host is a unique feature of the EIA virus. Understanding the mechanisms of the antigenic variation and developing methods of immunologic control will be the most important contribution that research on EIA virus can make.

SELECTED REFERENCES

1. Banks, K.L. and Henson, J.B. (1973). Infect. Immun. 8, 679.
2. Cheevers, W.P. and McGuire, T.C. (1985). Rev. Infect. Dis. 7, 83.
3. Issel, C.J. and Coggins, L. (1979). J. Am. Vet. Med. Assoc. 174, 727.
4. Kono, Y., Kobayashi, K. and Fukunaga, Y. (1973). Arch. Virus Forschung 41, 1.
5. McGuire, T.C. and Crawford, T.B. (1979). Adv. Vet. Sci. Comp. Med. 23, 137.
6. Montelaro, R.C., Parekh, B., Orrego, A. et al. (1984). J. Biol. Chem. 259, 10539.

IMMUNOLOGIC AND VIROLOGIC STUDIES ON BOVINE LEUKOSIS

R. D. Schultz*†
T. O. Manning

James A. Baker Institute for Animal Health
Cornell University, Ithaca, New York

J. C. Rhyan
B. A. Buxton
V. S. Panangala

*School of Veterinary Medicine
Auburn, Alabama

I. M. Bause
W. C. Yang*

†Department of Pathobiological Sciences
School of Veterinary Medicine
University of Wisconsin
Madison, Wisconsin

SEROLOGIC TESTS TO DETECT BOVINE LEUKOSIS VIRUS

The most commonly used serologic tests for the detection
of antibody to bovine leukosis virus (BLV) antigens, notably the
glycoprotein (gp)70 antigen and/or internal protein (p)24 antigen
are the agar-gel-immunodiffusion (AGID) test, radioimmunoassay
(RIA) and virus neutralization (VN) assay. Antibody is readily
detected by the three tests in BLV-infected animals. The major
difference among the tests is that the RIA and VN have the advantage of identifying positive animals earlier after infection than

does the AGID test, but both have the disadvantage of complexity and expense. The AGID test is routinely used as a diagnostic test, for seroepidemiologic studies, and is the official test of the United States Department of Agriculture for purposes of classifying the BLV infectivity status of animals for export. When serologic tests are used to determine infectivity, false positive results occur during the first 3 to 6 months of life because an animal may be antibody positive but not infected. The false positive test is due to antibody from the dam's colostrum. The infectivity status of young animals (<6 months) with maternal antibody must be determined with one of the infectivity assays. Many other serologic assays are used to detect antibody to BLV in infected animals. Enzyme-linked immunosorbent assays (ELISA) have been developed and are used for diagnostic and regulatory purposes in Europe and for research purposes in the United States. Our initial experience with an ELISA test we developed in 1976 using BLV antigen from the fetal lamb kidney (FLK) cells, standard cell line for production of antigen, was unacceptable false positive results due to contamination of the FLK line with bovine viral diarrhea (BVD) virus. We subsequently developed an ELISA with an antigen that was free of BVD virus. A comparative study between the AGID test and the ELISA suggested the ELISA was slightly more sensitive at 3 months post infection; however, at 5 months the AGID detected more positive animals than the ELISA (Table I). A number of AGID-positive and ELISA-negative animals were found in the study that were unexpected and are unexplained since we assumed the ELISA was more sensitive and was detecting antibody to the antigens detected by the AGID test. (See Refs. 1-8.)

SEROEPIDEMIOLOGIC SURVEY

A study was designed to compare the prevalence of animals with antibody to BLV in a random group of dairy cattle in New York with a random group of beef and dairy cattle in Alabama. Ten

TABLE I.   Comparison Between the AGID and ELISA Test
for Detection of Antibody at 3 Months and 5 Months
Post Infection with BLV

No. of animals	BLV antibody positive 3 months		BLV antibody positive 5 months	
	AGID	ELISA	AGID	ELISA
21	12/21	15/21	20/21	18/21

samples per herd were selected randomly from approximately 200
herds of New York dairy cattle, 200 herds of Alabama beef cattle
and 50 herds of Alabama dairy cattle. Similar techniques and
reagents were used for detection of antibody to a dual antigen
(gp and p24) by the AGID test. The results of this study were the
first to find the percentages of antibody-positive beef and dairy
cattle to be similar. Previous studies suggested that the ratio
of infected dairy to beef cattle was about 5 to 10:1. The overall
number of New York dairy cattle positive was 300 of 2000 tested
(15%); whereas 400 of 2060 Alabama beef cattle samples (19%) were
positive. The distribution of the number of positive samples per
herd was also similar between the diary cows in New York and beef
cows in Alabama. Of the 500 samples, 212 (42%) of the Alabama
dairy samples were positive, providing evidence of a significant
difference in the number of positive Alabama dairy samples compared with dairy cattle in New York and beef cattle in Alabama.

This study similar to previous studies found that antibody
to gp was more easily detected by AGID than was antibody to p24
antigen.

It was also found in this serologic survey that the relationship between history of clinical disease in the herd and numbers
of serologically positive animals in the same herd cannot always
be predicted. Although in general many animals in herds that had

TABLE II.   Unusual Relationship Between History
of Clinical Disease and Percentage
of Animals Positive to BLV

Herd	Clinical disease status	Percentage of animals positive in herd
A	2 cases in previous 2 years	12 (16/135)[a]
B	5 cases in previous 10 years	18 (18/100)
C	1 case in previous 2 years	22 (17/78)
D	9 cases in previous 5 years	33 (52/160)
E	1 case in previous 10 years	12 (26/220)
F	0 cases in previous 5 years	65 (67/103)
G	0 cases in previous 5 years	90 (54/60)
H	0 cases in previous 10 years	90 (54/60)
I	0 cases in previous 10 years	85 (77/90)

[a]Number of positive animals/total number in herd.

a history of clinical cases of disease would be BLV positive,
some herds with histories of numerous clinical cases were found
to have relatively few positive animals; and, conversely, certain
herds with no history of disease had significantly higher numbers
of serologically positive animals (Table II). However, it is
noteworthy that we have not found an animal with adult enzootic
clinical leukosis serologically negative by AGID test.

CELLULAR ASSAYS FOR BLV

In contrast to the experience with serologic tests being
easily applied to detect antibody in BLV-infected and diseased
cattle, few groups have successfully applied cellular assays for
detection of antigen-reactive T cells, killer (K) cells or
natural killer (NK) cells.

The results of cellular studies in our laboratory can be
summarized as follows: The lymphocyte blastogenesis test (LBT),
primarily a measure of T helper cells, is not regularly nor
consistently positive when a variety of BLV antigens (e.g.,

purified gp, crude antigen or infected cells) are used to stimulate lymphocytes from infected or diseased animals. The reason
for the difficulty in stimulating lymphocytes with BLV antigens
are not readily apparent, but does not appear to be caused by a
suppressive factor in the BLV preparations or by an abnormal
number or class of lymphocytes in infected animals.

The leukocyte migration inhibition factor assay for detection
of BLV-reactive lymphocytes has also not produced consistent
results and is regularly negative for BLV-infected animals.

Studies with cytotoxic T lymphocytes to BLV-infected target
cells remain to be done by enough laboratories to critically
assess their role in cellular immunity to BLV. Few studies have
critically evaluated the role of K cells in antibody-dependent
cellular cytotoxicity (ADCC) assays to BLV and to our knowledge
NK activity to BLV-infected cells or BLV-transformed cells has
not been reported. Thus, additional studies are required to
determine the role of cellular immunity in BLV-infected and
diseased animals.

IMMUNOSUPPRESSION IN BLV-INFECTED AND DISEASED CATTLE

Diseased Cattle

Infection of the mouse, cat and several other species with
leukemia viruses has been shown to cause suppression of cellular
and/or humoral immunity. Nonspecific immunosuppression has also
been associated with lymphoid malignancies of nonviral etiology.
Currently, little or no information exists on the role of BLV,
nor on adult enzootic bovine leukosis (lymphosarcoma), in causing
immunosuppression. We have estimated that 0.1% of the BLV-
infected cattle develop clinical leukosis. As part of our program
on BLV a study was undertaken to determine if nonspecific immunosuppression was present in cattle with clinical leukosis. Parameters of cellular and humoral immunity were tested in cows with

clinically diagnosed bovine lymphosarcoma and in healthy, age, breed and sex-matched control cattle. Cellular immunity was eval- uated using skin allograft rejection and the LBT. Humoral immu- nity was evaluated by: 1) radial immunodiffusion (RID) to quanti- tate IgG_1, IgG_2, IgM and IgA; 2) detection of antibody to BLV; 3) determination of antibody titers to infectious bovine rhino- tracheitis virus (IBR) and 4) immunization of cattle with chicken red blood cells (CRBC). The results of the studies suggested there were no significant differences in cellular and humoral immunity between healthy cattle and cattle with leukosis. Allo- graft rejection occurred by 14 days in both groups of cattle and the response to phytomitogens for lymphocytes from diseased cattle was not suppressed when compared to control cattle. Con- trol cultures without mitogen were often elevated for diseased cattle as were the lymphocyte responses to lipopolysaccharide (LPS). No significant deficiencies were found between the two groups of cattle in the quantity of serum IgG_1, IgG_2 or IgM; however, the quantity of IgA was lower in certain cattle with lymphosarcoma than the normal controls (Table III). The signifi- cance of this observation is not known since the quantity of IgA in normal cattle serum is very low and only minimal changes in concentration cause statistical, but perhaps not biological, dif- ferences to be found. All cows with clinical leukosis had anti- body to BLV, whereas only one of the control cows was antibody positive and antibody titers to IBR were similar in both groups. The antibody response of healthy and lymphosarcomatous cattle to inoculation with CRBC was also similar. These results suggest that significant immunosuppression does not occur in cattle with clinical leukosis. More recent studies have included assays to measure ADCC to CRBC and NK-like activity to parainfluenza-3 (PI-3) virus-infected vero cells in a limited number of diseased cattle. The K cell activity to CRBC and NK activity was not sup- pressed in cattle with clinical leukosis.

TABLE III. Comparison Between the Quantity mg/ml
of Immunoglobulins in Serum of Normal Cattle
and Cattle with Adult Enzootic Leukosis

	IgG_1	IgG_2	IgM	IgA
Normal	11.0 ± 3	7.5 ± 2	2.0 ± 0.8	0.2 ± 0.10
Diseased	7.3 ± 2	10.5 ± 3	1.6 ± 0.5	0.05 ± 0.05[a]

[a]Significant decrease p <0.05.

Therefore, the only significant difference in the immune
response between cattle with clinical leukosis and normal cattle
was the lymphocyte response to LPS. Peripheral blood lymphocytes
(PBL) from diseased animals readily respond to the LPS from a
number of gram-negative bacteria including: Escherichia coli,
Salmonella sp. and Brucella abortus. Presumably this is due to
an increased number of B lymphocytes in the blood.

Fetal Studies

Additional studies were designed to determine if the bovine
fetus experimentally infected at various times during gestation
could develop an antibody response to BLV and whether the BLV
infection during this critical period of immune system development caused immunosuppression. The methods used to assess the
immunologic competence of calves infected as fetuses in utero
were similar to tests used in cattle with clinical leukosis.

Cell-free BLV from FLK and bat lung cell (BAT)-BLV infected
monolayer cell cultures was used to inoculate bovine fetuses from
BLV serologically negative dams at various stages of gestation.
The fetuses were allowed to proceed to term. Cows were monitored
serologically with the AGID for the development of gp and p24
antibody. Certain aspects of the fetuses' cellular and humoral
responses were investigated. Precolostral sera from the calves

were tested for antibody to BLV. Their immunoglobulin concentrations were quantitated by RID and their lymphoproliferative
responses to nonspecific mitogens were assessed using the LBT.
Antibody responses to viruses commonly infecting cattle (e.g.,
IBR, BVD and PI-3) were also determined.

Twenty-four fetuses were inoculated in utero. Sixteen were
inoculated with FLK-BLV preparations, seven with BAT-BLV cell-
free virus and one with the lymphocytes from its BLV-positive
dam. Eight of 16 FLK-BLV fetuses survived to term. These fetuses
remained in utero from 21 to 209 days post inoculation. The
remaining eight FLK-BLV fetal inoculations terminated as abortions. Five of seven cows whose fetuses were inoculated in utero
with BAT-BLV had their calves 17 to 60 days post inoculation.

Results of this study support the theory that the bovine
fetus could be infected with the cell-free form of BLV. Although
we were unable to detect evidence of BLV antibody in precolostral
serum or serums from aborted fetuses, six of these calves maintained in isolation developed persistent BLV infections and
seroconverted between 25 to 85 days postparturition. The time
required for antibody to be detected after inoculation was as
short as 84 days for the older inoculated fetuses to as long as
162 days for the younger fetuses. It was found that the FLK-BLV
culture was contaminated with BVD virus. Most serum samples from
aborted fetuses, as well as precolostral serums from calves,
contained BVD neutralizing antibodies.

All newborn calves were tested by RID and LBT. BLV-inoculated
calves responded in both RID and LBT with values in the same
range as control calves inoculated in utero with antigens or
virus. These results suggest that BLV did not cause immunosuppression when inoculated at critical stage of immune system
development in these animals. Furthermore some of these animals
have now been studied for as long as 10 years post inoculation.
They have remained infected with BLV throughout that period, have

had persistence of antibody to BLV detectable by any of the known serologic assays and have remained remarkably healthy. Although never vaccinated they have all had subclinical infections with IBR, BVD, PI-3 and a variety of bacteria including Pasteurella sp., Haemophilus somnus and Leptospira sp. Serologic tests for each of the above microbes would suggest that the antibody responses of these cattle, infected as fetuses with BLV, are within the range of values found in non-BLV-infected cattle maintained in our "BLV experimental herd." Similarly, cellular immunity as determined by a variety of assays has remained in the normal range for the BLV-infected animals. Thus, our results suggest that there is little or no evidence of immunosuppression in BLV-infected animals.

Adult Cattle

Adult cattle naturally infected at various ages with BLV were also studied to 1) characterize the class of lymphocytes and relative numbers in cattle with and without persistent lymphocytosis (PL), 2) determine if a cytochemical stain for detection of purine nucleoside phosphorylase (PNP) could be used to identify specific lymphocyte classes in BLV-infected cattle and 3) determine lymphocyte reactivity to a variety of mitogens.

The results of the study to characterize cells from BLV-infected and control uninfected cattle suggested that PBL from normal and from various classes of bovine leukemia virus-infected cattle using surface immunoglobulin (sIg) immunofluorescence and peanut agglutinin (PNA) immunofluorescence were as follows: Fluorescein isothiocyanate-conjugated PNA (FITC-PNA) labeled the majority of sIg-PBL from normal cattle suggesting the marker labeled T lymphocytes. The largest percentage of PBL from BLV-infected animals with PL was sIg^+ PNA^- and there was no significant difference in the number of PNA^+ lymphocytes from that of normal animals. The percentage of sIg^+ and PNA^+ cells was similar for BLV-infected nonlymphocytosis animals and normal animals (Table IV). Also of interest was the observation that in animals with adult lymphosarcoma, the majority of PBL and tumor cells was not labeled with either marker. PBL from a single thymic lymphosarcoma case had normal proportions of B and T cells though there was a moderate increase in both cell populations.

A cytochemical stain for the detection of PNP was evaluated as a potential T lymphocyte marker in cattle. A double label study combining immunofluorescent demonstration of sIg and the PNP stain suggested that PNP is not specific for bovine T or B cells. PBL from normal, BLV-infected, BLV-infected persistent lymphocytotic and lymphosarcoma cattle were examined for sIg and PNP reactivity. PBL samples from most animals contained PNP reaction product. PBL from lymphosarcoma animals contained a greater than normal percentage of PNP-negative cells. Thymus, lymph node and lymphosarcoma cells were also examined for PNP. Lymph node and tumor cells were found to have percentages of PNP positive and negative cells similar to PBL from normal animals. Nearly all thymocytes were PNP negative. Serial samples of visceral trunk lymphocytes collected daily were found to have consistently lower percentages of PNP-positive cells than blood samples collected from the same animals.

Results of lymphocyte responses to various mitogens for cattle infected with BLV and uninfected cattle can be found in Table V. The results clearly demonstrate that responses to phytohemagglutinin (PHA), concanavalin A (con A) and pokeweed mitogen (PWM) are similar among the different groups of cattle, but the response to LPS is significantly different among the three groups of cattle. The B. abortus soluble antigen (BASA) preparation contains LPS that nonspecifically stimulates the B cells in some of the BLV-infected non-PL animals and the B cells in most of the BLV-infected animals with PL. These results suggest that BLV-infected cattle have an LPS-reactive class of lymphocytes in their blood, most likely a B cell subclass. (See Refs. 9-18.)

TABLE IV. Percentages and Absolute Numbers of B (sIg^+) and T (PNA^+)
Cells in Peripheral Blood from Normal, Lymphocytotic and Lymphosarcoma Cattle

Group	No. of animals	Lymphocytes ($\times 10^3/mm^3$ blood)	% B cells	% T cells	B cells ($\times 10^3/mm^3$ blood)	T cells ($\times 10^3/mm^3$ blood)
BLV^-, PL^-	10	3.5 ± 1.1	20.1 ± 7.7	73.2 ± 6.9	0.7 ± 0.4	2.5 ± 0.7
BLV^+, PL^-	10	4.7 ± 1.4	29.6 ± 13.6	67.4 ± 15.4	1.5 ± 1.0	3.1 ± 1.0
BLV^+, PL^+	10	14.8 ± 8.3[a]	70.6 ± 11.4[a]	24.3 ± 12.5[a]	10.7 ± 6.6[a]	3.3 ± 2.0

Data from groups expressed as mean ± standard error.

[a] Significantly different (p <0.01) from control (BLV^-, PL^-) group.

TABLE V. Lymphocyte Response to Mitogens for Cattle Infected
with BLV or Without PL and Uninfected Cattle

Group of cattle BLV status	No. cattle	Lymphocyte response (cpm × 10^{-3})					
		PHA	con A	PWM	$\frac{E.\ coli}{LPS}$	BASA
Uninfected	10	145 ± 40	180 ± 50	150 ± 50	1 ± 2	Neg.
Infected-Non-PL	10	125 ± 50	185 ± 65	160 ± 60	15 ± 10	3 ± 2
Infected-PL	10	150 ± 50	160 ± 70	170 ± 50	65 ± 20	30 ± 25

INFECTIVITY AND TRANSMISSION STUDIES--THE ROLE OF INSECTS

We have conducted the most extensive studies to date on the role of insects as mechanical vectors in the transmission of BLV. The results of infectivity studies demonstrate that certain infected animals were more infectious than others and that only very small quantities of blood were required for transmission of virus. Peripheral blood mononuclear cells were obtained from 13 BLV-infected cattle and inoculated subcutaneously into 29 recipient adult steers to determine 1) the number of mononuclear cells (equivalent amount of blood) necessary to cause infection and 2) factors influencing infectivity of mononuclear cells. A total of 55 inoculations were made. Inoculation of 1×10^4, 2×10^4 and 5×10^4 mononuclear cells caused seroconversion in 12%, 57% and 62% of steers, respectively. No infections occurred with 1×10^3 or 2×10^3 mononuclear cells. Cattle infected for longer than 24 months and those animals greater than 3 years of age had cells that were more likely to cause infection when 1 to 5×10^4 mononuclear cells were inoculated into susceptible cattle than were cattle infected for less than 24 months or animals less than 3 years of age. Lymphocytes from cattle with PL caused more infections when 1×10^4 or 2×10^4 mononuclear cells were inoculated than did lymphocytes from non-PL cattle; however, both groups were equally infectious when 5×10^4 mononuclear cells were inoculated. No differences were found in infectivity of leukocytes from experimentally vs. naturally exposed animals. A limited study designed to determine if beef calves were more resistant to infection than dairy calves suggested that there was no difference in susceptibility to experimental infection when 1×10^4 leukocytes from a BLV-infected animal were inoculated.

Although the most infectious animal in the study above required an equivalent of 1 to 2 μl of blood, our most highly infectious PL cow (not included in the above study) can cause

infection when as little as 0.1 μl of blood is inoculated
intradermally in susceptible cattle. Thus it is not surprising
that contaminated needles, surgical instruments, dehorning and
castrating equipment, hoof knives, nose leads and insects serve
as excellent vectors for the transmission of BLV-infected
leukocytes.

A variety of studies were designed to specifically determine
the role of insects in the transmission of BLV. A model system
using mosquitoes that were permitted to feed on blood from a
BLV-infected animal demonstrated BLV could be transmitted to
sheep in a simulated mechanical transmission experiment, using
the following species of mosquitoes: Anopheles freeborni,
A. stephensi, A. quadrimaculatus and A. albimanus. Mosquitoes
were fed on blood taken from a BLV-infected cow with PL. Mouthparts and heads of mosquitoes were removed immediately after
feeding, placed in RPMI-1640 medium and inoculated subcutaneously
into sheep. Nine sheep were inoculated with mouthparts and heads
from 37 to 122 mosquitoes. Infection was determined serologically. Three monthly serum samples were collected from the sheep
and were tested for the presence of antibodies to BLV using the
AGID test. Sera that were negative by AGID at 3 months were
tested by RIA. There was exact agreement between results obtained
by RIA and those obtained by AGID. Four of the nine sheep
developed antibody to BLV. Sheep that seroconverted were inoculated with mouthparts and heads from as few as 54 mosquitoes.

Although the results of the mosquito study are interesting
they have little or no relevance to natural transmission; therefore, studies were designed to determine the ability of stable
flies (Stomoxys calcitrans), horn flies (Haematobia irritans) and
tabanids (Diptera: Tabanidae) to transmit BLV. Stable flies and
horn flies were fed on blood collected from an infected cow, and
the flies' mouthparts were immediately removed, placed in RPMI-
1640 medium, ground and inoculated into sheep and calves.

Infection of sheep occurred with mouthparts from as few as 25
stable flies or 25 horn flies. However, sheep were not infected
when removal of stable fly mouthparts was delayed more than
1 hour after blood feeding. Infection of calves occurred after
inoculation of mouthparts removed immediately after feeding from
as few as 50 stable flies or 100 horn flies.

Infected blood, applied by capillary action to the mouthparts
(labella) of 15 deer flies (Chrysops sp.) and a single horsefly
(Tabanus astratus) caused infection in each of two sheep.

Infection did not occur in two calves inoculated daily for
5 days with mouthparts from 50 horn flies collected after feeding
on a BLV-infected steer. Four calves receiving bites from 75
stable flies interrupted from feeding on a BLV-positive cow also
were not infected. Seronegative cattle held for 1 to 4 months in
a screened enclosure with positive cattle in the presence of
biting flies were not infected with BLV. An important role for
stable flies, horn flies and tabanids in transmission of BLV is
probably limited to local areas of heavy fly infestations, such
as certain areas of the South, where the prevalence of BLV-
infected animals is significantly higher than the North. (See
Refs. 19-25.)

SEMEM AS A VECTOR IN THE TRANSMISSION OF BLV

Three studies were designed to determine the role for semen
in the transmission of BLV. In the first study semen was experimentally contaminated with cell-free BLV and/or lymphocytes from
a BLV-infected animal then used to breed heifers that were in
estrus. The second study employed semen experimentally contaminated with large numbers of BLV-infected lymphocytes that was
used to inseminate animals in luteal phase of estrus cycle. The
third study has been ongoing since 1974 and is designed to
determine if BLV-infected bulls in a commercial artificial

insemination cooperative shed infectious lymphocytes or virus in
their semen.

The results of the first study can be summarized as follows:
Semen experimentally contaminated with BLV or BLV-infected leukocytes was used to breed 16 serologically negative animals.
Infected semen was capable of causing conception in all of the
cows. With the exception of one cow bred with BLV contaminated
semen, none of the cows became serologically positive, suggesting
the cows did not become infected as a result of multiple insemi-
nations. Furthermore, it is probable that the one cow that did
become serologically positive did so as a result of previous
natural infection and not as a result of the infected semen
because she was positive less than 2 weeks after the first insemination. Fetuses and calves born to cows inseminated with contaminated semen were serologically negative and appeared normal.
Contaminated semen remained infectious for lambs; therefore, it
is suggested that the genital tract of cows in estrus is relatively resistant to infection with BLV. Thus, the results of this
study strongly suggested that semen would not be an important
vector in the transmission of BLV.

However, the results of the second study differ from the
first in that cattle in the nonluteal phase of estrus appear to
be highly susceptible to infection when inseminated with experimentally contaminated semen.

Transmission of BLV by inseminating extended semen containing
leukocytes from a BLV-infected cow was attempted in two experiments with a total of 27 cows at the luteal phase of the estrual
cycle. Five months post insemination 20 of the cows had antibodies to BLV by the AGID test suggesting that they were highly
susceptible, during this period of the estrus cycle, to infection
by the genital route. Although infection of cows in the luteal
phase was possible by experimentally inseminating large numbers
of BLV-infected leukocytes admixed with semen, it is doubtful

that semen from BLV-infected bulls would serve as a natural mode of transmission of the infection, since few if any BLV-infected leukocytes have been found in semen.

Results of the third study in which semen from BLV-infected bulls has been tested for BLV by direct inoculation of the semen into sheep to determine infectivity in this highly susceptible species suggest that after more than 10 years of testing every ejaculate from BLV-infected bulls, we have not found a semen sample with BLV.

Our studies have also demonstrated that leukocytes are more susceptible to killing by the freezing procedures routinely used to freeze semen for artificial insemination. Thus it is highly unlikely that semen used for artificial insemination is a vector for transmission of BLV. (See Refs. 26-30.)

IMMUNOMODULATION AND SUPPRESSION OF VIRUS RELEASE IN BLV-INFECTED CELLS

FLK cells, persistently infected with BLV, express a viral gp antigen on the surface in random circumferential distribution. Six bovine sera from naturally infected animals as well as three sera from experimentally infected sheep were used to culture FLK-BLV⁺ cells in the presence of BLV antibodies. After treatment, the viral antigen was redistributed on the cell membrane into patches or a unipolar cap, as demonstrated by indirect immunofluorescent assay. As a consequence of this immunomodulation the release of whole viral particles from infected cells into the culture supernatant was suppressed; but, the virus was accumulated within the cell. Suppression of virus release and intracellular accumulation of virus were shown by quantitation of purified ether-treated particles in a single RID test. This study offers an explanation for the absence of viral particles in the serum and the survival of infected lymphocytes carrying proviral DNA in BLV-infected cattle in the presence of a persistent antibody titer.

Preliminary studies in our laboratory have not confirmed the observations that there is a nonantibody factor in the plasma of BLV-infected cattle that blocks BLV transcription in proviral-infected cells. (See Refs. 31-39.)

BOVINE ACQUIRED IMMUNODEFICIENCY SYNDROME (BAIDS)

A model for BAIDS was developed that includes three critical factors: 1) semen, 2) BLV and 3) BVD virus.

Preliminary studies involved the inoculation of large quantities of semen only or insemination with semen experimentally contaminated with BLV and BVD virus.

Cattle inoculated intravenously and intranasally with large quantities of semen (100 ml) develop a transient immunosuppression detected by a number of in vitro assays of cellular immunity. Studies in progress have demonstrated that semen suppresses a number of cells including, but not limited to, T lymphocytes, neutrophils and macrophages. The mechanisms for the suppression, which has been found for a number of species, is complex and not completely understood, but may have natural survival advantages for the sperm in the immunologically hostile environment of the female genital tract.

Six cows, all BVD antibody positive and BLV antibody negative, were repeatedly inseminated with semen experimentally contaminated with BLV and BVD. One of the six cows developed a severe immunodeficiency, characterized by lymphocyte unresponsiveness, decreased immunoglobulins, lymphoid hypoplasia, lymph node atrophy and death.

Semen, BLV or BVD virus when given alone did not cause disease. However, semen contaminated only with BVD virus, a virus known to cause immunosuppression under certain circumstances, was not tested. Studies in progress will hopefully provide additional information on the mechanism in this bovine model for AIDS.

SUMMARY

The results of numerous studies on BLV from our laboratory were summarized in this chapter. Important findings in these studies are as follows:

1. Numerous serologic tests can be used to detect antibody to BLV; and except for a period of approximately 6 months after birth, a positive serologic test can be readily used to identify BLV-infected cattle.

2. Few if any assays of cellular immunity have been successfully applied to detect specific BLV-reactive lymphocytes. Limited attempts to correlate cellular assays with infectivity or protective immunity for BLV have been unsuccessful.

3. A large percentage of the dairy cattle in the United States are infected with BLV. A survey in the northeast (New York) and the southeast (Alabama) suggested that 15% of New York dairy cattle were positive; whereas 42% of Alabama dairy cattle were positive. These figures are likely to represent the extremes, and the national average for percentage of infected cattle will be approximately 25%. The prevalence of BLV-positive beef cattle in Alabama is similar to prevalence of BLV-positive dairy cattle in New York.

4. Significant immunosuppression does not occur when fetuses are infected with BLV during various periods of gestation nor does BLV infection of the adult cause clinically relevant immunosuppression. Furthermore, cattle with clinical leukosis (lymphosarcoma) are not immunosuppressed.

5. The total number of T cells in the peripheral blood of
   BLV-infected cattle with PL remains normal or slightly
   elevated; whereas the total number of B cells increases
   significantly.

6. PNA appears to be a reliable marker for T cells in
   cattle. PNP was not specific for cattle T or B cells.

7. PBL from BLV-infected cattle are more likely to respond
   to LPS than are lymphocytes from BLV-negative cattle.
   Lymphocytes from BLV-infected cattle with PL regularly
   respond to LPS from a variety of gram-negative bacteria,
   especially the LPS from B. abortus. This fact is especially significant to those studying the lymphocyte
   response to B. abortus, since a large percentage of
   dairy cattle (approximately 10%) have PL.

8. Cattle greater than 3 years of age, infected for longer
   than 24 months, with PL were the most infectious since
   1×10^4 to 2×10^4 of their mononuclear cells could cause
   infection in BLV-susceptible cattle. The most infectious
   animal in our herd is an 11 year old with PL that has
   been infected for approximately 9 years. Between 500 and
   1000 of her leukocytes cause infection in sheep and
   between 1000 to 5000 of her leukocytes regularly cause
   infection in cattle.

9. Insects including mosquitoes, stable flies, horn flies,
   deer flies and horseflies are capable of mechanically
   transmitting BLV. However, insects are only important as
   vectors for transmission of BLV in local areas where
   there is heavy fly infestations and a large cattle population with a number of highly infectious cattle.

10. Semen, especially when used in artificial insemination,
    was not an important vector for the transmission of BLV
    because a) the genital tract is relatively resistant to
    infection during estrus; b) leukocytes are more sensitive

to freezing than sperm, thus survival of BLV-infective lymphocytes is poor and c) BLV-infected bulls rarely if ever shed enough lymphocytes to cause infection when the semen is used for artificial insemination; however, under rare and unusual circumstances some bulls may have enough leukocytes to cause infection during natural service of a BLV-susceptible heifer.

11. Antibody to BLV inhibits the release of viral particles from infected cells causing a significant accumulation of virus within the cell. Since we have been unable to demonstrate the presence of a plasma factor that blocks BLV transcription we propose that the ability of antibody to inhibit viral release offers a partial explanation for the absence of virus in serum and secretions of BLV-infected cattle.

12. A bovine AIDS model was developed that is dependent on the simultaneous inoculation of semen, BLV and BVD virus.

SELECTED REFERENCES

1. Baumgartener, L.E., Olson, C., Miller, J.M. et al. (1975). Am. J. Vet. Res. 166, 249.
2. Ferrer, J.F., Piper, C.E., Abt, D.A. et al. (1976). Bibl. Haematologica 43, 235.
3. Ferrer, J.F., Piper, C.E., Abt, D.A. et al. (1977). Am. J. Vet. Res. 38, 1977.
4. House, C., House, J.A. and Glover, F.L. (1977). Cornell Vet. 67, 510.
5. Miller, J. and Olson, C. (1972). J. Natl. Cancer Inst. 49, 1459.
6. Miller, J.M. and Van der Maaten, M.J. (1976). Vet. Microbiol. 195.
7. Burny, A., Bex, F., Chantrenne, H. et al. (1978). Adv. Cancer Res. 28, 251.
8. Bex, F., Bruck, C., Mammerickx, M. (1979). Cancer Res. 39, 1118.
9. Essex, M. and Grant, C.K. (1979). In "Basic and Clinical Aspects of Veterinary Immunology" (B.I. Osburn and R.D. Schultz, eds.). Adv. Vet. Sci. Comp. Med. 23, 184.
10. Jarrett, W.F.H. (1975). Br. J. Cancer 31, 147.

11. Winkelstein, A., Mikulla, J.M., Sartiano, G.P. et al. (1974). Cancer 34, 549.

12. Dent, P.B. (1972). Prog. Med. Virol. 14, 1.

13. Muscoplat, C., Johnson, D.W., Pomeroy, K.A. et al. (1974). Am. J. Vet. Res. 35, 593.

14. Paul, P.S., Pomeroy, K.A., Castro, A.E. et al. (1977). J. Natl. Cancer Inst. 59, 1269.

15. Paul, P.S., Pomeroy, K.A., Johnson, D.W. et al. (1977). Am. J. Vet. Res. 38, 873.

16. Schultz, R.D. and Adams, L.S. (1978). In "Symposium on Practical Immunology" (R.D. Schultz, ed.). Vet. Clin. North Am. 8, 121.

17. Schultz, R.D. (1982). Am. J. Vet. Res. 181, 1169.

18. Trainin, Z. (1969). Am. J. Vet. Res. 30, 1475.

19. Ferrer, J.F. (1979). J. Am. Vet. Med. Assoc. 175, 1281.

20. Burridge, M.J., Puhr, D.M. and Henneman, J.M. (1981). J. Am. Vet. Med. Assoc. 179, 704.

21. Ohshima, K., Okada, K., Numakunai, S. et al. (1981). Jpn. J. Vet. Res. 43, 79.

22. Buxton, B.A., Schultz, R.D. and Collins, W.E. (1982). Am. J. Vet. Res. 43, 1458.

23. Miller, J.M. and Van der Maaten, M.J. (1979). J. Natl. Cancer Inst. 62, 425.

24. Burridge, M.J., Wilcox, C.J. and Henneman, J.M. (1979). Eur. J. Cancer 15, 1395.

25. Buxton, B.A., Hinkle, N.C. and Schultz, R.D. (1985). Am. J. Vet. Res. 46, 123.

26. Baumgartener, L.E., Crowley, J., Entine, S. et al. (1978). Lbl. Vet. Med. B 25, 202.

27. Lucas, M.H., Dawson, M., Chasey, D. et al. (1980). Vet. Rec. 106, 128.

28. Todd, O. and Adair, B.M. (1980). Vet. Rec. 107, 124.

29. Miller, J.M. and Van der Maaten, M.J. (1979). J. Natl. Cancer Inst. 62, 425.

30. Ressang, A.A., Gielkens, A.L.J., Quak, S. et al. (1978). Ann. Rech. Vet. 9, 663.

31. Kettman, R., Portetell, D., Mammerickx, M. et al. (1976). Proc. Natl. Acad. Sci. 73, 1014.

32. Boyse, E.A., Stockert, E. and Old L.J. (1967). Proc. Natl. Acad. Sci. 58, 954.

33. Ritz, J., Pesando, J.M., Notis-McConarty, J. et al. (1980). J. Immunol. 125, 1506.

34. Genovesi, E.V., Marx, P.A. and Wheelock, E.F. (1977). J. Exp. Med. 146, 520.

35. Aoki, T. and Hohnson, P.A. (1972). J. Natl. Cancer Inst. 49, 183.

36. Oldstone, M.B.A. and Tishon, A. (1978). Clin. Immunobiol. Immunopathol. 9, 55.

37. Driscoll, D.M., Onuma, M. and Olson, C. (1977). Arch. Virol. 55, 139.

38. Onuma, M., Olson, C. and Baumgartener, L.M. (1975). J. Natl. Cancer Inst. 54, 1199.
39. Gupta, P., Kashmiri, S.V.S. and Ferrer, J.F. (1984). J. Virol. 50, 267.

PATHOGENESIS OF SAIDS IN RHESUS MONKEYS INOCULATED WITH TISSUE HOMOGENATES OR SERUM

David L. Madden
Delia Budzko
William T. London
Maneth Gravell
John Sever

National Institute of Neurological
and Communicative Disorders and Stroke
National Institutes of Health
Bethesda, Maryland

Roy V. Henrickson
Donald Maul
Preston Marx
Murray Gardner

California Regional Primate Center
Davis, California

Simian acquired immunodeficiency syndrome (SAIDS) was first reported in 1982 (1,2). Epizootiological studies have indicated that the disease was present in the primate colony in Davis, California, for many years prior to that time (3). Studies have shown that tissue homogenates and serum from rhesus monkeys (Macaca mulatta) near death are infectious for other monkeys (4,5). A type D retrovirus has been isolated which when inoculated into the same species produces a similar disease syndrome (6-8). In this report we describe the pathogenesis of the disease as it occurs in laboratory raised rhesus monkeys using tissue homogenates or serum which was known to be highly infectious.

ANIMAL MODELS OF RETROVIRUS INFECTION
AND THEIR RELATIONSHIP TO AIDS

325

The 24 animals used in these studies were young juvenile
rhesus monkeys between 8 and 20 months of age. All animals have
been raised in small groups, two to three animals per cage, at
the National Institutes of Health, National Institute of Neurological and Communicative Disorders and Stroke, facilities. No
disease syndrome which is comparable to SAIDS has occurred in
this colony.

All animals were examined clinically for signs of disease.
Blood was obtained from the femoral vein. Total blood counts,
differential and blood chemistries were done before and after
inoculation. For the cellular immune studies blood was collected
in vacutainer tubes (Becton Dickenson). White cells were collected through a Percoll density gradient 1.077. Concanavalin A
(con A), pokeweed mitogen (PWM), phytohemagglutinin (PHA) and
formalinized Staphylococcus aureus Cowan I (SAC) were used as
T and B nonspecific mitogens. All mitogen studies were performed
in RPMI containing 50 IU penicillin, 50 μg streptomycin, L-
glutamine and 5% fetal bovine serum. The presence of T4, T8,
T11 and Ia markers were detected using an indirect fluorescent
antibody technique with Ortho antihuman monoclonal antibodies
and an Ortho FC 200/4800 cytofluorograph.

SAIDS was readily transmitted with tissue homogenates or
serum from acutely ill animals. All 24 animals developed signs
of SAIDS. SAIDS was diagnosed if the animal had four or more of
the following signs: anemia, neutropenia, persistent lymphopenia,
weight loss, diarrhea unresponsive to treatment, splenomegaly,
lymphadenopathy, histological evidence of lymphoid depletion,
chronic infection unresponsive to treatment, opportunistic
infections, tumors and death.

The source of the SAIDS virus used at NIH is presented in
Table I. Davis 1 and 2 were tissues from two different monkeys
with SAIDS and were received from the California Primate Research
Center, Davis (CRPC) in November, 1982. Each inoculum represents

TABLE I.   SAIDS Inocula Virulence Used at NIH

Inoculum	No. dead/ No. inoculated
Tissue Homogenates	
Davis 1	1/2
Davis 1 into NIH monkey (pool 748)	6/8
Davis 2	2/2
Serum	
Davis 3	2/2
Davis 3 into NIH monkey (pool A)	6/10

tissue obtained from a monkey near death. Individual homogenates were made from tissues and each inoculated into two monkeys. One monkey inoculated with Davis 1 (monkey 748) died, and tissue obtained from this monkey was homogenated and inoculated into eight monkeys, six of which died within 1 year after inoculation. The other two monkeys inoculated with this pool and the other monkey inoculated with Davis 1 have remained healthy for over 24 months. Both of the monkeys inoculated with Davis 2 died.

Davis 3 was obtained from CRPC as fresh serum in April, 1983, from an animal dying of acute SAIDS disease. This serum was inoculated into two monkeys and both developed acute signs of disease. In the terminal stages, both animals were exsanguinated, serum collected, dispensed into 1 ml amounts and stored at -70°C. This serum was labeled pool A. Aliquots from pool A were inoculated into 10 monkeys, six of which have died. In total, 70% of the 24 animals inoculated have died.

The time interval from inoculation until death is presented in Table II. Ten of the 24 inoculated monkeys (41.6%) died within 3 months after inoculation. Five of 24 (20.8%) died 4 to 6 months after inoculation. Two monkeys of 24 (8.2%) died 6 to 12 months

TABLE II.   Interval Until Death of Rhesus Monkeys
Inoculated with SAIDS

Months post inoculation	No. of animals that died	No. of animals alive	% of total dead	Cumulative % dead
1-3	10	0	41.6	41.6
4-6	5	0	20.8	62.5
7-9	1	2	4.1	66.6
10-12	1	0	4.1	70.8
>12	0	5	0	70.8

after inoculation and 8 of 24 (30%) of the inoculated monkeys
have survived over 1 year. The inoculum used did not influence
the death rate.

Three types of disease syndrome were recognized and are presented in Table III. Acute disease occurred in 41% of the animals. These monkeys died within 3 months. Death was associated
with anemia, acute septicemia or other viral infections. The
animals with subacute disease (29%) developed acute signs of illness which was followed by a slow progressive disease with death
occurring 4 to 12 months after inoculation. The initial signs did
not appear to be as severe as these animals developed several
relapses with chronic or opportunistic diseases before death.
Eight of the animals (30%) developed a chronic disease form. They
recovered from the initially mild disease and for over 1 year
they had only minimal evidence of clinical disease such as
splenomegalia or lymphadenopathy.

The hematological changes associated with these three types
of disease are shown in Figures 1 to 3. Leukocytopenia, lymphocytopenia, neutropenia and anemia were characteristic in all
three types of disease. The degree of involvement, especially
anemia, was associated with the severity of infection. Animals

TABLE III. Response of Rhesus Monkey
to Inoculation of Virulent Virus

1. Acute disease with rapid death

2. Subacute disease with late death

3. Chronic disease with long time survival and minimal
    evidence of clinical disease

that died shortly after inoculation with an acute disease
developed severe anemia and the anemia was one of the primary
causes of death (Fig. 1). Animals which died with a subacute
disease developed severe anemia but seemed to recover from the
anemia and died of secondary infections 4 to 12 months after
inoculation. Other hematological changes such as leukocytopenia
and neutropenia were also less severe (Fig. 2). Animals that
developed the chronic disease had minimal hematological changes.
They recovered rapidly and resisted secondary infections
(Fig. 3).

Alterations in lymphocyte helper/suppressor markers similar
to that observed in AIDS were not found in infected rhesus
monkeys. The T4/T8 ratios remained normal in infected animals
regardless of clinical outcome. The total number of T11 cells
decreased in direct proportion to the total white cells. The
number of lymphocytes with the Ia markers decreased significantly
in monkeys that were near death.

All animals tested developed an impaired cellular immune
response 4 to 6 weeks after inoculation. The T cell nonspecific
mitogen response stimulated by PHA and con A, the T cell-
dependent B cell responses stimulated by PWM and the B cell
response stimulated by SAC were all reduced. For animals that
died in the acute stage of the disease, the cellular immune
reactions remained decreased. In those animals that survived the

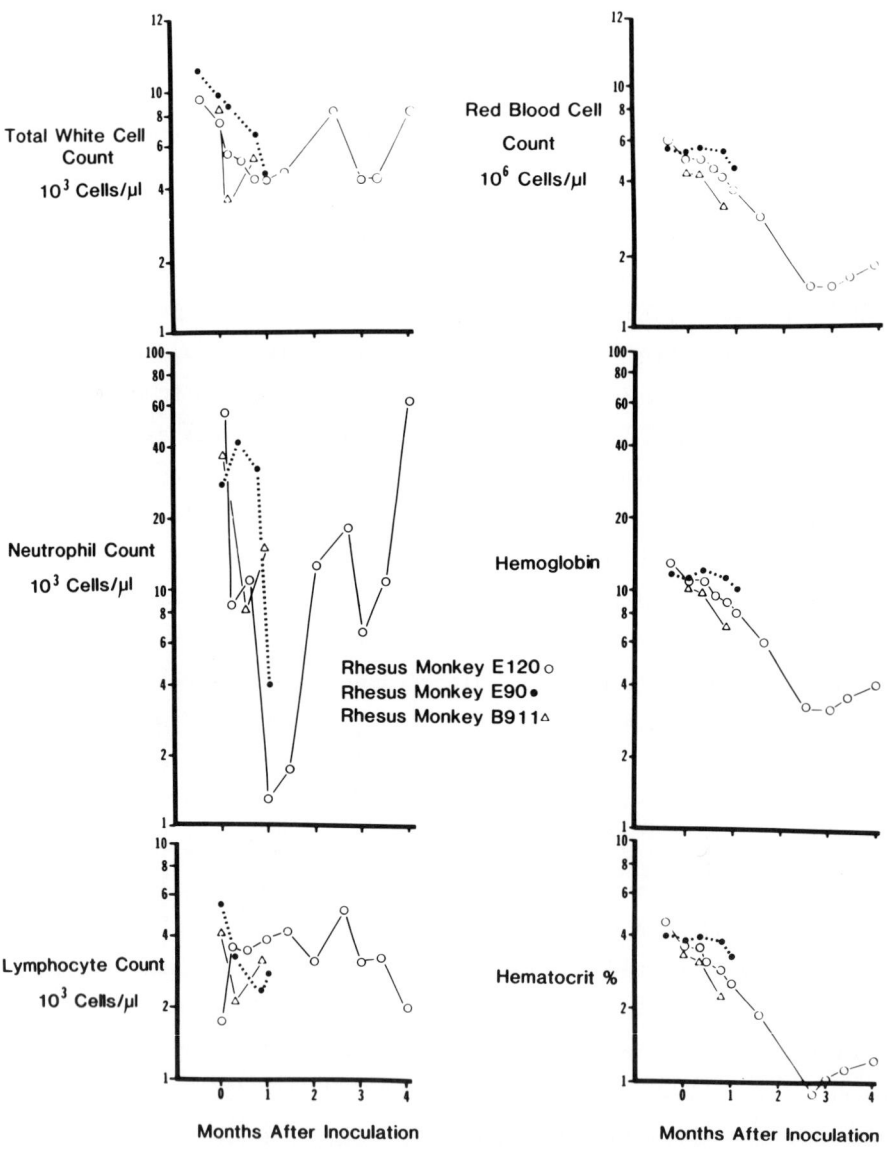

Fig. 1. Hematological values of SAIDS monkeys which developed <u>acute</u> disease.

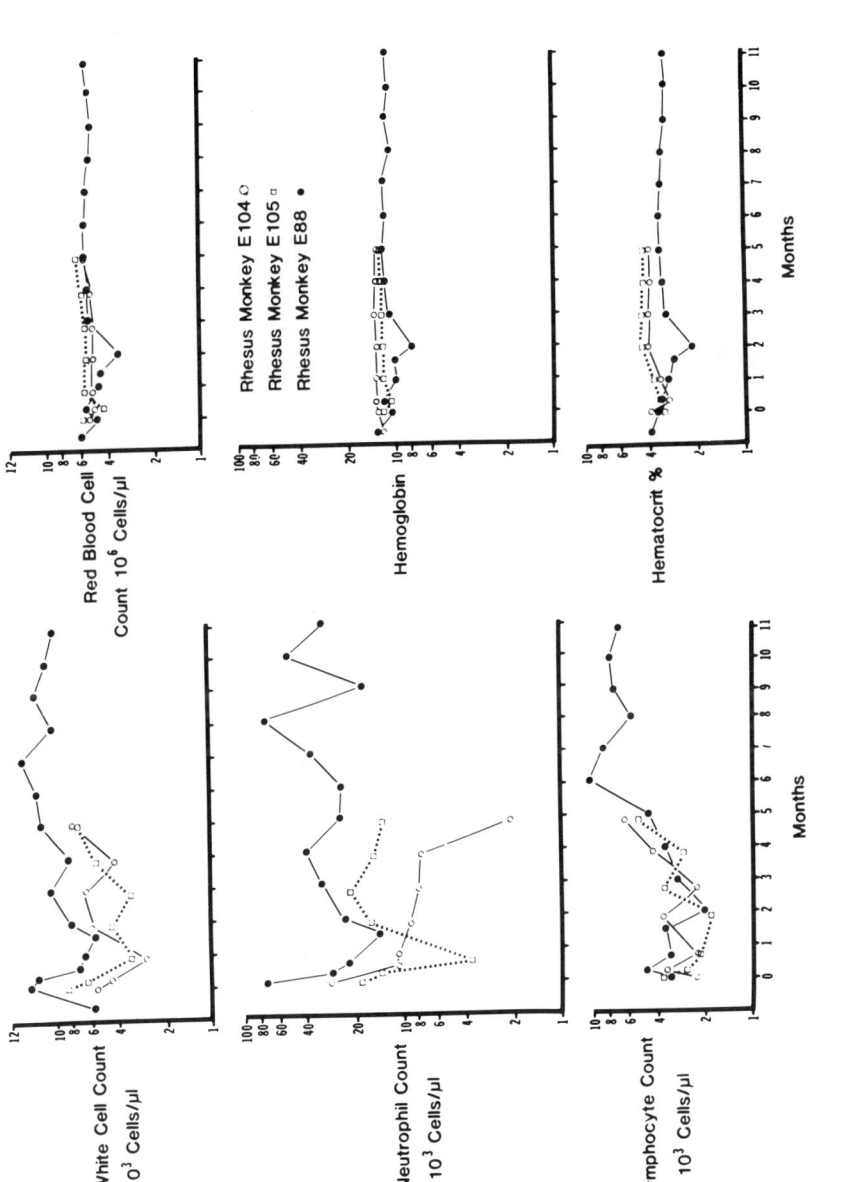

Fig. 2. Hematological values of SAIDS monkeys which developed subacute disease.

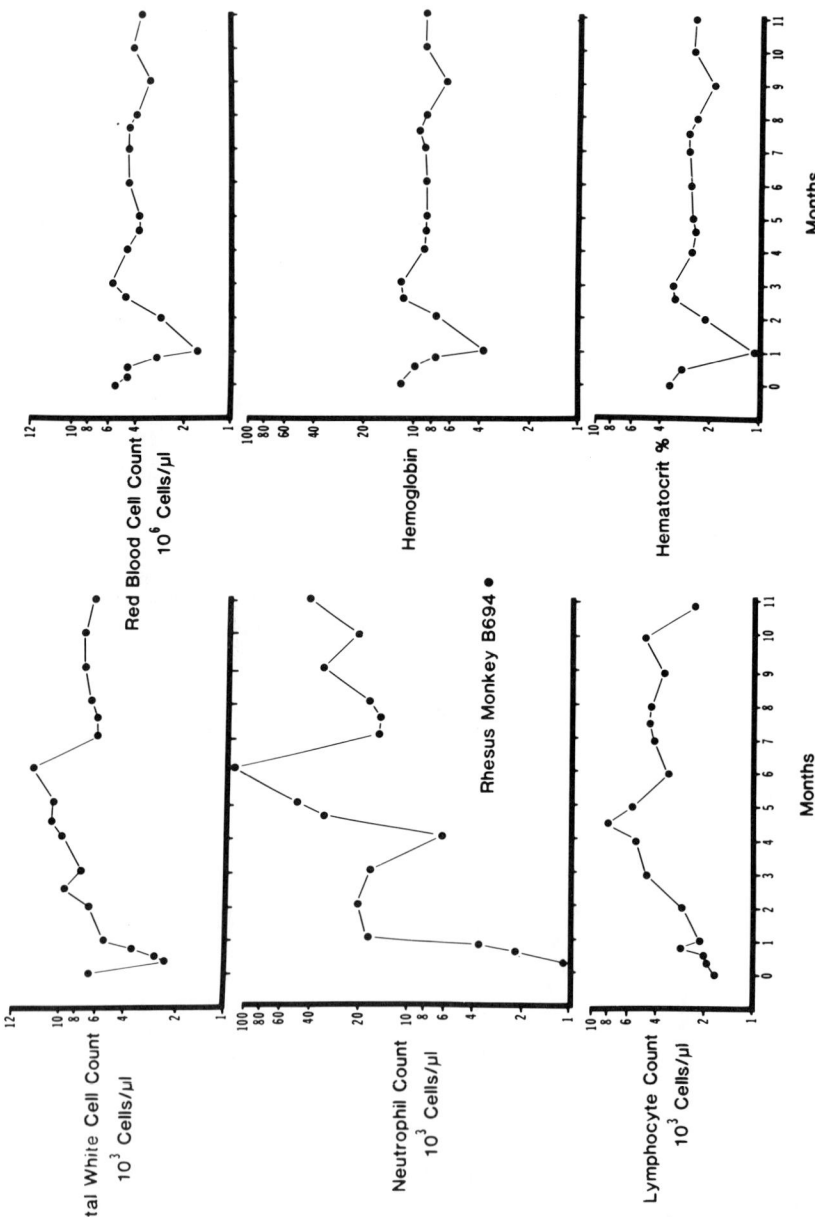

Fig. 3. Hematological values of SAIDS monkeys which developed chronic disease.

initial disease process, the cellular immune response returned
to a normal response level. The cellular immune response would
again decrease only when the animals were acutely ill and near
death. Because of wide variation in individual monkeys, random
determination of the number of cells with lymphocyte markers
could not be accurately interpreted until the animals reached a
terminal stage and gross signs of disease were evident.

From these studies we can conclude that 70% of the monkeys
died within 1 year after inoculation. Three stages of disease
could be recognized: 1) an acute disease with rapid death, 2) a
subacute disease with death occurring 4 to 6 months after the
initial stage and 3) a chronic disease in which the animals survived for 1 year. All of the animals developed anemia, leukocytopenia, neutropenia and impaired cellular immunity 2 to 4 weeks
after inoculation. The more severe the hematological changes the
more acutely the animals died. The reason why some animals survived and others showed acute or subacute disease has not been
identified.

REFERENCES

1. Henrickson, R.V., Maul, D.H., Osborn, K.G. et al. (1983).
   Lancet 1, 388.
2. Letvin, N.L., Eaton, K.A., Aldrich, W.R. et al. (1983). Proc.
   Natl. Acad. Sci. 80, 2718.
3. Henrickson, R.V., Maul, D.H., Lerche, N.W. et al. (1984).
   Lab. Anim. Sci. 34, 140.
4. London, W.T., Madden, D.L., Gravell, M. et al. (1983). Lancet
   2, 869.
5. Gravell, M., London, W.T., Houff, S.A. et al. (1984). Science
   223, 74.
6. Gravell, M., London, W.T., Hamilton, R.S. et al. (1984).
   Lancet 1, 334.
7. Marx, P.A., Maul, D.H., Osborn, K.G. et al. (1984). Science
   223, 1083.
8. Daniel, M.D., King, N.W., Letvin, N.L. et al. (1984). Science
   223, 602.

ASSOCIATION OF RETROPERITONEAL FIBROMATOSIS WITH TYPE D RETROVIRUSES

Raoul E. Benveniste
Kurt Stromberg

Laboratory of Viral Carcinogenesis
National Cancer Institute
Frederick Cancer Research Facility
Frederick, Maryland

William R. Morton
Che-Chung Tsai

Regional Primate Research Center
University of Washington
Seattle, Washington

W. Ellis Giddens, Jr.

Division of Animal Medicine and Department of Pathology
School of Medicine, University of Washington
Seattle, Washington

INTRODUCTION

Retroviruses have been implicated in several recent outbreaks of neoplastic disease accompanying immunosuppressive syndromes at various regional primate centers. All of the known endogenous and infectious primate retroviruses are listed in Table I. Endogenous retroviruses have been obtained from six species of primates; the properties of this class of viruses is shown in Table II. The infectious retroviruses include a type C isolate obtained from a

TABLE I. Endogenous and Infectious Primate Retrovirus Isolates

	New World monkeys	Old World monkeys		Apes
		Cercopithecinae	Colobinae	
Endogenous				
Oncornavirus type C	Owl	Baboon Macaques	Colobus	
Oncornavirus type D	Squirrel		Langur	
Infectious				
Oncornavirus type C	Woolly			Gibbon
Oncornavirus type D		Macaques		
Lentivirus		Macaque		Man
Spumavirus	Spider Squirrel	Macaques African Green		Chimpanzee

TABLE II.   Characteristics of Endogenous Retroviruses

---

1. Present in the cellular DNA of all somatic and germ cells of all animals of the species of origin.

2. Vertically transmitted from parent to offspring; may be used as an evolutionary index of genetic distance.

3. Present as multigene families--10 to 100 copies per haploid genome. These multiple copies seem to evolve more rapidly than other cellular genes; useful as an indicator of taxonomic relationships among closely related species.

4. Generally not infectious for cells of the same species but may replicate readily in cells of heterologous species.

5. Retroviruses have been transmitted between vertebrate species that are only remotely related phylogenetically, with subsequent incorporation into the germ line. They may, thus, serve to transfer genes between sympatric species.

6. Not pathogenic.

---

woolly monkey fibrosarcoma (1), and a group of closely related type C viruses isolated from gibbons (2,3) which have been shown to cause myelogenous leukemias and lymphosarcomas in these apes (4). Infectious type D isolates include the Mason-Pfizer monkey virus (MPMV) from the rhesus monkey carcinoma (5), and related isolates obtained from various species of macaques with an acquired immunosuppression syndrome (6-8). The infectious human viruses include the human T cell lymphotropic virus type I (HTLV-I) and -II isolates, which have been obtained predominantly from patients with T cell malignancies (9), and isolates from patients with the acquired immune deficiency syndrome (AIDS): lymphadenopathy-associated virus (LAV) (10) and HTLV-III (11). These AIDS viruses are classified in the lentivirus class of retroviruses (12). Primate viruses closely related to HTLV-I have also been obtained from Old World monkey species (13,14), and a lymphotropic virus related to HTLV-III (STLV-III) has recently

been isolated from a rhesus with malignant lymphoma (6,15). In
addition, various serotypes of foamy virus have been isolated
from primates (reviewed in Ref. 16). The general properties of
these infectious retroviruses are listed in Table III.

This report will focus on the infectious type D retroviruses
that have been isolated at the University of Washington primate
center and on their association with disease in that colony.

DISEASE AT THE WASHINGTON PRIMATE RESEARCH CENTER (WPRC)

The WPRC was established in 1962, and in 1976, a peculiar
fibroproliferative syndrome called retroperitoneal fibromatosis
(RF) was first recognized (17-19). RF at WPRC is characterized
by an aggressive proliferation of highly vascular fibrous tissue
subjacent to the peritoneum and usually involving the ileocecal
junction and associated mesenteric lymph nodes (Table IV). The
fibrous tissue may regress, remain localized or extend throughout the abdominal and pleural cavities. Some animals develop
multiple lesions subcutaneously rather than in the usual abdominal location. Despite the aggressive local infiltration, the
cellular morphology of most lesions lack the characteristic
anaplasia and high mitotic index seen in fibrosarcoma (19).

RF has been observed in 82 macaques from 1976 to 1983
(Table V), including pigtailed macaques (M. nemestrina, the
principal species maintained in the colony) M. fascicularis,
M. fuscata and M. mulatta (18-20). The incidence of RF was
approximately 1% in all four species of macaques and there were
no differences in the incidence by sex (20). RF occurs predominantly in younger animals; the incidence is 5.7% in macaques
1 to 2 years old, and 3.4% in animals 2 to 3 years old, but less
than 1.0% in age groups of under 1 year and over 3 years.

Macaques affected with RF show a syndrome characterized by
recurrent diarrhea, progressive weight loss, lymphocytopenia,

TABLE III. Properties of Infectious Retroviruses

1. Present only in the cellular DNA of infected animals.

2. Present as only a few (1 to 2) copies of proviral DNA per cell.

3. Horizontally transmitted among members of a species.

4. Generally infectious for cells of the same species.

5. Often pathogenic.

TABLE IV. Retroperitoneal Fibromatosis

1. Aggressive proliferation of highly vascular fibrous tissue in the abdominal cavity or, rarely, in the subcutis.

2. Often accompanied by profound immunodeficiency with lymphocytopenia, thymic and lymphoid atrophy, persistent diarrhea and wasting.

TABLE V. Retroperitoneal Fibromatosis
Washington Primate Research Center
1976-1983

Species	Cases RF	Incidence
M. nemestrina	77/8620	0.9%
M. fascicularis	2/1700	0.1%
M. fuscata	1/104	1.0%
M. mulatta	2/491	0.4%

TABLE VI.   Clinical Observations in 36 Cases of RF
and 36 Matched Controls

	RF cases		Controls	
Category	No.	%	No.	%
Diarrhea	34	94	11	30
Mesenteric lymphadenopathy	34	94	0	
Hypoproteinemia (protein <6 gm/100 ml)	24	67	3	8
Weight loss (>10%)	18	50	0	
Pneumonia (clinical)	15	42	6	17
Lymphocytopenia (<2000 cells/ml)	13	36	1	3
Necrotic/ulcerative gingivitis (noma)	5	14	0	

lymphadenopathy and unusual opportunistic infections (predominantly bacterial pathogens) (Table VI; 19). Histologically, there
is marked thymic atrophy, follicular and paracortical atrophy of
lymph nodes and variable myeloid and lymphoid hyperplasia in
bone marrow. Most animals in the latter stages of illness showed
marked immunodeficiency as evidenced by depressed mitogen
responses of peripheral blood mononuclear cells, as well as failure to mount normal antibody responses to the T cell-dependent
antigen, bacteriophage ϕX 174 (8,21). These animals are thus
similar in many ways to patients with AIDS (22,23), and also
resemble macaques with similar syndromes at the New England (24,
25) and California (26) primate centers. RF has similarities to
Kaposi's sarcoma which is often present in AIDS (27).

The case fatality rate of RF was 98% with a course of about
2 years. The leading cause of death was due directly to RF
lesions in 43% of cases, to enterocolitis in 36%, septicemia in
12%, amyloidosis in 5% and malignant lymphoma in 2% (19). A

comparison of the occurrence of RF in colony-born and feral
animals imported into the colony reveals that the minimum incubation period for natural exposure is about 9 months.

INOCULATION OF MACAQUES WITH RF TISSUES

Experimental intraperitoneal inoculation of M. nemestrina and
M. fascicularis in two separate experiments with suspensions of
RF tissue resulted in an immunosuppressive syndrome in 5 of 16
macaques and RF in 3 of 16 animals (19). Inoculation of RF tissue
into nude mice, hamsters and marmosets (Saguinus labiatus) did
not result in disease. These studies suggested that an infectious
agent might be involved in RF and immunosuppression among
macaques at WPRC.

ISOLATION AND CHARACTERIZATION OF TYPE D RETROVIRUSES FROM THE
WPRC

In order to isolate the etiologic agent of RF at the WPRC,
RF tissue from immunodeficient rhesus monkey was cocultivated
with mammalian cells known to support the replication of a wide
variety of primate viruses. A retrovirus, which morphologically
resembled a type D isolate, was obtained after cocultivation with
canine, human, rhesus, bat and mink cells (8). Viral replication
was detected by assaying for an Mg^{2+}-dependent reverse transcriptase activity in cell culture supernatant fluids. Electron
microscopic examination of the virus revealed typical type D
viral particles, similar to the prototype type D virus MPMV (8).
Type D retroviruses, also related to MPMV, have been isolated
from the New England (28), California (7) and Oregon (29) primate
centers (see also Table VII).

The host range of all known type D retroviruses was compared
to that of retrovirus-D/Washington (R-D/W) (Table VIII). As is

TABLE VII.   Retrovirus Isolates
Regional Primate Research Centers

Location	Species	Disease Immuno-deficiency	RF	Isolate
University of Washington	M. nemestrina	+	+	Type D
	M. mulatta	+	+	Type D
	M. fascicularis	+	+	Type D
	M. fuscata	+	+	Type D
University of California	M. mulatta	+	-	Type D
New England	M. cyclopis	+	-	Type D
	M. mulatta	+	-	Type D
	M. mulatta	+	-	STLV-III
Oregon	M. nigra	+	+	Type D

TABLE VIII. Host Range of Type D Retroviruses

Cell line	R-D/W	MPMV	Langur	SMRV
Monolayer				
Human adenocarcinoma (A549)	+	+	+	+
Canine thymus (FCf2Th)	+	+	+	+
Mink lung (MvlLu)	+	+	+	+
Bat lung (TblLu)	+	+	+	+
Rhesus lung (DBS)	+	+	-	+
Cat fibroblasts (FeC)	-	-	-	-
Lymphocytes				
Macaque PBL	+	+	-	NT[a]
Baboon PBL	+	+	+	NT
Marmoset (70N2)	-	-	-	NT
Human T cell (HUT 78)	+	+	-	NT
Human B cell (RAJ1)	+	+	-	NT

[a]Not tested.

TABLE IX.   Nucleic Acid Homology Primate Type D Retroviruses

| Viral RNA | [^{3}H]DNA transcripts--% hybrids | | | |
	R-D/W	Langur	MPMV	SMRV
R-D/W	100	33	36	4
Langur	37	100	35	3
MPMV	39	30	100	4
SMRV	2	2	3	100

evident, this isolate replicates well in a wide variety of mammalian monolayer cell lines, in peripheral blood lymphocytes isolated from macaques and baboons and in several human lymphocyte lines such as RAJI (a human Burkitt lymphoma cell line) and Hut 78, a T cell tumor line, although titers are much lower in this latter cell line.

Molecular hybridization experiments performed with a [^{3}H]DNA probe prepared from the R-D/W isolate and the other type D retroviruses revealed that R-D/W, the endogenous langur type D virus and MPMV are all partially related to each other (Table IX), but do not share any detectable homology, under the hybridization conditions employed, with the squirrel monkey retrovirus, an endogenous type D virus of New World monkeys (30). The cellular DNA of several primate species was also tested for nucleic acid sequence homology to the R-D/W virus. Table X shows that the highest degree of homology was obtained with DNA from the Colobinae subfamily of Old World monkeys, especially langur DNA. The cellular DNA from all Old World monkeys belonging to the subfamily Cercopithecinae (macaques are members of this subfamily) hybridize approximately 35% to the viral probe. Cellular DNA extracted from the RF tissue of a M. nemestrina with RF hybridized 92%, revealing the presence of R-D/W viral sequences in RF DNA

TABLE X. R-D/W—Related Sequences in Primate DNA

Species	Tissue	% Hybrid
Old World Monkeys		
Colobinae		
Langur	Testes	51
Colobus	Liver	42
Cercopithecinae		
Pig-tailed macaque	Liver	35
Rhesus	Liver	34
Lion-tailed macaque	Spleen	33
African green	Spleen	38
Baboon	Testes	36
Pig-tailed macaque	RF	92
Apes and Man		
Gibbon	Spleen	2
Human	Spleen	1
New World Monkeys		
Squirrel	Spleen	3
Nonprimates		
Mouse	Liver	2
Dog	Liver	6
Cow	Thymus	1

superimposed on the baseline level of partially related endogenous sequences that are present in normal macaque cellular DNA.

PROBABLE ORIGIN OF R-D/W

The high extent of hybridization of R-D/W viral DNA to
langur DNA suggests that this virus, like MPMV, may have arisen
from an endogenous langur virus or another closely related Asian
Colobinae (31). Southeast Asia, where both macaques and langurs
reside, may thus be a reservoir for these retroviruses (Table
XI).

TABLE XI.   Probable Origin of R-D/W

---

1. Related virogene sequences in <u>all</u> Old World monkeys (Cercopithecinae and Colobinae subfamilies).

2. Highest final extent of hybridization to Colobinae subfamily (especially langur cellular DNA).

3. Related endogenous type D virus isolated from langurs.

4. R-D/W originated from Asian Colobinae--now horizontally
   transmitted among certain Asian primates.

During the course of evolution, retroviruses have been transferred between vertebrate species that are only remotely related
phylogenetically (32). There have now been several documented
examples of retrovirus transfer, including transfers from ancestors of primates to ancestors of carnivores, from rodents to carnivores, from rodents to primates, from rodents to artiodactyls,
from primates to primates and from primates to birds (for a
review, see Ref. 33). In those cases where the tranferred virus
is incorporated into the germ line and transmitted as normal
cellular genes, the viruses no longer seem to produce disease
(Table XII). In those cases where the acquired retrovirus is
still infectious and not genetically transmitted, the viruses
often cause disease. The type D viruses discussed here and the
AIDS retroviral isolates (HTLV-III and LAV) are examples of
transmitted retroviruses that have not yet become endogenous.

ASSOCIATION OF RF AND RETROVIRUS ISOLATION AT THE WPRC

A total of 41 separate type D retroviruses have now been
obtained from the WPRC (Table XIII). Twenty-one of these isolates
were from RF tissues or plasma obtained from four species of
macaques (<u>M</u>. <u>nemestrina</u>, <u>M</u>. <u>fascicularis</u>, <u>M</u>. <u>mulatta</u> and

TABLE XII. Transmission of Retrovirus Genes Between Species

Donor	Recipient	Genetically transmitted in recipient	Disease
Primate (Old World monkey)	Cat ancestor (RD-114)	Yes	—
Primate (New World monkey)	Skunk ancestor	Yes	—
Rodent (mouse ancestor)	Pig ancestor (PK-15)	Yes	—
Rodent (? ancestor)	Mink ancestor	Yes	—
Rodent (rat ancestor)	Cat ancestor (FeLV)	No	Leukemia
Rodent (Asian Mus species)	Primates (gibbon)	No	Lymphosarcoma
Primate (Old World monkey)	Primates (MPMV)	No	Immunosuppression
	(R-D/w)	No	RF
?	Cattle (BLV)	No	Lymphosarcoma
?	Sheep (VISNA)	No	CNS, pneumonitis
?	Goats (CAEV)	No	CNS, arthritis
?	Horses (EIAV)	No	Anemia
?	Man (HTLV-I, -II)	No	T cell malignancies
?	(AIDS viruses)	No	AIDS

TABLE XIII. Type D Retroviruses Isolated
at the Washington Primate Research Center

Species	Disease	No. of animals	No. viral isolates
M. nemestrina	None (feral imports)	63	0
	RF	18	18
	Lymphoma	4	3
	Immunosuppressive syndrome[a]	8	8
M. fascicularis	RF	1	1
	Immunosuppressive syndrome[a]	2	2
M. mulatta	RF	1	1
	Immunosuppressive syndrome[a]	2	2
M. fuscata	RF	1	1
	Immunosuppressive syndrome[a]	5	5
		(Total)	41

[a]These animals had one or more of the following: significant weight loss, recurrent diarrhea, lymphadenopathy.
M. fuscata, in addition, also frequently had marked petechial
hemorrhages.

M. fuscata). The additional 20 isolates have been obtained from
macaques with recurrent diarrhea, significant weight loss or
lymphadenopathy. Molecular hybridization experiments reveal that
the nonrepetitive cellular DNA of 11 RF tissues tested contain
sequences homologous to R-D/W. This virus has not been isolated
from 63 healthy feral M. nemestrina imported into the colony from
Southeast Asia.

This association between RF and type D retroviruses suggests
that this class of viruses might be responsible for RF in

macaques. A biologically cloned virus, originally isolated from
a rhesus monkey with RF (8) was therefore inoculated intravenously into six 1-year-old M. nemestrina. Four animals have
developed high titers of antibodies to the virus as measured by
radioimmunoassay (RIA) to the major core antigen p27, and have
remained virus free and healthy 16 months after inoculation. The
two other macaques became viremic (10^4 virus particles/ml of
plasma) soon after inoculation. One of these animals died at
5 weeks after experiencing weight loss, enterocolitis, candidiasis and cryptosporidiosis. Histologically, the mesenteric
lymph nodes revealed lymphoid depletion and capsular fibrosis, an
early histological manifestation of RF. The other viremic animal
had palpable abdominal nodes 15 weeks after inoculation; a biopsy
at 26 weeks confirmed the presence of RF. These studies thus
showed that in macaques not mounting a protective antibody
response, RF could be induced after R-D/W inoculation.

A preliminary screening of the healthy macaques at WPRC shows
that the majority of the colony animals have antibodies to the
type D virus (Table XIV). This, together with the fact that feral
animals imported into the colony are antibody and virus negative,
suggests that the type D retroviruses are endemic in the colony
at WPRC and are not being introduced by feral animals on a frequent basis.

CHARACTERIZATION OF TYPE D ISOLATES ISOLATED AT VARIOUS PRIMATE
CENTERS

To better establish the relationship of R-D/W to MPMV, six
structural proteins obtained from each virus have been purified
and compared (34). The proteins purified from each type D retrovirus included p4, p10, p12, p14, p27 and a phosphoprotein designated pp18 for MPMV and pp20 for R-D/W. Amino acid composition
and N-terminal amino acid sequence analysis show that these six

TABLE XIV.   Antibody to R-D/W
Washington Primate Research Center

Species		No. of animals	% Antibody (R/D-W p27)[a]
M. nemestrina	Normal (feral)	63	0
	Normal (colony born)	160	67
	Viremia	8	0
	Viremia + RF	11	0
	Viremia + lymphoma	3	0
M. mulatta	Viremia + RF	1	0
M. fascicularis	Viremia + RF	1	0
M. fuscata	Viremia	7	0

[a]Antibodies to the major viral core antigen (p27) was
measured in plasma by RIA.

proteins of R-D/W are distinct from the homologous proteins of
MPMV but that these proteins from the two viruses share a high
degree of amino acid sequence homology. These results agree with
those obtained by liquid hybridization (8) and by restriction
endonuclease analysis (35) that suggest that these retroviruses
are still distinct members of a closely related family.

The purified proteins from R-D/W were iodinated and used in
RIA to compare the various isolates to each other. Several of the
structural proteins can be shown to be antigenically distinct
among the retrovirus D isolates from the various primate colonies, and can therefore be used to type these isolates
(Benveniste, R.E. and L.O. Arthur, unpublished data).

SUMMARY

Tumors and immunosuppressive disease have occurred in several
species of macaques at various primate centers in the United
States. An outbreak of lymphoma occurred 15 years ago in the
California colony; cases of lymphoma have also been at the New
England, Washington and in other primate colonies. RF has been
observed in large numbers of macaques primarily at the Washington
colony among all their macaque species, and at the Oregon center
among Celebes macaques. At the Washington primate center, the
type D retrovirus present in the colony is strongly associated
with RF. In addition, the ability to cause RF by inoculation of
macaques with biologically cloned virus suggests that this retrovirus may be responsible for RF in macaques.

The recent isolation of a lymphotropic lentivirus at the New
England primate center (6) suggests that this virus may be an
important factor in disease in that colony and perhaps at other
primate centers as well. The role of these and other viruses such
as the primate viruses related to HTLV-I in the etiology of
lymphoma and other primate immunosuppressive diseases remains to
be determined.

The type D retrovirus isolates from the California colony are
associated with an acute form of immunosuppressive disease and
mortality (36), whereas the isolates from the New England primate
center are more often associated with a transient lymphadenopathy
and a decrease in lymphocyte blastogenic responsiveness (37). No
cases of RF have been obtained after inoculation of macaques with
viruses from these two primate colonies. The Washington primate
center isolates, on the other hand, which have been shown to
transform various rodent fibroblast cell lines in vitro, are
strongly associated with RF. Their role in immunosuppression has
not been clearly established. These three isolates, which are
molecularly distinct, are thus associated with different patho-

genicities in vivo. Detailed analyses of molecular clones of these retroviruses may allow the identification of the molecular basis for the heterogeneity in pathogenicities seen in this class of viruses.

REFERENCES

1. Theilen, G.H., Gould, D., Fowler, M. et al. (1971). J. Natl. Cancer Inst. 47, 881.
2. Kawakami, T.G., Huff, S.D., Buckley, P.M. et al. (1972). Nature (New Biol.) 235, 170.
3. Todaro, G.J., Lieber, M.M., Benveniste, R.E. et al. (1975). Virology 67, 335.
4. Kawakami, T.G. and Buckley, P.M. (1974). Transplant. Proc. 6, 193.
5. Chopra, H.C. and Mason, M.M. (1970). Cancer Res. 30, 2081.
6. Daniel, M.D., Letvin, N.L., King, N.W. et al. (1985). Science 228, 1201.
7. Marx, P.A., Maul, D.H., Osborn, K.G. et al. (1984). Science 223, 1083.
8 Stromberg, K., Benveniste, R.E., Arthur, L.O. et al. (1984). Science 224, 289.
9. Poiesz, B.J., Ruscetti, F.W., Gazdar, A.F. et al. (1980). Proc. Natl. Acad. Sci. 77, 7415.
10. Barre-Sinoussi, I.F., Chermann, J.C., Rey, F. et al. (1983). Science 220, 868.
11. Popovic, M., Sarngadharan, M.G., Read, E. et al. (1984). Science 224, 497.
12. Gonda, M.A., Wong-Staal, F., Gallo, R.C. et al. (1985). Science 227, 173.
13. Yamamoto, N., Hinuma, Y., zur Hausen, H. et al. (1983). Lancet 1, 240.
14. Komuro, A., Watanabe, T., Miyoshi, I. et al. (1984). Virology 138, 373.
15. Kanki, P.J., McLane, M.F., King, N.W., Jr. et al. (1985). Science 228, 1199.
16. Hooks, J.J. and Gibbs, C.J., Jr. (1975). Bacteriol. Rev. 39, 169.
17. Giddens, W.E., Jr., Bielitzki, J.T., Morton, W.R. et al. (1979). Lab. Invest. 40, 294.
18. Giddens, W.E., Jr., Morton, W.R., Hefti, E. et al. (1983). In "Viral and Immunological Diseases in Nonhuman Primates" (S.S. Kalter, ed.), p. 249. Alan R. Liss, Inc., New York.
19. Giddens, W.E., Jr., Tsai, C.-C., Morton, W.R. et al. (1985). Ann. J. Pathol. (in press).

20. Tsai, C.-C., Giddens, W.E., Jr., Morton, W.R. et al. (1985).
    Lab. Anim. Sci. (in press).
21. Tsai, C.-C., Giddens, W.E., Jr., Ochs, H.D. et al. (1985).
    Lab. Anim. Sci. (in press).
22. Fauci, A.S. (1982). Ann. Intern. Med. $\underline{96}$, 777.
23. Levy, J.A. and Ziegler, J.L. (1983). Lancet $\underline{2}$, 78.
24. Letvin, N.L., Eaton, K.A., Aldrich, W.R. et al. (1983). Proc.
    Natl. Acad. Sci. $\underline{80}$, 2718.
25. King, N.W., Hunt, R.D. and Letvin, N.L. (1983). Am. J.
    Pathol. $\underline{113}$, 382.
26. Henrickson, R.V., Maul, D.H., Lerche, N.W. et al. (1984).
    Lab. Anim. Sci. $\underline{34}$, 140.
27. Gottlieb, G.J. and Ackerman, A.B. (1982). Hum. Pathol. $\underline{13}$,
    882.
28. Daniel, M.D., King, N.W., Letvin, N.L. et al. (1984). Science
    $\underline{223}$, 602.
29. Shiigi, S.M., Wilson, B.J., Malley, A. et al. (1985).
    J. Clin. Immunopathol. (in press).
30. Heberling, R.L., Barker, S.T., Kalter, S.S. et al. (1977).
    Science $\underline{195}$, 289.
31. Benveniste, R.E. and Todaro, G.J. (1977). Proc. Natl. Acad.
    Sci. $\underline{74}$, 4557.
32. Benveniste, R.E. and Todaro, G.J. (1974). Nature $\underline{252}$, 456.
33. Benveniste, R.E. (1985). In "Molecular Evolutionary Genetics"
    (R.J. MacIntyre, ed.), p. 359. Plenum Publishing Corp., New
    York.
34. Henderson, L.E., Sowder, R., Smythers, G. et al. (1985).
    J. Virol. (in press).
35. Desrosiers, R.C., Daniel, M.D., Butler, C.V. et al. (1985).
    J. Virol. $\underline{54}$, 552.
36. Gardner, M.B. and Marx, P.A. (1985). Adv. Viral. Oncol. $\underline{5}$,
    57.
37. Letvin, N.L., Daniel, M.D., Sehgal, P.K. et al. (1984).
    J. Virol. $\underline{52}$, 683.

NOVEL MECHANISM FOR INDUCTION OF INTERFERON
BY VISNA LENTIVIRUSES: POSSIBLE ROLE OF
THE INTERFERON IN RESTRICTED "SLOW"
REPLICATION AND CHRONIC DISEASE[1]

Opendra Narayan

Departments of Neurology and Comparative Medicine
Johns Hopkins University School of Medicine
Baltimore, Maryland

ABSTRACT

"Slow" diseases caused by lentiviruses in sheep and goats are
associated with an unusual restricted type of virus replication
in macrophages. We show here that the viruses induce an interferon during a unique synergistic interaction between the lenti-
virus-infected macrophages and lymphocytes. No interferon was
produced when either cell type alone was inoculated. The interferon caused a profound restriction of lentivirus replication in
macrophages.

Interferons (INF) are a family of small regulatory proteins
which modify a variety of biologic functions including cell differentiation and proliferation, immune responses and control of
intracellular parasitic replication. Cells produce alpha- and
beta-INF in response to various stimuli including infection
with certain viruses. A third type, gamma-INF, is produced by

---

[1]These studies were supported by grants NS12127, NS15145 and
RR00130 from the National Institutes of Health.

lymphocytes after mitogen stimulation of peripheral blood mononuclear cells (PBMC) and requires interaction of mitogen, monocytes and lymphocytes (1,2).

Although cell cultures infected with retroviruses do not produce INF, we nevertheless considered the ruminant lentivirus subgroup as INF-inducing candidates because these viruses replicate
productively in cell cultures (3), whereas in their animal hosts
they cause persistent infections and replicate at a restricted
level for an indefinite period (4,5) in cells of the macrophage
lineage (6-8). We show here that these lentiviruses do indeed
induce an INF but production occurred only during interaction
between infected macrophages and lymphocytes. Further, the
induced INF was effective 1) in restricting replication in macrophage cultures, 2) in prevention of maturation of monocyte to
macrophages and 3) in prevention of lentivirus-induced fusion of
cell cultures.

Lentiviruses are nononcogenic retroviruses that cause slowly
progressive diseases after unusually long incubation periods.
Visna-maedi virus of sheep and caprine-arthritis-encephalitis
(CAE) virus of goats are prototypes of this group of agents and
cause paralysis, pneumonia, arthritis and mastitis months to
years after initial infection (9). Visna virus shares genetic
sequences with the AIDS lentivirus of humans (10) and has several
parallels in virus host interactions, such as dissemination by
exchange of body fluids, persistent infections (4,11,12), poor
neutralizing antibody responses against the viruses (13,14) and
antigenic variability of the viruses (13-15). Infection with
the ruminant viruses in nature is exogenous and is widespread
although only few animals develop disease (11,16,17). Disease may
occur acutely in newborn animals (18) but more usually it is slow
in onset and progression, manifests as paralysis, dyspnea and
arthritis in adults. Histologic lesions in newborn and adult
animals consist of accumulation of large numbers of macrophages

and mononuclear cells in target organs that include the central
nervous system, lungs and joints (9).

   In preliminary tests to determine the IFN-inducing capacity
of lentiviruses, we inoculated visna and CAE viruses into cultures of sheep choroid plexus (SCP) fibroblasts, goat synovial
membrane cells (GSMC), PBMC and cultures of sheep or goat macrophages. PBMCs were purified from freshly collected blood of sheep
and/or goats by centrifugation on Ficoll-Hypaque gradients and
primary cultures of macrophages were obtained by cultivating
PBMCs in Dulbecco's minimum essential medium (MEM) plus 20% lamb
serum from 1 week during which time the monocytes in the PBMC
matured into monolayers of adherent macrophages (7). A cell line
of sheep alveolar macrophages, transformed with SV40 (T MØ), was
also used (19). Supernatant fluids from inoculated cultures were
tested for IFN activity by determining whether they could protect
cultures of GSMC and T MØ against the lytic effects of challenge
vesicular stomatitis virus (VSV). Table I shows that visna and
CAE viruses did not induce IFN in any of the inoculated cultures.
Positive controls in this experiment included inoculation of
macrophage cultures with parainfluenza virus type 3 (PI-3), a
member of the paramyxovirus group which is used extensively for
production of alpha-IFN (20), and treatment of PBMC suspensions
with concanavalin A (con A) at a concentration of 10 µg/ml, a
procedure commonly used for protection of gamma-IFN (21,22).
After 48 hours of incubation at 37°C, supernatant fluids from the
PI-3 virus/T MØ culture had developed an acid-resistant IFN and
the con A/PBMC culture, an acid-labile IFN (typical of alpha- and
gamma-IFNs, respectively). This confirmed that the cell cultures
infected with lentiviruses did not produce IFN.

   We next attempted to transpose conditions that exist in the
inflammatory lesions in the animal to a cell culture setting to
determine whether IFN could be produced. Since lesions contain
infected macrophages closely associated with lymphocytes, we

TABLE I. Culture Requirements for Lentivirus Induction of IFN

Inducer	Cells	IFN indicator system		Sen. to pH2[a]
		VSV/GSMC	VSV/T MØ	
Visna/CAEV	SCP/GSMC	0	0	
Visna/CAEV	T MØ	0	0	
Visna/CAEV	PBMC	0	0	
PI-3	T MØ	1/160[b]	1/20	1/80
con A	PBMC	1/160	0	1/10
Visna/CAEV	MØ + Lym	1/320	1/320	1/320
Visna/CAEV	GSMC + Lym	0	0	
0	MØ + Lym	0	0	

Various cell cultures (sheep choroid plexus [SCP] fibroblasts, goat synovial membrane cells [GSMC], SV40-transformed
sheep alveolar macrophages [T MØ] or sheep or goat peripheral
blood mononuclear cells [PBMC]) were inoculated with inducers
lentiviruses (visna and caprine-arthritis encephalitis [CAE]
virus), parainfluenza 3 virus (PI-3) or concanavalin A. Supernatant fluids were examined periodically 2 to 10 days later
for IFN activity in the two indicator systems listed.

[a]The pH of supernatant fluids was lowered to pH2 with HCl
overnight at 4°C then returned to neutrality with NaOH before
testing for IFN activity. The lentivirus-IFN, although produced
in part by lymphocytes, was unlike typical gamma-INF in its
resistance to pH2.

[b]Fractions indicate the highest dilution of the fluid which
protected cells in the particular indicator system from lysis
by vesicular stomatitis virus (VSV). The two lentiviruses
induced IFN only in macrophage (MØ)-lymphocyte (Lym) cultures;
the lentivirus-IFN was protective to both GSMC and T MØ cells.

inoculated macrophage cultures with lentiviruses and added fresh
nonadherent lymphocytes to the cultures 2 to 10 days later. As
noted above, no IFN was produced in infected macrophage cultures
and none was produced when normal lymphocytes were added to normal macrophage cultures. However, large amounts of IFN were found
in the supernatant fluids of infected macrophage cultures to
which lymphocytes were added (Table I). The IFN was acid-
resistant and, further, was distinct from IFNs induced by PI-3

virus and con A because it protected macrophages from VSV-induced
lysis. Biological activity of the latter two IFNs was minimal in
the VSV/macrophage system (Table I). Subsequent experiments
showed that other field strains of ovine-caprine lentiviruses
described in a previous report (6) were as efficient as visna and
CAE viruses in IFN induction provided ovine-caprine macrophages
(including T MØ) were used for inoculation and lymphocytes from
either species were added. No IFN was produced if the ruminant
lentiviruses were substituted with bovine leukemia virus. Similarly, no IFN was produced if macrophages or lymphocytes were
substituted with similar types of cells from bovine or other
species. Histocompatibility between sheep-goat cell donors was
not important because goat macrophages reacted with sheep lymphocytes and vice versa. Macrophages were indispensible because
addition of lymphocytes to lentivirus producing GSMC or SCP
fibroblasts did not result in IFN production.

The IFN produced during the interaction between lentivirus-
infected macrophages and lymphocytes occurred in a quantal
manner and depended on synergism between the two cell types
(Fig. 1). IFN was first detected approximately 8 hours after
addition of the lymphocytes and reached peak values between 24
and 48 hours. No new IFN was produced between 48 and 72 hours.
In order to determine whether macrophages or lymphocytes were
the IFN-producing cells, we separated the two cell types at different intervals after co-cultivation and cultured each separately for a further 24 hours. As shown in Figure 1, IFN was
produced in dishes containing either of the separated cell types
but at much lower levels and for a shorter duration than when the
two cell types were cultured continuously together. Although IFN
was produced in the macrophage dishes, this may have been due to
lymphocytes which had become trapped by macrophages and could
not be separated off. Nevertheless, the data show that the production of IFN was most efficient when infected macrophages and

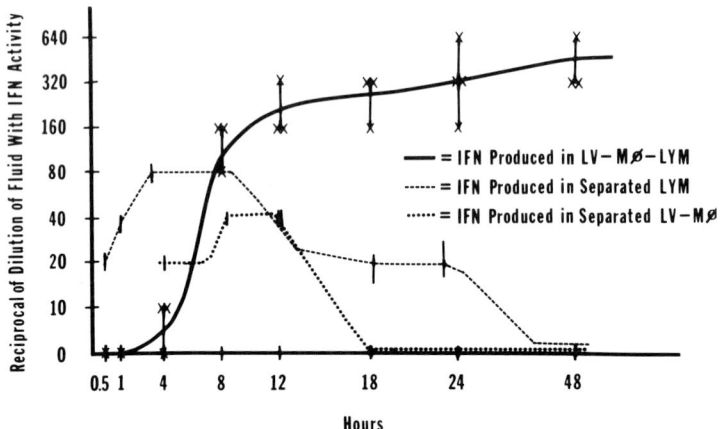

Fig. 1. Shows a burst of INF production in lentivirus (LV)-
infected macrophage (MØ) cultures, hours after lymphocytes (Lym)
were added. Peak production occurred 24 to 48 hours after addition of Lym. In parallel co-cultures, Lym were removed from MØ
cultures at indicated intervals after co-cultivation and cultured
for a further 24 hours. IFN levels in supernatant fluids of each
cell type are indicated at time points when the cultures were
separated. Note synergism between MØ and Lym cultures and low
short-lived production of IFN by individual cell types after
separation.

lymphocytes were in continuous contact. Addition of spent lympho-

cytes (removed from infected macrophage cultures 48 hours after

co-cultivation) to "new" infected macrophages did not result in

IFN production. However, addition of new lymphocytes to "old"

infected macrophages resulted in a new wave of IFN production.

Thus, the IFN-inducing signal acquired by macrophages after

infection with lentiviruses was apparently produced continuously,

and lymphocytes responded to this signal with a single burst of

IFN.

Preliminary investigations of the effect of the lentivirus-

induced IFN on replication of lentivirus showed restriction in

three areas. First, treatment of PBMC with the IFN retarded the

maturation of monocytes to macrophages (Fig. 2A,B). A similar

phenomenon had been observed previously after treating PBMCs
with alpha-IFN (23). This is a potential point of blockade in the
virus replication cycle because patent lentivirus infection in
monocytes becomes productive during the maturational process of
monocytes to macrophages (7). Second, the IFN inhibited fusion of
cells by visna and CAE viruses (Fig. 2C,D). This is a natural
cytopathic effect of lentiviruses in vitro whose pathogenic significance in vivo may be important for virus dissemination from
cell to cell. IFN inhibition of virus-induced fusion has been
reported previously (24,25) for other viruses. Third, the IFN
restricted replication of the virus in macrophages. For example,
in CAE virus-infected cultures, the infectivity titer in supernatant fluids was reduced from 5×10^5 $TCID_{50}$/ml to 1×10^2
$TCID_{50}$/ml when the IFN was added to the culture medium. This supports previous studies by Friedman and coworkers (26,27) showing
that although retroviruses do not induce IFN in infected cell
cultures, replication of the viruses is nevertheless sensitive
to exogenously added IFN.

These studies suggest new insights into the role of INF in
viral diseases. We report a new mechanism for virus induction of
IFN whose production was dependent on, and limited to, a cooperative syngerism between macrophages and lymphocytes. This indirect
system of IFN induction (in which the lentivirus infects a macrophage, which does not produce IFN, but rather produces a signal
for IFN production by lymphocytes) is particularly relevant for
the in vivo environment because it has a potential for amplification and continuity in production (one infected macrophage can
stimulate many lymphocytes to produce IFN) without requirement
for massive production of extracellular virus. In this system,
virus production by the macrophage was not essential for IFN production. Although both virus production and the IFN-inducing
signal by the macrophage were dependent on infection, the two
processes are independent on each other. Maintenance of infection

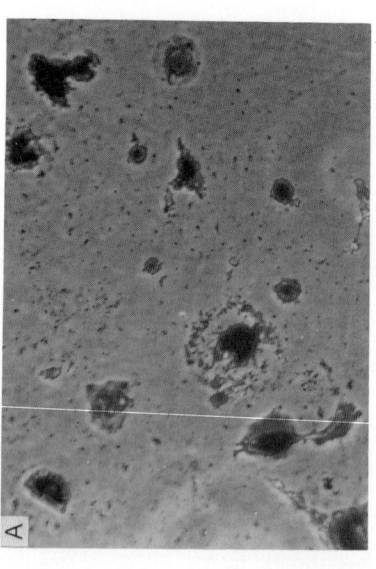

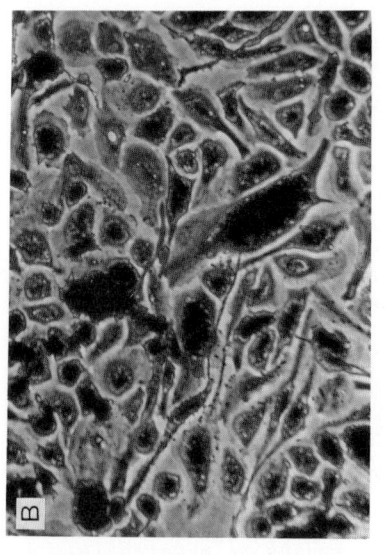

Fig. 2. Peripheral blood mononuclear cells (PBMC) were suspended in Dulbecco's MEM plus 20% heated lamb serum and equal numbers of cells seeded in tissue culture dishes and incubated at 37°C in a CO_2 incubator. Cultures in (A) were given 40 units (1 unit = highest dilution which protected VSV/T MØ cells) of lentivirus-induced IFN preheated at 56°C for 10 minutes to inactivate virus. Note scant macrophage maturation-differentiation in contrast to normal maturation of monocytes to macrophages in (B), 10 days after culture. (C) Extensive fusion in CAE virus-infected GSMC 10 days after inoculation with virus. Parallel cultures treated with 40 units of heated lentivirus-IFN (D) did not develop fusion although the amount of virus infectivity in the two cultures was the same.

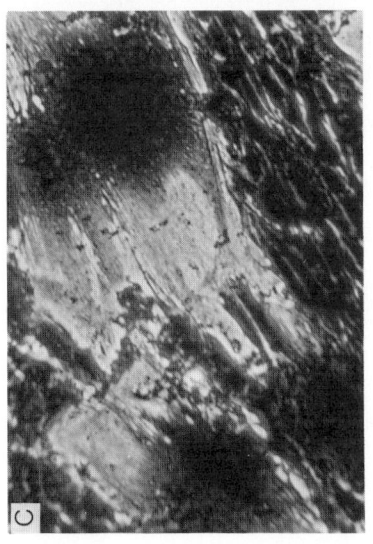

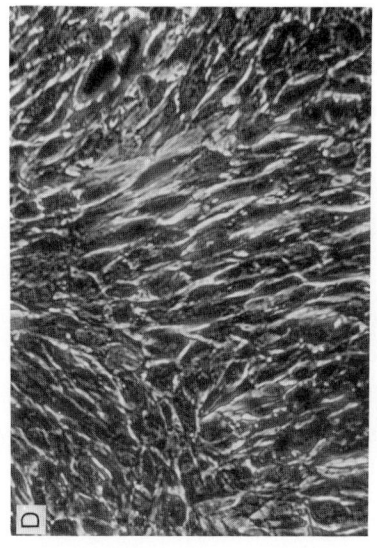

Fig. 2C,D

in macrophages was not dependent on cell-free virus but rather on division and maturation of latently infected pro-macrophages in the bone marrow (8). Presumably, bone marrow cells become infected by circulating, infected macrophages. While IFN that was produced locally may lead to dampening of virus replication in vivo (restricted replication), the IFN could also lead to disturbances in normal immune regulation and cause disease as exemplified by persistent inflammatory lesions in the animal.

Although the cellular interactions leading to IFN production are not understood fully, the requirement for macrophage-lymphocyte cooperation in this new scheme of virus-induced IFN closely resembles conditions required for mitogen-induced gamma-IFN, in contrast to the direct induction of alpha- and beta-INFs in virus-infected cells. The specificities of these cellular reactions and further characterization of the IFN are currently being investigated. The relevance of the study, however, is that if the combined effects of the IFN (restriction of monocyte maturation, prevention of virus-induced fusion and restriction of virus replication in macrophages) were applied in vivo, virus replication in tissue cells would probably be restricted to a level not unlike that found in nature. Since severity of pathologic lesions varies with the extent of lentivirus replication (28), and since all infected animals do not become ill (9), it is conceivable that the fate of the infected animal—whether it develops no disease, slowly progressive disease or rapid onset disease—may depend on its ability to produce IFN of the type described here. Similar mechanisms may be involved in the control of virus replication and pathogenesis of human retrovirus infections. The relevance of this is heightened by the recent isolation of a unique IFN from patients with AIDS (29), a disease also associated with infection with a lentivirus (30).

ACKNOWLEDGMENTS

I thank Darlene Sheffer for technical assistance and Linda Kelly for preparation of the typescript.

REFERENCES

1. Pestka, S. and Baron, S. (1978). Methods Enzymol. 78, 3.
2. Preble, O.T. and Friedman, R.M. (1983). Lab. Invest. 49, 4.
3. Haase, A.T., Stowring, L., Harris, J.D. et al. (1982). Virology 119, 399.
4. Gudnadottir, M. (1974). Prog. Med. Virol. 18, 336.
5. Narayan, O., Griffin, D.E. and Silverstein, A.M. (1977). J. Infect. Dis. 135, 800.
6. Narayan, O., Wolinsky, J.S., Clements, J.E. et al. (1982). J. Gen. Virol. 59, 345.
7. Narayan, O., Kennedy-Stoskopf, S., Sheffer, D. et al. (1983). Infect. Immun. 41, 67.
8. Gendelman, H.E. et al. Proc. Natl. Acad. Sci. (in press).
9. Narayan, O. and Cork, L.C. (1985). Rev. Infect. Dis. 7, 89.
10. Gonda, M., Wong-Staal, F., Gallo, R.C. et al. (1985). Science 227, 173.
11. Crawford, T.B. and Adams, D.S. (1981). J. Am. Vet. Med. Assoc. 178, 713.
12. Popovic, M., Sarngadharen, M.G., Read, E. et al. (1984). Science 224, 497.
13. Narayan, O., Sheffer, D., Griffin, D.E. et al. (1984). J. Virol. 49, 349.
14. Ho, D. et al. (1985). N. Engl. J. Med. 312, 649.
15. Narayan, O., Griffin, D.E., Chase, J. et al. (1977). Science 197, 376.
16. Cutlip, R.C., Jackson, T.A., Laird, G.A. et al. (1977). Am. J. Vet. Res. 38, 2091.
17. DeBoer, G.F. et al. (1979). Res. Vet. Sci. 26, 202.
18. Cork, L.C., Hadlow, W.J., Crawford, T.B. et al. (1974). J. Infect. Dis. 129, 134.
19. Gendelman, H.E. et al. Lab. Invest. (in press).
20. Marcus, P.I., Svitlik, C. and Sekellick, M.J. (1983). J. Gen. Virol. 64, 2419.
21. Wheelock, E.F. (1965). Science 149, 310.
22. Green, J.H. et al. (1969). Science 164, 1415.
23. Lee, J.H.S. and Epstein, L.B. (1980). Cell. Immunol. 50, 177.
24. Chatterjee, S. and Hunter, E. (1980). Virology 104, 487.
25. Chatterjee, S., Cheung, H. and Hunter, E. (1982). Proc. Natl. Acad. Sci. 79, 835.

26. Friedman, R.M. and Ramseur, J.M. (1974). Proc. Natl. Acad.
    Sci. 71, 354.
27. Friedman, R.M., Chang, E.H., Ramseur, J.M. et al. (1975).
    J. Virol. 16, 569.
28. Narayan, O. et al. (1984). In "Symposium on Viruses and
    Demyelineating Diseases" (C.A. Mims, M.L. Cuzner and R.E.
    Kelly, eds.), p. 125. Academic Press, New York.
29. Eyster, M.E., Goedert, J.J., Poon, M.C. et al. (1983).
    N. Engl. J. Med. 309, 583.
30. Vilmer, E., Barré-Sinoussi, F., Rouzioux, C. et al. (1984).
    Lancet 1, 753.

VACCINES AND IMMUNOTHERAPY

IMMUNOLOGICAL MECHANISMS
IN RETROVIRAL LEUKEMOGENESIS[1]

James N. Ihle

NCI-Frederick Cancer Research Facility
Frederick, Maryland

INTRODUCTION

The potential approaches for immunological manipulation of
retroviral infections are many, and the potential effects are
equally varied. In this chapter I would like to take the opportunity to review briefly some of the experiments in murine model
systems and to consider in some detail the mechanisms that appear
to be involved in some of the unexpected effects associated with
immune responses against retroviruses.

Several years ago, in collaboration with Drs. W. Schaffer,
D. Bolognesi and P. Fischinger, a series of experiments were
initiated to examine the effects of immunizing mice with the
major envelope glycoprotein of Friend murine leukemia virus
(FLV). In BALB/c mice, immunization resulted in the induction of
a transient, antigen-specific T cell response which was detectable in blastogenesis assays and subsequently the induction of
neutralizing antibodies. When these mice were subsequently challenged with FLV-spleen focus-forming virus (SFFV) they were found

[1]Research sponsored by contract N01-CO-23909 at Litton
Bionetics, Inc., Frederick, Maryland.

to be completely resistent to erythroleukemia induction (1).
Although the best protection was observed with gp70, some protection was also obtained by immunization with p15E or p30. The
results therefore were those expected and demonstrate that protective immunity can be induced against murine retroviruses.

   In the same series of experiments, C57BL/6 mice were immunized with FLV gp70 and were shown to develop an immune response
which was comparable to that observed with BALB/c mice (2). When
these mice were irradiated, to induce leukemia, there was no
detectable affect of the immunization on the incidence or latency
of leukemia. This was unexpected based on the hypothesized role
of endogenous retroviruses in radiation-induced leukemia and
consequently supported the concept that there is no etiological
relationship between endogenous retroviruses and radiation-
induced leukemia.

   Finally, the effects of immunizing AKR mice with FLV gp70
were examined (3). In these mice, FLV-specific antibodies were
detectable following immunization. In contrast to the expected
result, however, immunization of these mice dramatically accel-
erated the appearance of spontaneous leukemias by 2 to 3 months.
From these studies, therefore it became apparent that immunization with retroviral proteins could have quite different consequences on leukemogenesis. In the next sections I would like to
focus on the possible mechanisms in the latter result. Namely,
the ability of an immune response to exacerbate conditions that
predispose for leukemia.

Immune Response as a Determinant of Leukemogenesis

   The ability of an immune response to be a determining factor
in leukemogenesis has been most clearly demonstrated in studies
using CBA/N mice. In the initial studies (4,5) it was observed
that CBA/N mice were resistant to leukemia induction by Moloney
leukemia virus (MoLV). In contrast MoLV induces a high incidence

TABLE I.   Correlation of Immune Responses and Leukemia

Parameter examined	BALB/c	CBA/N
Parental virus (FFU/ml)	3.6×10^5	1.7×10^6
Recombinant virus (FFU/ml)	2.1×10^3	1.1×10^4
T cell response to gp70 (no./total)	8/10	1/10
T cell response to p12 (no./total)	6/10	1/10
Fold increase in lymphokine responsive cells	20-500	<2
Leukemia incidence at 9 months	10/10	0/10

of leukemia with a short latency in BALB/c mice. In comparing the virological parameters, the resistence of CBA/N mice was found to not be due to lack of replication of the parental or recombinant viruses as summarized in Table I. The only correlation which existed was the apparent absence of an immune response against MoLV as evaluated by the lack of either antibodies against the virus or helper T cells which could be detected in blastogenesis assays against viral proteins. These results therefore suggested the unusual possibility that the resistance to leukemia was due to the inability to develop an immune response and conversely suggested that an immune response may be required for leukemogenesis.

The possible ways in which an immune response can contribute to leukemogenesis have come from studies characterizing the function of antigen-specific helper T cells. In MoLV-inoculated BALB/c mice, $Thy-1^+$, $Lyt-1^+,2^-$ helper T cells which react with gp70 and p12 are detectable in blastogenesis assays. The conditions and concentrations of viral proteins required are comparable to those observed in viremic mice. Moreover viral antigen-reactive T cells are present until the onset of leukemia. Over

TABLE II. Properties of T Cell-Derived Lymphokines

Property	IL-2	IL-3	GM-CSF
Apparent molecular weight	15, 30 kd	28 kd	23 kd
Protein molecular weight	16 kd	15 kd	14 kd
Chromosomal location (murine)	——	11	11
Primary source of production	T cells	T cells	T cells
Lineages affected	T, B	G, M, mast, E, T	G, M

the past several years, one of the primary functions of helper
T cells has been shown to be the production of lymphokines as a
consequence of antigen stimulation. Indeed, in the case of gp70-
induced blastogenesis, it has been shown that the majority of
the proliferation observed is due to the response of secondary
cells to the lymphokines produced (6). Consequently in vivo in
viremic mice the high levels of viral antigens might be expected
to chronically stimulate helper T cells to produce lymphokines.

The properties of some of the lymphokines produced by activated T cells are summarized in Table II. Perhaps the best known
lymphokine is interleukin 2 (IL-2). This factor was detected by
its ability to support the proliferation of mitogen-activated
T cells and was initially termed T cell growth factor (7). Both
murine and human IL-2 have been purified to homogeneity and their
complete structures have been deduced from cDNA clones (8,9).
Murine IL-2 is a homodimer with an apparent molecular weight of
30 kd, whereas human IL-2 has an apparent molecular weight of
15 kd. The primary function of IL-2 is to support the proliferation of antigen-activated, mature T cells and through this effect
causes an amplification of functional T cells. More recently IL-2

has also been shown to stimulate the proliferation of mature
B cells.

Antigen-activated helper T cells also produce colony stimulating factor (CSF) activity, the majority of which is due to a
lymphokine termed CSF-2 or granulocyte macrophage CSF (GM-CSF).
Both human and murine GM-CSF have been purified to homogeneity
and their structures have been deduced from cDNA clones (10,11).
Murine GM-CSF is a glycoprotein with an apparent molecular weight
of 23 kd and a protein molecular weight of 15 kd. In mice it is
coded for by a single gene which has been mapped to chromosome
11. As discussed below, GM-CSF primarily supports the proliferation and terminal differentiation of cells committed to the
myeloid lineage. It should also be noted that GM-GSF is structurally distinct from other CSFs including CSF-1 and G-CSF which are
not produced by T cells.

In addition, activated T cells produce IL-3. This lymphokine
has been purified to homogeneity and the structure has been
deduced from cDNA clones. IL-3 is a glycoprotein with an apparent
molecular weight of 28 kd and has a protein component of 15 kd
(12-14). It is coded for by a single gene in mice which has been
mapped to chromosome 11 (Ihle, J.N., Gilbert, D., Silver, J. et
al., manuscript submitted). How closely IL-3 is genetically
linked to GM-CSF is not known. The human homologue of the murine
IL-3 has been identified. The function of IL-3 is to promote the
differentiation of early stem cells as described below. Finally
T cells produce factors which affect the proliferation and differentiation of B cells. In general these factors have not been
purified to homogeneity and have not been cloned. For these reasons they will not be considered here.

As noted above, viral antigen-specific helper T cells might
be expected to be chronically stimulated to produce lymphokines
in viremic mice. It has not been possible, however, to detect
circulating levels of these lymphokines in viremic mice. Since

all the factors cause proliferation and an amplification of
their target populations, we examined the effects of viremia and
the presence of an immune response on the frequencies of lymphokine responsive cells. As noted in Table I, there was a 50- to
200-fold increase in the frequency of lymphokine responsive cells
in viremic BALB/c mice (5). In contrast, in CBA/N mice, in the
absence of viral antigen-specific T cells, there was no increase
in the frequencies of cells responding to lymphokines. These
results therefore support the concept that in the presence of an
immune response and viremia there is an increase in the production of lymphokines. More importantly, however, the results suggest that the increased numbers of cells responding to lymphokines may constitute an important "target" cell population for
viral transformation.

Biological Properties of IL-3

The relationship between immunological increases in potential
target cell populations and transformation has, in part, come
from understanding the biological activities of IL-3. Our interest in IL-3 initially came from studies designed to identify factors which controlled the early differentiation of T cells. For
this, we took advantage of the observation that the enzyme 20αSDH
was expressed at high levels in T cells (15) and initially identified IL-3 as a T cell factor which could induce 20αSDH in cultures containing lymphoid stem cells (16). When IL-3 had been
purified to apparent homogeneity, however, it became obvious that
this lymphokine could mediate a variety of effects in vitro (17).
A listing of some of the relevant activities is given in Table
III.

In addition to the ability to induce 20αSDH in cultures of
bone marrow cells, IL-3 is the only lymphokine known which can
induce the expression of Thy-1 in cultures of Thy-1-depleted bone
marrow cells. In such cultures, 20 to 40% of the cells can be

TABLE III. Biological Activities of IL-3

Activity	Reference
20αSDH	16
Thy-1-inducing factor	18
Mast cell growth factor	19
P cell-stimulating factor	17
Histamine cell-producing stimulating factor	17
Colony stimulating factor	17
WEHI-3 growth factor	20
Hematopoietic growth factor	20

induced to express Thy-1 at levels which are comparable to those found on thymocytes. IL-3 has also been shown to be equivalent to mast cell growth factor, histamine cell-producing factor and P cell-stimulating factor. These names were initially given to T cell factors affecting the differentiation and proliferation of mast cells. In addition, IL-3 has a CSF activity and accounts for approximately 5% of the CSF activity detected in conditioned media from T cells. Lastly, IL-3 has been shown to be equivalent to WEHI-3 growth factor or hematopoietic growth factor, which were initially defined as growth factors for cell lines derived from long-term bone marrow cultures.

The relationship of the multiple activities associated with IL-3 has come from studies of the sequence of differentiation induced by this factor. A summary of these results is shown in Figure 1. IL-3 initially induces the differentiation of a stem cell and induces the expression of 20αSDH. This stem cell appears to be initially noncycling and in a stochastic manner acquires the ability to respond to IL-3 (21). At this point the cell is committed to differentiation and its continued proliferation and differentiation is dependent upon growth factors.

The second detectable event in differentiation is the induction of the expression of Thy-1. At this point the cells begin

Proposed Sequence of IL-3-Induced Differentiation

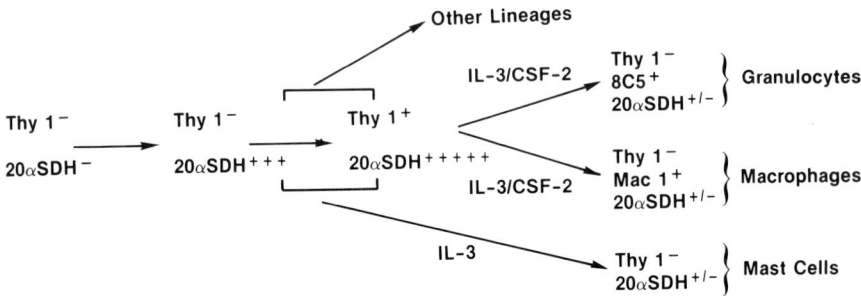

Fig. 1.   Proposed sequence of IL-3-induced differentiation.

to undergo lineage restrictions which include macrophages,
granulocytes and mast cells. Although not directly demonstrated,
indirect evidence exists to suggest that some of the Thy-1[+] cells
also become committed to the T cell lineage and to the erythroid
lineage. In the tissue culture systems we have used, the mature
functional phenotypes that can be identified are myeloid and mast
cells. Those cells which become committed to the mast cell lineage continue to be dependent on IL-3 for their continued differentiation and proliferation. During differentiation the cells
lose Thy-1 but retain a low level of expression of 20αSDH. The
mast cells are unique in that unlike granulocytes or macrophages,
functionally differentiated cells retain the ability to proliferate in vitro and can be maintained in tissue culture for several
months.

The Thy-1[+] cells which become committed to the myeloid lineage will continue to proliferate and differentiate in the presence of IL-3 or GM-CSF. The inability of GM-CSF to induce 20αSDH
or Thy-1 suggests that the ability to respond to this lymphokine
may constitute part of the commitment to the myeloid lineage. In
the presence of either IL-3 or GM-CSF, the cells lose Thy-1 and
20αSDH as they continue to differentiate. In culture, the differentiated cells lose the ability to proliferate and subsequently

lose viability and die off. The differentiation of granulocytes can also be followed by the induction of the expression of a cell surface marker detected by the monoclonal antibody 8C5. As indicated, this marker is expressed by fully differentiated granulocytes and is acquired late in differentiation, subsequent to the expression of Thy-1.

Within the context of the effects of an immune response on leukemogenesis, the ability of IL-3 to induce the proliferation and differentiation of stem cells for a variety of lineages has considerable significance. In particular, in viremic BALB/c mice there is a 50- to 200-fold increase in the frequencies of cells which proliferate in response to IL-3 and therefore undergoing the differentiation shown. If this population is indeed a target for transformation, then it would be expected that some of the primary leukemias would have the properties of the above normal cells. To address this aspect we have characterized primary leukemias for phenotypic and functional properties related to IL-3-regulated cells.

Characteristics of IL-3-Dependent Leukemias

In initial experiments we have demonstrated that approximately half of the MoLV-induced splenic lymphomas in BALB/c mice expressed 20αSDH (22). To further characterize these tumors, we looked at the expression of receptors for IL-3 and the ability of primary tumors to proliferate in response to IL-3 (23). The properties of several primary tumors are summarized in Table IV. In addition to the expression of 20αSDH several of the tumors also expressed receptors for IL-3. Of particular significance, however, was the observation that many of the tumors proliferated in vitro to IL-3 and could be readily established as cell lines in the presence of IL-3. In contrast relatively few of the primary tumors could be established in tissue culture in the absence of IL-3.

TABLE IV. Phenotype and Growth Properties
of Primary Lymphomas

Tumor no.	Thy-1	20αSDH	IL-3 receptors	Growth
118	++	46	0.65	-
119	++	29	0.43	-
120	++	62	0.95	-
121	+/-	404	3.93	+
122	+	483	1.25	+
123	++	2736	1.30	+

All lymphomas were induced in BALB/c mice by MoLV. Thy-1 expression was assessed by fluorescence. 20αSDH activity is given as pmoles conversion/hr/10^8 cells. The binding of iodinated IL-3 was used to assess the expression of receptors for IL-3. The values represent the percentage binding by 10^7 cells. Growth in vitro is in the presence of IL-3. + indicates that a long-term cell line was established.

In addition to the primary tumors induced in BALB/c mice by MoLV, IL-3 has also been used to establish cell lines from tumors induced by Rauscher MuLV (Pierce, J. and J.N. Ihle, unpublished data) and Gross MuLV (Fischinger, P. and J.N. Ihle, unpublished data). In more recent experiments FLV-induced erythroleukemias have been shown to grow in tissue culture in a source of IL-3 (24). To determine whether IL-3 responsiveness was associated with certain types of leukemias, we also examined tumors induced by a wild mouse ecotropic virus (Cas-Br-M-MuLV). This virus was of interest since it had been shown to induce a variety of types of tumors (25). In examining approximately 60 tumors, the majority of the myeloid and erythroid leukemias were found to be IL-3 responsive (26). In contrast, the majority of the B cell and thymic T cell leukemias did not respond to IL-3.

From the above studies a variety of cell lines have been established. The majority of these lines continue to require IL-3 for growth and many of the lines have been continuously

maintained in tissue culture for several years without losing the
requirement for IL-3 for growth. The concept that primary leukemias require T cell-derived lymphokines for growth has potentially interesting therapeutic implications. In particular, therapies directed at eliminating the T cell factors might be expected
to be beneficial. One approach to accomplishing this is the use
of cyclosporin A. This drug, which was initially identified by
its immunosuppresive properties (27), specifically blocks the
antigen-induced production of lymphokines including IL-3, IL-2
and GM-CSF (28).

With the establishment of IL-3-dependent cell lines from
retrovirus-induced tumors it has been possible to study in detail
the properties of the cells and their relationship to normal
IL-3-induced differentiation. The properties of several of the
lines established from myeloid leukemias are summarized in Table
V. Morphologically, the cell lines have the general appearance
of immature myeloblasts. Within the cultures there is little evidence of differentiation to mature granulocytes or macrophages.
Whether morphological differentiation can be induced by agents
such as phorbal esters has not been evaluated.

The most striking property of the lines is their dependence
on IL-3 for growth and the maintenance of viability. To assess
the latter, we have used experiments which measure the loss of
the ability to recover IL-3 responsiveness as a function of time
in the absence of IL-3. The results demonstrate that the cells
lose the ability to recover in a biphasic manner. This is related
to the cell cycle dependence for IL-3. During the first 6 to
8 hours there is a relatively slow loss of viability. After this
the cells begin to lose viability with first order kinetics such
that half the population loses viability every 2 to 4 hours
depending upon the cell line. Therefore, unlike fibroblasts, the
IL-3-dependent cells do not appear to have a 60, nondividing

TABLE V.   Properties of IL-3-Dependent and
Independent Myeloid Leukemias

Cell line	Lymphokines		Mitogenic activity	20αSDH	IL-3 receptors	Thy-1
	IL-3	GM-CSF				
NFS-58 D	++	+	<0.1	9,450	++	+/-
NFS-60 D	++	+	<0.1	21,000	++	+
NFS-78 D	++	+	<0.1	1,680	++	+/-
NFS-107 D	++	+	<0.1	479	++	+/-
DA-3 D	++	+	<0.1	3,500	++	+/-
DA-8 I	ND[a]	ND	<0.1	<100	-	-
NFS-61 I	ND	ND	<0.1	<100	-	-
NFS-124 I	ND	ND	<0.1	<100	-	-
WEHI-3 I	ND	ND	100	150	-	++

The cell lines were obtained from either MoLV-induced lymphomas in BALB/c mice or from Cas-Br-M-MuLV-induced tumors in NFS mice. D indicates factor-dependent lines and I indicates factor-independent lines. The response to lymphokines was determined in thymidine incorporation assays. The presence of mitogenic activity in conditioned media was assayed on DA-1, IL-3-dependent cells. The levels of 20αSDH are given in pmoles conversion/hr/10^8 cells. The presence of receptors for IL-3 was assessed by binding of iodinated IL-3. The expression of Thy-1 was assessed by immunoflouresence. +/- indicates that both positive and negative cells were present.

[a]Not done.

state. The mechanisms which are responsible for the rapid loss of viability of the cells in the absence of IL-3 are not known.

As indicated above, the commitment of cells to the myeloid lineage is associated with the acquisition of the ability to respond to GM-CSF. As indicated in Table V, all the IL-3-dependent myeloid cell lines examined also proliferated in response to GM-CSF. In contrast, a number of lines, which were not myeloid in origin, did not respond to GM-CSF (data not shown). In all the cases examined, the response of the myeloid leukemia lines to GM-CSF was less than that observed with IL-3.

In additional studies (29), GM-CSF has been shown not to compete for the binding of IL-3 by its receptor, indicating that the cells have receptors for both factors. In this context it should also be noted that there is no apparent sequence homology between IL-3 and GM-CSF.

Another property associated with cells early in myeloid differentiation is the expression of Thy-1. As indicated in Table V, all of the myeloid cell lines expressed Thy-1. In many cases, however, only a subpopulation of cells was positive. By sorting experiments, using a flourescence-activated cell sorter, it has been found that most of the proliferation is associated with the Thy-1$^+$ cells which continually give rise to Thy-1 cells. In all the cases examined, when the cells are cultured in GM-CSF, Thy-1 expression is lost. When the cells are returned to IL-3, Thy-1 expression is reinduced. The significance of this effect is not known but may indicate that the expression of Thy-1 is affected by the rate of proliferation. In spite of this phenotypic change, however, when the cells are cultured in GM-CSF there is no morphological indication of differentiation of the cells.

Lastly, as shown in Table V, all the IL-3-dependent myeloid cell lines express high levels of 20αSDH. Taken together the data suggest that the cells are blocked in their ability to differentiate. More specifically the cells appear to be blocked at a point in differentiation when lineage restrictions are normally occurring and shortly after the commitment to the myeloid lineage. Although the cells are altered or transformed with regard to their ability to differentiate, there is no indication that there is an affect on the growth factor responsiveness or dependency of the cells. With regard to normal differentiation, this observation suggests that regulation of growth and differentiation are distinct components. Factors such as IL-3 are required for growth while the cells have genetic programs which control differentiation.

The possible mechanisms that may be involved in transformation are largely unknown. However one of the cell lines (NFS-60) has recently been found to contain a rearrangement of the c-myb locus. The myb gene was initially identified as the oncogene of the avian myeloblastosis virus and induces myeoblastic tumors in chickens (30). In the case of the NFS-60 cell line, a retrovirus has intergrated into the c-myb locus resulting in the transcription of a truncated mRNA of approximately half the normal size. Whether this is necessary and sufficient for the transformation of the NFS-60 cells is not known but is currently being addressed. The absence of comparable events in the other myeloid cell lines would suggest that other transforming genes can give rise to comparable phenotypes.

In addition to the factor-dependent cell lines, three factor-independent myeloid cell lines were also obtained. One possible mechanism for the acquisition of independence is the ability to produce a necessary growth factor autonomously. As indicated in Table V, however, this does not appear to be the case for these tumors. In particular the cells do not produce mitogenic factors for the factor-dependent cell lines nor is their growth inhibited by an antiserum against IL-3. More strikingly, however, the cells lack detectable receptors for IL-3 and phenotypically are quite distinct in lacking detectable 20αSDH activity or Thy-1. Therefore it is not clear that the factor-independent leukemias are related in a simple way to the factor-dependent cell lines.

Within the context of the above results, however, the properties of the WEHI-3 cell line are of interest. This cell line was isolated from a myeloid leukemia which had been passaged in vivo for a number of generations (31). Like the IL-3-dependent cells the WEHI-3 cells express Thy-1 at high levels. Of particular interest however is the observation that the WEHI-3 cells uniquely and constitutively produce IL-3 at high levels (32). By Southern blot analysis, the WEHI-3 cell line contains a rearrangement in the 5' region of one of the IL-3 alleles which is not found in any other cell lines examined (unpublished data). These results suggest the possibility that at one point in its derivation the WEHI-3 cell line may have been dependent on IL-3 for growth and may have had a phenotype which is comparable to that of the IL-3-dependent cell lines. There was a subsequent selection for a variant either in vivo or during adaptation to tissue culture capable of expressing IL-3. However, at this point in time the cells do not appear to require IL-3 since their proliferation is not inhibited by an antiserum to IL-3 nor do the cells express receptors for IL-3.

Taken together, the properties of the IL-3-dependent leukemias support the concept that one of the properties of transformation of myeloid cells is the loss of the ability to terminally differentiation. In one case, this may be due to rearrangements in the c-myb locus. The properties of the cells are consistent with a block in the sequence of differentiation normally promoted by IL-3 and therefore support the concept that the expanded populations, resulting from chronic immunological stimulation, can represent a target for transformation. Moreover the results further suggest that an immune response may contribute to the growth of the tumor, after transformation, by producing the growth factors necessary for proliferation.

SUMMARY

In the past there has been a general assumption that in viral diseases immunization provides the best approach to control. For the most part this concept is correct and can be generally applied to situations in which immunization is used to anticipate an encounter with viruses. In terms of murine retroviruses, there is considerable evidence that immunization, particularly with viral glycoproteins, can protect against subsequent challenge.

The situation becomes somewhat more complex however when considering the potential effects of immunizations in animals that harbor the virus. Within this context it is imperative to consider the levels of virus that are being expressed and the capability of an immune response to deal with those levels.

The expression of high levels of virus present unique problems. In AKR mice, it is clear that the simple concept of viral immunization as a therapeutic approach is inaccurate and conversely only serves to exacerbate the problem. A more realistic approach in this situation is passive immunotherapy to attempt to reduce the viral burdens to levels that can be dealt with by the hosts immune response. Indeed, this approach has been shown to have beneficial effects (33).

In situations in which the virus persists, particularly in the face of cellular immune responses, the consequences of manipulating the immune response become more difficult to predict. As illustrated here, the altered regulation of the production of lymphokines can have a variety of effects which can contribute to adverse effects such as leukemia. In other situations altered production of lymphokines, either systemically or locally, may contribute to pathological effects that are not related to transformation. As more is learned concerning the effects of lymphokines in regulating the differentiation and function of various cell types it may be possible to further predict and deal with the secondary effects of manipulating an immune response.

REFERENCES

1. Ihle, J.N., Collins, J.J., Lee, J.C. et al. (1976). Virology 75, 74.
2. Ihle, J.N., Lee, J.C., Collins, J.J. et al. (1976). Virology 75, 88.
3. Ihle, J.N., Collins, J.J., Lee, J.C. et al. (1976). Virology 75, 102.
4. Lee, J.C. and Ihle, J.N. (1981). Nature 209, 407.

5. Lee, J.C. and Ihle, J.N. (1981). Proc. Natl. Acad. Sci. 78, 7712.
6. Enjuanes, L., Lee, J. and Ihle, J.N. (1981). J. Immunol. 126, 1478.
7. Morgan, D.A., Ruscetti, F.W. and Gallo, R.C. (1976). Science 193, 1007.
8. Taniguchi, M., Matsui, H., Fujita, T. et al. (1983). Nature 302, 305.
9. Kashima, N., Nishi-Takaoka, C., Fujita, T. et al. (1985). Nature 313, 399.
10. Gough, N.M., Gough, J., Metcalf, D. et al. (1984). Nature 309, 763.
11. Wong, G.G., Witek, J.S., Temple, P.A. et al. (1985). Science 228, 810.
12. Ihle, J.N., Keller, J., Henderson, L. et al. (1982). J. Immunol. 129, 2431.
13. Fung, M.C., Hapel, A.J., Ymer, S. et al. (1984). Nature 307, 233.
14. Yokota, T., Lee, F., Rennick, D. et al. (1984). Proc. Natl. Acad. Sci. 81, 1070.
15. Weinstein, Y. (1977). J. Immunol. 119, 1223.
16. Ihle, J.N., Pepersack, L. and Rebar, L. (1981). J. Immunol. 126, 2184.
17. Ihle, J.N., Keller, J., Oroszlan, S. et al. (1983). J. Immunol. 131, 282.
18. Ihle, J.N., Keller, J. and Palaszynski, E.W. (1983). In "Interleukins, Lymphokines, and Cytokines" (J.J. Oppenheim and S. Cohen, eds.), p. 113. Academic Press, New York.
19. Razin E., Ihle, J.N., Seldin, D. et al. (1983). J. Immunol. 132, 1479.
20. Ihle, J.N., Keller, J., Greenberger, J.S. et al. (1982). J. Immunol. 129, 1377.
21. Suda, T., Suda, J., Ogawa, M. et al. (1984). J. Cell. Physiol. (in press).
22. Pepersack, L., Lee, J.C., McEwan, R. et al. (1984). J. Immunol. 124, 279.
23. Ihle, J.N., Rein, A. and Mural, R. (1984). In "Advances in Viral Oncology" (G. Klein, ed.), vol. 4, p. 95. Raven Press, New York.
24. Oliff, A., Oliff, I., Schmidt, B. et al. (1984). Proc. Natl. Acad. Sci. 81, 5464.
25. Frederickson, T.N., Langdon, W.Y., Hoffman, P.M. et al. (1984). J. Natl. Cancer Inst. 72, 447.
26. Holmes, K., Palaszynski, E., Frederickson, T.N. (1985). Proc. Natl. Acad. Sci. (in press).
27. Borel, J.F., Feurer, C., Magnee, C. et al. (1977). Immunology 32, 1017.
28. Hess, A.D., Tutschka, P.J. and Santos, G.W. (1982). J. Immunol. 128, 355.

29. Palaszynski, E.W. and Ihle, J.N. (1984). J. Immunol. 132, 1872.
30. Klernpnauer, K.-H., Gonda, T.J. and Bishop, J.M. (1982). Cell 31, 453.
31. Warner, N.L., Morre, M.A.S. and Metcalf, D. (1969). J. Natl. Cancer Inst. 43, 963.
32. Lee, J.C., Hapel, A.J. and Ihle, J.N. (1982). J. Immunol. 128, 2393.
33. Schwarz, H., Fischinger, P.J., Ihle, J.N. et al. (1979). Virology 93, 159.

EQUINE INFECTIOUS ANEMIA VACCINE

David T. Shen

Veterinary Micropathology
Washington State University
Pullman, Washington

Equine infectious anemia (EIA) presents a serious problem to
the 12 million horses in the People's Republic of China, 2 million of which are in the Heilongjiang Province. In some regions
of the People's Republic of China, the rate of the EIA infection
has been as high as 30%.

The EIA Research Laboratory at Harbin has 23 employees—12
scientists, six technicians and five animal caretakers. Currently, they are studying both the humoral and cell-mediated
immune responses to EIA in an effort to develop an effective EIA
vaccine. They are also working on new diagnostic assays for
detecting EIA in horses. Laboratory tests routinely used for EIA
studies include complement fixation, cytopathic effect (CPE) in
donkey leukocyte culture (DLC), horse inoculation, agar-gel
immunodiffusion (ID) and the enzyme-linked immunosorbent assay
(ELISA). Electron microscopy is also available for morphological
studies. The fluorescent antibody technique is not routinely
used for EIA viral detection. The ID test used at Harbin was
designed after the Coggins method. In the United States, the
Coggins test is the only assay currently available for detecting
EIA in horses. The tissue culture-grown antigen used in China's

ID test has not been compared with the EIA antigen used in the
United States and Japan.

The scientists at Harbin followed the Kobayashi method of
propagating EIA virus in a horse leukocyte culture (HLC) system.
Because of the difficulty in propagating EIA virus in HLC, alter-
native methods were sought. The scientists found that the DLC was
an easier system to cultivate, maintain and use for propagation
of EIA virus. After 10 years of hard work, they attenuated EIA
virus through a series of passages in DLC, yielding an effective
modified live EIA vaccine.

The basic scheme of EIA attenuation was as follows:

1.   The virus was isolated from a horse with EIA.
2.   The isolate was passaged 5 to 10 times in horses to
     yield a titer 10^6 $TCID_{50}$ per ml.
3.   The EIA isolate was subsequently passed 45 times in
     donkeys. At this time the isolate was highly virulent to
     both horses and donkeys. This virulent strain of EIA is
     a stock virus used to challenge the immunized animals in
     subsequent studies.
4.   The virulent strain of virus was then passed 120 times
     in DLC, yielding an attenuated strain of EIA virus which
     remained antigenic but not pathogenic to the animals.
     Three isolates have been obtained in the blood of horses
     with EIA. These have been designated the L, H and Y
     strains of virus. These three isolates show no differ-
     ences in antigenicity or pathogenicity. The Chinese iso-
     lates have not been compared with the isolates from other
     countries.

Susceptible horses used for this study were obtained from
EIA-free areas, isolated for 3 months before use and shown to be
EIA-negative by ID. The EIA virus was initially isolated by
inoculating infective serum onto DLC. Once CPE appeared, subsequent passages were made by freeze-thawing the infected cells

twice to release the cell-associated virus and inoculating the
infected supernatant medium onto uninfected DLC. Parallel negative controls were run with normal donkey serum.

The following observations were made during passages of EIA
virus on DLC:

1. The CPE was seen in 5 to 6 days after inoculation in
    lower passages and in 3 to 4 days in higher passages.

2. The CF titers were consistently high from the 70th
    passage on.

3. Titration at various numbers of passages in DLC revealed
    that the virus titer of the culture was 10^6 $TCID_{50}$ per ml
    before the 100th passage, and 10^7 $TCID_{50}$ per ml at the
    170th passage.

4. The virulence for horses and donkeys decreased as the
    number of passages increased. No clinical signs were
    observed in animals inoculated with cultures at the 120th
    and 150th passage. Modes of inoculation included intra-
    venous, intradermal and subcutaneous.

The cultured virus was back-passed in horses and donkeys:

1. Fourteen horses were inoculated with virus from the 95th
    to 105th passage. The horses were bled at days 30, 48,
    97 and 175 after inoculation. Blood (200 ml) from each
    bleeding was inoculated into susceptible donkeys (one
    donkey per horse). All donkeys remained clinically nor-
    mal after inoculation. Donkeys were then challenged with
    a virulent strain of EIA virus, and all became sick or
    died after challenge, demonstrating the lack of
    protection.

2. Eight donkeys were inoculated with 10 ml of stock virus
    at the 125th passage level. At the days 45, 60, 80 and
    90 after inoculation, two donkeys were killed, and their
    blood and internal organs (spleen, lymph nodes, liver

and bone marrow) were collected, pooled and inoculated
into susceptible donkeys. All donkeys remained normal
after inoculation. All became infected or died after
challenge with virulent virus.

3. Attenuated virus was back-passaged in horses and don-
    keys. Results in several trials indicated that the atten-
    uated virus could not be propagated for more than three
    passages. Whole blood (5-15 ml) and internal organs were
    used as passage materials. Passage intervals ranged from
    2 to 4 months. The criteria for the presence of the
    attenuated virus were performance in complement-fixation
    tests and virulent virus challenge.

4. Attenuated virus from various DLC passages (90, 95, 96,
    100, 105, 115, 118, 119, 122, 124, 125, 129, 131 and 135)
    was inoculated into a total of 62 horses by various
    routes and in various dilutions. After 2 to 4 months, the
    vaccinated horses were challenged with virulent virus.
    After challenge, 42 horses remained normal, four showed
    moderate signs, three were "suspicious" and 13 showed
    clinical signs of EIA. Five of the 13 horses with clini-
    cal signs died. The total protection rate was 79%. In the
    nonvaccinated control group, 100% showed clinical signs
    and 70% died after challenge. Vaccinated horses that
    showed signs after challenge had significantly longer
    incubation periods and lower death rates than horses of
    the nonvaccinated control group. Intravenous challenge
    of virulent virus should be avoided because the Chinese
    strain of EIA virus will be pathogenic regardless of the
    effectiveness of the vaccine. The highest dilution of
    attenuated virus from cell culture which produced immun-
    ity in horses or donkeys was 10^5. Similar results were
    obtained from the vaccine trials on donkeys, except that
    the protection rate reached 100%.

5. Immunity begins about 2 months after vaccination. Sub-
    cutaneous inoculation of the vaccine seems to be more
    effective than any other route. For up to 3 months after
    vaccination, the animal will have a positive antibody
    titer by the ID test. Thereafter, the EIA antibody is
    undetectable by this method.

6. Stability of the attenuated virus at various tempera-
    tures has been studied. The virus is stable at 15 to 20°C
    for 7 days, at 0°C for at least 60 days and at -50°C for
    at least 400 days.

7. Two million doses of vaccine have been tried in various
    parts of the People's Republic of China. The EIA infec-
    tion rate has dropped to 1 to 2% in Heilongjiang Prov-
    ince. The duration of immunity is currently under study.

The pathology laboratory has begun the study of the immunologic mechanisms involved in effectively vaccinating horses
against EIA. Preliminary data indicate that cellular immunity is
important in controlling replication of EIA virus. The total number of lymphocytes decreased greatly immediately after vaccination but returns to normal 3 to 5 months after vaccination. The
vaccinated horses exhibit a marked leukocyte migration inhibition
(LMI) 10 days after inoculation. The LMI persists for an indeter-
minate amount of time; one horse has exhibited LMI for 4 years.

For 75 years, EIA has been recognized as an animal virus
disease. As with several other slow virus diseases, the mechanism that causes the persistent virus infection is a fundamental
biological phenomenon that remains to be explained. Not long ago,
scientists in Japan obtained some evidence suggesting that antigenic drift may occur in an EIA-infected horse, but no one has
confirmed their observations. The vaccine data do not necessarily
disagree with the Japanese observations. After 120 passages in
DLC, the Chinese may have indeed selected out a strain that is
perfect for a vaccine. Other scientists may be skeptical about

the EIA vaccine at this time. The vaccine's effectiveness must be further evaluated before a conclusion can be made.

If the vaccine data are accurate and the EIA vaccine can protect the animal, then studies on other slow virus vaccines should begin. Perhaps EIA can serve as a model in the basic understanding of the immunological processes involved in slow virus infection.

The Chinese scientists as well as the government officials fully realize the need of basic research to substantiate their observations. They are eager and willing to cooperate with United States scientists in equine research. The United States-People's Republic of China cooperative research on EIA will be mutually beneficial.

FELINE LEUKEMIA VACCINE

Richard Olsen

The Ohio State University
Department of Veterinary Pathobiology
Columbus, Ohio

Feline leukemia is an attractive model to study a retrovirus vaccine from several points of view. First of all, the agent is well characterized and, most importantly, the etiologic (feline retrovirus) is horizontally transmitted. Theoretically, immuno-prophylaxis should block the transmission of this horizontally transmitted agent in the host's natural setting. Indeed, there is a need for such a vaccine in veterinary medicine in that the cat is a companion animal to man, and there certainly has been an interest in the cat over and beyond the interest in cat disease as a model to develop a vaccine for retroviral diseases.

INACTIVATD FELINE LEUKEMIA VIRUS VACCINE

Early studies at the Ohio State University to develop a feline leukemia virus (FeLV) employed the classical regimen of killed virus. The objective was to inactivate FeLV by formalin treatment or ultraviolet radiation treatment. In principle, cats immunized with said inactivated FeLV should respond by develop-ing an active immunity which should protect the cat from subse-quent FeLV disease. In actuality, however, we found that immunized cats when challenged with virulent FeLV were more

ANIMAL MODELS OF RETROVIRUS INFECTION
AND THEIR RELATIONSHIP TO AIDS

393

susceptible to FeLV disease than nonvaccinated controls (1). The
parameters were well controlled. Not only did the immunized
animals die faster as a result of the challenge with a malignant
tumor, but the number of progressor and regressor tumors clearly
showed that the vaccinated animals were more susceptible to
disease than controls.

We and others (2) attempted to immunize animals with FeLV
gp70, the glycosylated envelope protein of feline leukemia. It
was found that the FeLV gp70 isolated from feline leukemia virus
would elicit a neutralizing antibody in a guinea pig; but, when
used as an immunogen in cats, not only was the virus neutralized
and antibody very low, but protection was nil.

TUMOR CELL FeLV VACCINE

Jarrett et al. (3) a number of years ago evaluated a tumor
cell vaccine prepared from an FeLV-transformed cell line. We also
tried this system and found that this tumor cell vaccine would
indeed induce potent antibody and apparently would protect
against FeLV challenge (4). In our hands, however, this type of
vaccine (tumor cell vaccine) was not adequate for protecting
against persistent FeLV viremia. In an attempt to prevent tumor
development and FeLV viremia we coupled the tumor cell vaccine
with inactivated FeLV (5). Our objective was to induce active
immunity to the tumor-associated antigen (FOCMA [feline
oncornavirus-associated cell membrane antigen]) and to develop an
antiviral immunity and avoid viremia. Cats that received the dual
vaccine of inactivated virus and tumor cells were not protected
from persistent FeLV viremia. In addition these cats produced
lower levels of FOCMA antibody than did cats that received tumor
cell alone and the cats that received the dual vaccine were more
susceptible to FeLV disease.

It became quite evident that the presence of inactivated FeLV is immunotoxic and contributes to disease enhancement. In subsequent studies, an envelope-associated 15,000 dalton peptide (FeLV p15E) was found to be responsible for the immunosuppressed properties of FeLV. In in vitro studies, FeLV p15E was found to have a deleterious effect on T cell functions. Moreover, by administering FeLV p15E into cats, enhancement of FeLV disease was observed (6). Subsequent work with FeLV p15E indicated the relevance of immunosuppression associated with feline leukemia and certainly had a very striking effect on the development of an FeLV vaccine.

FeLV SUBUNIT VACCINE

It was our contention that due to the peculiar immunosuppressive properties in killed FeLV that a subunit FeLV vaccine however novel was required for prevention of FeLV disease. Our initial studies with cell cycle suggested that FeLV peptides and FOCMA could be obtained from FeLV persistent antigens by infected cells, synthesized and shed FOCMA antigen and virion antigens as the cell proceeded through certain stages of the cell cycle (7). The release of FeLV antigens was by various assays, including a cytotoxic inhibition assay (8).

The recovery of FeLV-associated peptides from persistently infected cells was basically the scheme used to develop the feline leukemia vaccine that the Nordin Corporation is presently marketing. The vaccine production method consists of growing FL-74 cells to near saturation density and then placing the cells in serum-free media. As in the cell cycle studies, the cells placed in serum-free medium release FeLV immunogens that can be detected serologically and which appear to be FeLV-specific. The cells we use in the vaccine production are persistently infected with the kairakami-thelon strain of virus containing the A, B and C

serotypes. Serum-free supernatant fluids when collected were
mixed with enzyme inhibitors to stabilized the vaccine. As a
result of placing the FeLV-infected cells in serum-free media we
were able to demonstrate that virus production ceased; however,
immunogens were continually synthesized and released. Though the
viable cell numbers decreased, up to 90% of the cells remained
viable. These cells can be used over and over again in a fer-
menter for developing or harvesting FeLV vaccine.

The subsequent FeLV vaccine was evaluated in a number of ways
(9). The animals were vaccinated. We were interested, at that
time, in the FOCMA antibody response. In our vaccinates, before
challenge, there was a reasonable FOCMA antibody response on both
FL-74 cells and FeLV-infected mink cells (CCL-64). As expected,
in the specific-pathogen free (SPF) controls there was no antibody before challenge. After challenge with an oral-nasal challenge, 100% of the control animals became viremic. Those animals
eventually showed all the classic signs of feline leukemia. Control infected cats became immunosuppressed, developed a persistent viremia and, when held long enough, some cats would develop
tumors. In the vaccinated group, we found that protection was
greater than 80%. These animals, after challenge, would maintain
their FOCMA antibody status. These animals were held for a good
number of months, for way over a year and they still did not show
evidence of a persistent viremia or indications of AIDS
(immunosuppression).

Mark Lewis, in our laboratory, subsequently showed that at
the time of challenge the vaccinated animals developed a very
good antibody response to FeLV gp70, a fair response to both the
p27 and p12 core and a reasonable titer to p15E which, of course,
the control animals did not develop. Essentially similar results
were obtained in studies conducted by the group at Nordin Laboratories. The Nordin Labs adapted the FL-74 cell to large fer-
menters, where all parameters, including pH oxygen and carbon

dioxide, are maintained at optimum levels. The number of cells
which can be generated is very high. They found, as we did, that
it was necessary to stabilize this material with enzyme
inhibitors.

In one 20-cat experiment conducted at Nordin Laboratories
with the vaccine, immunizing twice a couple of weeks apart,
boosting several months later and then challenging after that
booster, at the end of a 2 year period, virtually 100% of the
controls broke with disease. The controls were kept in an environment where they were not exposed to conventional cats so there
should be no feline infectious peritonitis (FIP) or other secondary agents interfering. These animals showed classic signs of
acquired immune deficiency. Many of these control animals eventually developed the lymphosarcoma and died. At the end of this
2 year period, all the controls died. In the 20 vaccinates, protection is far exceeding what we demonstrated. It is greater than
90%. At the end of this 2 year period, there is no evidence of
viremia, no evidence of suppression. In essence, the vaccine is
fulfilling all the criteria that are necessary for feline leukemia, protecting against malignant disease. It is apparently protecting against all those facets of AIDS. Though the challenge
virus was also the Rickard, there is no evidence of anemia. That
data is a little soft because more extensive studies need to be
done with the KT challenge. Those studies have not been as
thorough as the ones done with the Rickard virus. Neutralizing
antibody titers are fairly weak before challenge. There was fair
activity to gp70, but the focus-forming units were not impressive. The weak response which has been obtained repeatedly is
real. The most important thing, of course, is the resistance to
challenge.

We have had a lot of fun with this vaccine. In central Ohio
we came upon a household where at one time there were over 300
cats (10). What made this particular environment a little

different from most of the multiple cat houses you read about in the newspaper is that this young couple actually tried to go at this in a very scientific way. They built a new house and built a wing on the side of the house, approximately 30 x 50. The cats were housed in this wing. The animals had very good veterinary care. The feed bill for these cats was at least $500 a month and, at times, the veterinary bill would top a thousand dollars. As you would suspect, they were not careful in introducing cats into the group. They did not raise cats for show or hire. They just had big hearts for any stray cat and they had the Fort Dix of the cat world. By the time we got to know these people, a good number of the cats had died and the attending veterinarian certainly confirmed that many of these cats were dying of FIP and feline leukemia.

We looked at the surviving cats in this multicat household and were able to break them up into two groups, one group included cats that were GSA-negative and viremia-negative by the criteria that Dr. Hardy described in his test. The other group included cats that were viremic with or without clinical signs. Obviously, we were interested in the first group as far as cats to vaccinate. More importantly, we were interested in the animals that possessed no FOCMA antibody titer, because we felt that those would be the susceptible animals. This is a biased experiment and were this the only thing done, it would not hold water. The transmission of the virus requires physical contact. You cannot have a cat over here and a cat over there and have the virus walk across. The more sociable the animal is, the more contact between cats in the multicat household, the greater the likelihood that these animals would be exposed to feline leukemia and either be placed in this group that would develop a FOCMA protective antibody or this group that would become persistently infected. In spite of that, we did the experiment because it was a lot of fun to go see this household. We were only interested

in vaccinating the one group, those 45 animals that represented
what we considered the susceptible population, but the woman
insisted we vaccinate the whole group. We did, but after vaccination, we followed the 45 cats of interest. All developed FOCMA by
the immunofluoresence criteria. After 52 weeks, 73% of those animals remained free of viremia and free of disease. During the
experimental period, we tried introducing some of our own SPF
cats into the house and at first this turned out to be a disas-
ter. It was like taking the kid off the farm in Nebraska and
putting him in New Jersey. These cats died instantly. Not only
was it a harsh environment as far as the pecking order was concerned, but it was also harsh in terms of the actual diseases to
which the cats were exposed. Larry Mathis and Wayne Halse at Ohio
State developed a clever way of conditioning our SPF cats. The
animals were first vaccinated against all the things that they
would be exposed to immediately. They were introduced into a
screened area in the household so that they could be exposed, but
not in an overwhelming fashion. Fortunately, 10 cats were able to
be conditioned in this way and could enter into this household
and not die instantly. These 10 cats were followed as sentinel
animals. Four of these cats died within 4 weeks when placed in
the household, two confirmed as having FeLV disease. The vaccinated animals that survived beyond this period, all died with
FeLV disease. They were constantly exposed to the persistently
infected animals. Over 80% of 10 other animals that were subsequently vaccinated and conventionalized in the same way survived
a year of this harsh environment and remained viremia-negative.

What can the vaccine do and what can it not do? First of all,
will the vaccine have an effect upon the animal that is already
viremic and has early signs of FeLV disease? There is absolutely
no evidence that it changed the course of that disease. Will the
vaccine have a deleterious effect upon a cat that has been
exposed to and may have one of the subclinical infections that

was described earlier? Such cats fit the model of a regressor/
progressor situation. If the challenge is high enough and the
host is an appropriate one, obviously a persistent disease can
develop. The bone marrow cells were studied in a radioimmunoassay
and very early development of FOCMA antibody was seen. The antibody persisted for a long time, although the cats are starting to
die. It is the other group that we found very interesting. It was
different from what we expected. The group that is infected with
FeLV never develops overt viremia. The animals remain virus-free
as far as one can determine by the conventional methods. There is
also no pathology. The bone marrow cells also expressed the FOCMA
antibody, and, much to our surprise, it persists for a long, long
time. There conceivably could be in this group, persistent virus,
though its expression may be somewhat repressed. It could be
activated by various manipulations. It is obvious that the vaccine has no effect upon this particular group. It is not going
to reverse the disease and, apparently, the effect is none. There
is an anamnestic response as far as serologic parameters but no
evidence that the response is going to activate virus.

In the animals that are vaccinated, challenged and remain
disease free, could persistent disease develop after challenge?
For the most part, we do not know. I think this would be an
important issue to resolve because it is important to find out
if the animals are still susceptible to disease. They may not be
susceptible right away but might be later on if environmental
things change.

I would like to highlight a few things we are doing at Ohio
State to characterize the p15 effect. In our hands, p15E from
the FeLV appears to be very T cell-specific. It will interfere
with almost all of the in vitro assays that involve T cell activity, such as mixed lymphocyte reactions to both recall immunogens
and mitogens. There has been controversy about whether p15 is
interfering with macrophage function or accessory cell function

and T cell functions. Synderman and others were able to demonstrate in North Carolina that p15 apparently interfered with
macrophage function. Most of their assays dealt with an inflammatory response. In our hands, p15 has no effect on the macrophage; it does not interfere with interleukin-1 (11) functions or
production; it apparently interferes with the T cell's ability to
either produce interleukin-2 or respond to interleukin-1 itself
(12). So we feel that not only would p15 have a very pronounced
influence on how to develop the vaccine since it may play a very
important role in abrogating the immune response, but also p15
release as a result of persistent infection may contribute, at
least in part, to the acquired immune deficiency that we associate with FeLV.

REFERENCES

1. Schaller, J.P., Hoover, E.A. and Olsen R.G. (1977). J. Natl.
   Cancer Inst. 59, 1441.
2. Salermo, R.A., Lehman, E.D., Larson, V.M. et al. (1978).
   J. Natl. Cancer Inst. 61, 1407.
3. Jarrett, W., Jarrett, O., Mackey, L. et al. (1975). Int. J.
   Cancer 16, 134.
4. Olsen, R.G., Hoover, E.A., Mathes, L.E. et al. (1976). Cancer
   Res. 36, 3642.
5. Olsen, R.G., Hoover, E.A., Schaller, J.P. et al. (1977).
   Cancer Res. 37, 2082.
6. Mathes, L.E., Olsen, R.G., Hebebrand, L.E. et al. (1978).
   Nature 274, 687.
7. Olsen, R.G., Milo, G.E., Schaller, J.P. et al. (1976).
   In Vitro 12, 37.
8. Wolff, L.H., Mathes, L.E. and Olsen R.G. (1979). J. Immunol.
   Methods 26, 151.
9. Lewis, M.G., Mathes, L.E. and Olsen, R.G. (1981). Infect.
   Immun. 34, 888.
10. Olsen, R.G., Hoover, E.A., Mathes, L.E. et al. (1979). Feline
    Pract. 9, 16.
11. Copeland, E.A., Rinehart, J.J., Lewis, M. (1983). J. Immunol.
    131, 2017.
12. Orosz, C., Zunn, N.E., Olsen, R. et al. (1985). J. Immunol.
    134, 3396.

EXTRACORPOREAL PERFUSION OF PLASMA OVER IMMOBILIZED
STAPHYLOCOCCUS AUREUS PROTEIN A AS A TREATMENT FOR FeLV
INFECTION AND LYMPHOSARCOMA: PROSPECTS FOR TREATMENT
OF RETROVIRAL INFECTION AND AIDS IN MAN[1]

Harry W. Snyder, Jr., Mitra C. Singhal, Nancy R. Ernst,
Chris K. Grant, Susan M. Cotter,* Lois H. Yoshida
and Frank R. Jones

Immune Response Program
Pacific Northwest Research Foundation
Seattle, Washington

*Department of Veterinary Medicine
Tufts University School of Veterinary Medicine
Boston, Massachusetts

INTRODUCTION

The feline leukemia virus (FeLV) is a contagious T cell
lymphotropic retrovirus which productively infects lymphoid and
myeloid cells in approximately 30% of exposed pet cats (1-3).
The inability of some exposed cats to produce a protective titer
of FeLV neutralizing antibody allows progression of the primary
localized infection to a persistent viremia (1,2). Cats rarely
overcome persistent FeLV viremia--one study showed that only
three of 144 cats were able to clear their infections spontaneously (3). After the onset of viremia, death usually results

---

[1]This work was supported by grants CA-16599, CA-24608, CA-
34394, CA-36678 and CA-38845 from the National Cancer Institute
and by grants from the Cancer Research Institute, Inc., and IMRE
Corporation.

403

within 3 months to 3 years due to degenerative bone marrow
disease, leukemia, lymphosarcoma (LSA) or, more likely, opportunistic infections secondary to an FeLV-acquired immune deficiency syndrome (FAIDS) (4-6).

There are numerous similarities between FAIDS and human
acquired immune deficiency syndrome (AIDS). Both syndromes are
characterized by lymphopenia, reduced lymphocyte response to
mitogens and allogeneic cells, cutaneous anergy, impaired antibody responses and secondary infections (3,7-10). Furthermore,
AIDS also appears to be caused by a retrovirus termed human T
cell lymphotropic virus type III (HTLV-III), lymphadenopathy-
associated virus (LAV) or AIDS-related retrovirus (ARV) (11-13).
Thus, studies of the natural history of FeLV infection, natural
and induced immune responses to virion and viral-associated antigens and potential therapies affecting the FeLV status of cats
should be of value in understanding AIDS and should assist in
the development of diagnostic and treatment procedures for that
disease.

For several years our laboratories have been interested in
the biochemistry and immunology of FeLV and FeLV-induced LSA.
Recently we have also been assessing the value of viral cell
surface antigens as targets for immunotherapy. The results of
our studies and their potential applications for the treatment
of AIDS are discussed in this chapter.

FeLV PROTEINS WHICH FUNCTION AS CELLULAR ANTIGENS

A variety of FeLV virion and viral-associated antigens are
expressed in the membranes of infected cells. The major immunogenic components are viral envelope antigens. The FeLV envelope
consists of a basement membrane with a 15,000 dalton virally
encoded protein p15E embedded within the membrane, and a 70,000
dalton glycoprotein (gp70) linked by disulfide bonds to p15E and

expressed on the external surface of the membrane (14). There is
antigenic polymorphism among gp70s from different natural isolates of FeLV. On the basis of viral interference and neutralization tests, which are dependent upon viral gp70, three broad
subgroups of FeLV (termed A, B and C) have been defined (15-17).
FeLV of subgroup A can be isolated from all viremic cats; in
approximately 50% of these viremic cats FeLV-B is also present.
In contrast, FeLV of subgroup C is only found in approximately
1% of viremic cats (2,15-17). LSA cells in viremic cats express
membrane antigens corresponding to the envelope antigens of the
subgroup(s) of FeLV initiating the infection. In addition, all
LSA cells express antigens related to the envelope glycoprotein
of FeLV-C, even though infectious FeLV-C is rarely found in LSA
cats (18,19).

Current thinking is that the FeLV-C gp70-related antigens
are encoded by variants of FeLV which arise following genetic
recombinations between exogenous genes for the envelope (env)
proteins derived from the infectious virus and endogenous FeLV-
related sequences in the cat genome. Such events can give rise
to LSA cells which express highly type-specific antigenic determinants in addition to antigens which are crossreactive with
prototype strains of infectious FeLV. Collectively, these highly
tumor-specific antigens have generally been referred to as the
feline oncornavirus-associated cell membrane antigen (20-22).

During a natural infection a cat may produce antibodies to
any of the viral gp70 or gp70-like antigens. These antibodies
may have the capacity to block infectivity of FeLV for feline
fibroblasts (2,17) and/or they may mediate complement-dependent
lysis of LSA cells in vitro (23). Thus the FeLV envelope antigens offer a multiplicity of potential targets for immunotherapy.

IMMUNOLOGICAL INTERVENTION IN FELINE RETROVIRUS INFECTIONS

The most effective means of immunological intervention in
retrovirus infections is to prevent the primary infection by
effective immunization. Progress in the development of a vaccine
for the prevention of natural FeLV infections is reported by
Richard Olsen ("Feline Leukemia Vaccine") in this volume.

Immunological intervention is also sometimes possible in cats
which are already infected with the virus. Passive immunotherapy
has been shown to be an effective means of protecting kittens
from feline sarcoma virus (FeLV/FeSV) challenge (3,24-27). Under
natural conditions, passive transfer of antibody from immune dams
to suckling kittens occurs and maternal antibodies remain detectable for up to 2 months (24-26). Experimental passive serotherapy
with autologous immune IgG has been shown to prevent fatal metastases of FeLV/FeSV fibrosarcomas in challenge cats (28,29).
Treatment with heterologous (goat) anti-FeLV gp70 serum was shown
to protect cats against both FeSV-induced fibrosarcomas and the
development of persistent FeLV viremia subsequent to challenge
with FeLV/FeSV (27,30).

Passive serotherapy against spontaneous feline lymphosarcomas
with immune cat serum has been successful in inducing short-term
remissions in some cats (2,3). However, Cotter et al. (31)
demonstrated with mediastinal lymphoma that passive serotherapy
is effective in prolonging remissions induced by chemotherapy
(cyclophosphamide/vincristine/prednisone). Chemotherapy alone
induced 16 complete remissions in 23 cats. The cats receiving no
other therapy lived for an average of 40 days while cats receiving autologous immune IgG lived for an average of 63 days. Two of
the serotherapy recipients lived 156 and 300 days, respectively.
However, in no case was the FeLV infection cleared due to
treatment.

A more controlled approach to serological intervention in feline retrovirus infections would involve the use of monoclonal antibodies (MAbs) against FeLV gp70s. Grant et al. (32) have described a number of such antibodies which are widely cross-reactive with gp70s from different subgroups of FeLV, and which function in complement-dependent lysis of cultured FeLV LSA cell lines. Preliminary studies with viremic but otherwise asymptomatic cats have shown that the recipients tolerate at least 250 mg of FeLV gp70 MAbs injected intravenously over a 14 day period. Using a pool of five MAbs with cytotoxic and virus neutralizing functions, we have been able to detect transient fluctuations in FeLV-related proteins in the sera of most recipients following infusions. The effects are relatively short-lived, however, and so far we have failed to permanently reduce FeLV burdens. Mouse IgG does persist in the blood of viremic recipients for up to 30 days, whereas when MAbs are injected into normal cats the murine IgG is cleared within 10 days. Following injection of mouse MAbs into viremic recipients, an antimouse IgG response is detected with peak titers at between days 28 and 36. This response is preceded by a peak of detectable circulating immune complexes (CIC) of cat and mouse IgG. A fraction of the total cat antimouse Ig response is anti-idiotype.

In contrast to the resilience of entrenched viremia, some leukemias and lymphomas appear to be relatively sensitive to MAb serotherapy. We have treated three tumor-bearing cats in the terminal stages of disease with 100 to 150 mg of a pool of cytotoxic MAb. The first cat presented with anterior mediastinal lymphoma which was radiosensitive. Three months later the cat relapsed with a grossly enlarged spleen and metastases throughout the duodenum and kidneys. After two MAb infusions renal function ceased and the cat was euthanised; autopsy revealed a normal-sized spleen and complete absence of tumor in the peritoneal cavity. The second cat had leukemia and, although it died within

hours of receiving the MAb infusion, there was marked evidence
of pernecrosis in the solid tumor deposits. The third cat presented with multicentric leukemia and enlarged lymph nodes up to
3.0 cm × 1.5 cm in size. Three infusions of 50 mg of MAb at daily
intervals reduced the size of all lymph nodes by 30 to 50%. The
effect was transient however; and within 7 days of the final
infusion, size increases were again noticed in all lymph nodes.

There are several potential problems associated with passive
serotherapy as a treatment for persistent FeLV infections and LSA
in the natural setting. The major problem is one of specificity.
The amount of polymorphism associated with the env proteins of
FeLV, and the fact that variants of these proteins appear to
arise during infection, make the choice of an appropriate serum
for treatment difficult. A large pool of MAbs directed at different specificities, however, and the ability to screen this pool
against cells or virus from specific cats, may enable us to
choose specific MAb pools to treat individual animals. Second,
it appears that to be effective against viremia per se passive
therapy should be administered before or shortly after exposure
to the virus. This is impractical in the natural setting. Another
potential problem is that there is a large amount of viral antigen circulating in plasma which may prevent immunoglobulin from
reaching a target cell expressing virus. Finally, a host immune
response to the exogenously administered immunoglobulin may ren-
der it ineffective by neutralization. These findings may account
for the observation that long-term protection depends upon the
ability of cats to develop their own immune response (27). For
these reasons, a therapy which would enhance the ability of the
cat's immune system to produce antibodies against the particular
serotypes of viruses in its circulation may have the best opportunity to produce a long-lasting effect.

TREATMENT OF FELINE LSA AND PERSISTENT FeLV INFECTION BY EXTRA-
CORPOREAL IMMUNOADSORPTION OF PLASMA OVER STAPHYLOCOCCUS AUREUS
COWAN I (SAC)

Immunoadsorption of plasma over SAC is a treatment which
has been shown to result in stimulation of the immune response to
FeLV antigens as well as development of antibodies which lyse LSA
cells (33,34). This procedure has also been used to remove IgG
and CIC, by virtue of binding to SAC-derived protein A (SpA),
from plasma of humans and dogs with tumors (35,36). In some
cases, treatment resulted in clinically measurable antitumor
responses. IgG and CIC containing FeLV and other antigens were
also shown to be removed from cat plasma by the extracorporeal
immunoadsorption procedure (37-39). In theory, such treatment may
remove "specific serum blocking factors" (SBF), associated with
CIC, which would otherwise aid tumor escape from immunological
control (40). Whether removal of SBF or other possible explana-
tions (Table I), alone or in concert, account for the LSA regres-
sions and FeLV clearances obtained in some treated cats (33,34,
41) is currently unknown.

Jones et al. (34) have treated 16 FeLV-infected cats with
LSA by extracorporeal immunoadsorption. Each cat was treated a
minimum of 10 times on a biweekly schedule and was monitored for
persistence of the FeLV virion antigens and for regression of
LSA. Cats were considered to have cleared the FeLV infection when
their peripheral blood leukocytes were negative for FeLV antigens in repeated immunofluorescent antibody tests over a 2 week
period. Regression of LSA was determined by clearance of lymphoblasts from the blood (when present) or by reduction of the proportion of bone marrow lymphocytes to 20% in the absence of
lymphoblasts. On the basis of these criteria, nine cats were
determined to have cleared their viremias and to have regressed
their LSAs during treatment. Two other cats regressed their LSA
but remained persistently viremic and the remaining five cats

TABLE I. Extracorporeal Immunoadsorption with SAC:
Possible Biological Effects

Removal of IgG and CIC

Reduction in immunologic "suppressor factor(s)"
Reduction in antigen concentration

Release of Protein A

Activation of complement system
Blast transformation of B and T lymphocytes
Polyclonal activation of antibody synthesis
Potentiation of NK cell activity
Induction of interferon
Induction of rapid clearance of CIC

Release of Endotoxin

Leukopenia, leukocytosis
Hemorrhagic necrosis of tumors
Stimulation of immune response
Fever, diarrhea, shock

---

failed to respond by either FeLV clearance or tumor regression.
Most responses observed were long term, with several responder
cats remaining free of FeLV infection and in complete tumor
remission for several years.

In a retrospective analysis of three responder cats, one cat
cleared the viremia after 14 treatments, a second cat required
22 treatments and a third cat needed 45 treatments (34,38). Three
other cats, given 14, 19 and 22 treatments, respectively, failed
to clear their infections. These results led to a search for useful prognostic indicators for the treatment in order to help predict, prior to therapy, how many treatments may be necessary to
achieve FeLV clearance and/or LSA regression and to identify cats
which would be good candidates for treatment.

ANTIBODY RESPONSES AGAINST LSA AND FeLV IN CATS TREATED BY EXTRA-
CORPOREAL IMMUNOADSORPTION OF PLASMA OVER SAC

Quantitative analyses were performed to determine the levels
of peripheral blood leukocyte-associated viral antigens, soluble
viral antigens, FeLV-specific and LSA-specific antibodies and
FeLV antigen-containing CIC in cats with different responses to
extracorporeal immunoadsorption treatments (34,38,39). Data
obtained from two representative cases, one cat which regressed
its LSA but not the FeLV infection (#205) and one cat which
regressed both its tumor and cleared its viremia (#248) are shown
in Table II.

In general, clearance of LSA from cats preceded clearance of
FeLV. In the cats we have studied, the difference in time varied
from approximately 4 to 12 weeks. During a period of 5 to 6 weeks
prior to tumor regression, precipitating antibodies crossreacting
with FeLV-C gp70, but not with FeLV-A or FeLV-B gp70, were found.
These antibodies co-existed with tumor cells for 4 to 5 weeks and
persisted long after the tumors were cleared. In contrast, cytotoxic antibodies which lysed cultured LSA cells were not detected
until near the time at which there was clinical evidence of tumor
regression. We hypothesize that the antibodies which crossreacted
with FeLV-C gp70 were induced by immunogens on early emerging LSA
cells whose antigenic phenotype changed over time; antibodies
crossreactive with FeLV-A or FeLV-B gp70 were absorbed out by the
accompanying viremia. Early during the immune response against
the established tumor the antibodies to FeLV-C gp70 were not
cytotoxic, although they were an indicator of an eventual tumor
regression. Later during the immune response more type-specific
cytotoxic antibodies which lysed the established tumor appeared.
Titers of these cytotoxic antibodies could be detected long after
the tumors disappeared.

In the case of clearance of FeLV, a different specificity of
antibody was involved—precipitating antibodies against FeLV-A

TABLE II

Cat no.	Weeks of treatment	LSA status	FeLV status		Antibody status						
					Ab to gp70 of FeLV subgroup		Cytotoxic Ab for LSA cells:				
			PBL	gp70 in serum (μg/ml)	C	A + B	FL74	F422	3272	3281	FeLV-CIC (μg/ml)
205	0	+	+	550	<1:10	<1:10	1.5	<1	<1	1.7	12
	1	+	+	600	1:80	<1:10					9
	3	+	+	450	1:160	<1:10	1.1	1.6	1.2	4.6	2
	7	+	-	250	1:20	<1:10	8.7	3.7	3.7	12.5	13
	9	-	+	350	1:20	<1:10	6.1	4.9	2.7	12.0	17
	13	-	+			<1:10	21.5	18.5	1.9	22.0	
	21	-	+	350		<1:10	34.0	29.0	2.3	47.0	32
248	0	+	+	700	<1:10	<1:10	<1	<1	<1	<1	3
	3	+	+	850	1:40	<1:10	3.0	9.5	2.6	5.7	
	6	+	+	750	1:40	<1:10	4.3	14.5	2.1	5.1	21
	14	-	+	400	1:40	<1:10					
	18	-	+	50		1:10	13.5	21.0	5.9	6.1	5
	20	-	+	350		1:20					4
	22	-	+	250		1:40					4
	24	-	-	<50		1:10	14.3	20.1	6.9	5.9	2
	26	-	-	<50		1:40					
	28	-	-	<50		1:80	22.0	27.0	6.5	24.0	25

(continued)

TABLE II (continued)

Antibody (Ab) responses in two cats with LSA and FeLV infection after treatment by extra-corporeal immunoadsorption of plasma over SAC. Antibody to purified gp70s from different sub-groups of FeLV were measured in radioimmunoassays (38). Antibody titers (1:X) are shown. Anti-bodies for LSA cells were measured in a complement-dependent cytotoxicity assay (23). The num-bers represent absolute antibody titers (1:X). Levels of antibody killing four different LSA target cell lines (FL74, F422, 3272 and 3281) were determined by ^{51}Cr-release. Levels of CIC containing only FeLV antigens were measured in an assay described by Snyder et al. (38,39). Levels of FeLV gp70-related antigens in cat serum were determined in a competition radio-immunoassay (38). FeLV antigen expression in peripheral blood leukocytes (PBL) were deter-mined by immunofluorescence (1).

413

and FeLV-B gp70. Low titers of antibodies to these gp70s in sera
from responder cats were first detected at times when FeLV antigens were beginning to be cleared from blood leukocytes and
higher titers were found in samples taken after the blood leukocytes became persistently FeLV-negative. There was an inverse
correlation between the levels of soluble antigen and antibody in
serum (38,39).

In order to determine whether the induced antibodies were
involved in clearing at least a portion of the viral antigens, a
quantitative method for measuring FeLV-specific CIC was developed
(39). It was necessary to develop an FeLV-specific CIC assay
since the levels of total complement-fixing CIC as measured in
the Raji cell assay (42) did not correlate with the fluctuating
levels of viral antigen and antibody in the sera of responder
cats. Using the specific assay, levels of FeLV-CIC were found
which were a reflection of the levels of corresponding antigen in
serum (39). Levels of FeLV-CIC remained high until all detectable
circulating viral antigen had disappeared from the serum.

The conclusion from these studies is that extracorporeal
immunoadsorption of plasma from FeLV-infected LSA cats using SAC
stimulates existing low level antibody responses (often detected
only in the form of FeLV-CIC in plasma) against FeLV envelope
antigens. These antibodies mediate tumor cell lysis and, in some
cases, also mediate clearance of viral antigens and virus
infection.

TREATMENT OF FELINE LSA, LEUKEMIA AND PERSISTENT FeLV INFECTION
USING PURIFIED SpA

We (unpublished data) and others (41) have demonstrated
that extracorporeal removal of IgG and CIC from plasma of FeLV-
infected cats with LSA or leukemia by perfusion of plasma over
columns containing purified SpA crosslinked to an inert solid
matrix also leads to regression of tumors and clearance of

viremia. These effects were associated with development of antiviral antibodies in responder cats. While these columns represented a considerable improvement over the previous columns
(which contained whole heat-killed and formalin-fixed SAC) in
terms of specificity of removal of proteins from plasma, the
question whether leaching of SpA into plasma or the presence of
contaminants of SpA preparations (e.g., enterotoxin) also play
a role in tumor regression remained unanswered.

To address the question of possible effects of introduction
of leached SpA into the circulation, two groups have infused
purified SpA intravenously into normal cats and FeLV-infected
cats with LSA or leukemia (43,44). Objective antitumor effects
were observed in some cats with LSA and leukemia in both studies.
Harper et al. (44) found no antiviral responses and the antitumor
effects were transient. In contrast, Liu et al. (43) found some
long-term remissions and clearance of FeLV. These effects were
correlated with an increase in serum interferon levels and
development of FeLV-specific antibodies. It is possible that the
differences in the results of these two studies can be attributed
to the preparations and/or the dosages of SpA used.

Overall, these results suggest that some of the antitumor and
antiviral effects noted during extracorporeal immunoadsorption
treatments might result from introduction of SpA or a copurifying
contaminant of SpA preparations into the circulation of cats. It
is also possible, and we hypothesize, that both a removal from
plasma of products which may modulate immune responses (such as
CIC or other molecules) may play a necessary role in achieving
long-lasting responses.

APPLICATION OF EXTRACORPOREAL IMMUNOADSORPTION OF PLASMA OVER SpA
COLUMNS AS A TREATMENT FOR KAPOSI'S SARCOMA ASSOCIATED WITH AIDS

The responses of FeLV clearance and tumor regression achieved
in cats with FAIDS and persistent FeLV infection using extracorporeal immunoadsorption therapy suggest that it may have applica-
ion in the treatment of human AIDS and persistent HTLV-III/LAV/
ARV infection. In a pilot study, Kiprov and coworkers (45,46)
treated four AIDS patients with Kaposi's sarcoma three times per
week for a minimum of 4 weeks. There were no other antitumor or
antiviral treatments given during the extracorporeal immunoadsorption treatment period. Three of the patients exhibited partial responses against Kaposi's sarcoma lesions. While all three
patients presented with progressive disease involving daily
appearance of new skin lesions, no new lesions appeared while
the patients were being treated. A reddish halo developed around
40 to 50% of the existing lesions in all three patients. Between
20 to 30% of the lesions showed slight decreases in size along
with central umbilication. Approximately 10% of the lesions disappeared completely. Subsequent to 12 treatments one of the
patients has developed no new skin lesions for more than
6 months.

Biopsies were performed before, during and after the treatments. Pretreatment tissues revealed characteristic histological
features of Kaposi's sarcoma. Post treatment microscopic examinations revealed decreases in tumor cell density, reduction in
tumor size and increased deposition of collagen and C3 between
tumor cells. Grossly identifiable changes in the lesions were
observed during the first week of treatment. Necrosis and lymphocytic infiltration were not observed. It will be of interest to
determine whether immune responses to HTLV-III/LAV/ARV, to other
viruses such as cytomegalovirus or to Kaposi's sarcoma-associated
antigens are affected by extracorporeal immunoadsorption treatments. At present we are investigating these parameters.

ACKNOWLEDGMENTS

Grateful appreciation is extended to Dr. W. D. Hardy, Jr. and the National Veterinary Laboratory, Franklin Lakes, New Jersey, for the FeLV tests of peripheral blood leukocytes.

Harry W. Snyder, Jr. is a Scholar of the Leukemia Society of America.

REFERENCES

1. Hardy, W.D., Jr., Hirshaut, Y. and Hess, P. (1973). In "Unifying Concepts of Leukemia" (R.M. Dutcher and L. Chieco-Bianchi, eds.), p. 778. Karger, Basel.
2. Hardy, W.D., Jr., Hess, P.W., MacEwen, E.G. et al. (1976). Cancer Res. 36, 582.
3. Hardy, W.D., Jr. (1980). In "Feline Leukemia Virus" (W.D. Hardy, Jr., M. Essex and A.J. McClelland, eds.), p. 3. Elsevier/North Holland, New York.
4. Dorn, C.R., Taylor, D.O.N. and Hubbard, H.H. (1967). Am. J. Vet. Res. 28, 993.
5. McClelland, A.J., Hardy, W.D., Jr. and Zuckerman, E.E. (1980). In "Feline Leukemia Virus" (W.D. Hardy, Jr., M. Essex and A.J. McClelland, eds.), p. 211. Elsevier/North Holland, New York.
6. Essex, M. (1980). In "Viral Oncology" (G. Klein, ed.), p. 205. Raven Press, New York.
7. Anderson, L.J., Jarrett, W.F.H., Jarrett, O. et al. (1971). J. Natl. Cancer Inst. 44, 339.
8. Perryman, L.E., Hoover, E.A. and Yohn, D.S. (1972). J. Natl. Cancer Inst. 49, 1357.
9. Mathes, L.E., Olsen, R.G., Hebebrand, L.C. et al. (1978). Nature 274, 687.
10. Trainen, Z., Wernicke, D., Unger-Waron, H. et al. (1983). Science 220, 858.
11. Barre-Sinoussi, F., Chermann, J.C., Rey, F. et al. (1983). Science 220, 868.
12. Popovic, M., Sarngadharan, M.G., Read, E. et al. (1984). Science 224, 497.
13. Levy, J.A., Hoffman, A.D., Kramer, S.M. et al. (1984). Science 225, 840.
14. Pinter, A. and Honnen, W.J. (1983). J. Virol. 46, 1056.
15. Sarma, P.S. and Log, T. (1971). Virology 44, 352.
16. Sarma, P.S. and Log, T. (1973). Virology 54, 160.
17. Jarrett, O., Laird, H.M. and Hay, D. (1973). J. Gen. Virol. 20, 169.

18. Snyder, H.W., Jr., Singhal, M.C., Zuckerman, E.R. et al. (1983). Virology 131, 315.
19. Vedbrat, S.S., Rasheed, S., Lutz, H. et al. (1983). Virology 124, 445.
20. Essex, M., Klein, G. and Harrold, J.B. (1971). Nature 233, 295.
21. Essex. M., Cotter, S.M., Stephenson, J.R. et al. (1977). Cold Spring Harbor Conf. Cell Prolif. 4, 1197.
22. Hardy, W.D., Jr., Zuckerman, E., MacEwen, E.G. et al. (1977). Nature 270, 249.
23. Grant, C.K., DeBoer, D.J., Essex, M. et al. (1977). J. Immunol. 119, 401.
24. Essex, M., Klein, G. and Harrold, J.B. (1971). Int. J. Cancer 8, 384.
25. Essex, M. and Snyder, S.P. (1973). J. Natl. Cancer Inst. 51, 1007.
26. Hoover, E.A., Schaller, J.P., Mathes, L.E. et al. (1977). Infect. Immun. 16, 54.
27. deNoronha, F., Schafer, W., Essex, M. et al. (1978). Virology 85, 617.
28. deNoronha, F., Grant, C.K., Essex, M. et al. (1980). In "Feline Leukemia Virus" (W.D. Hardy, Jr., M. Essex and A.J. McClelland, eds.), p. 253. Elsevier/North Holland, New York.
29. Essex, M., Sliski, A.H., Worley, M. et al. (1980). Cold Spring Harbor Conf. Cell Prolif. 7, 589.
30. deNoronha, F., Baggs, R., Schafer, W. et al. (1977). Nature 267, 54.
31. Cotter, S.M., Essex, M., McLane, M.F. et al. (1980). In "Feline Leukemia Virus" (W.D. Hardy, Jr., M. Essex and A.J. McClelland, eds.), p. 219. Elsevier/North Holland, New York.
32. Grant, C.K., Ernisse, B.J., Jarrett, O. et al. (1983). J. Immunol. 131, 3042.
33. Jones, F.R., Yoshida, L.H., Ladiges, W.C. et al. (1980). Cancer 46, 675.
34. Jones, F.R., Grant, C.K. and Snyder, H.W., Jr. (1984). J. Biol. Response Mod. 3, 286.
35. Bansal, S.C., Bansal, B.R., Thomas, H.L. et al. (1978). Cancer 42, 1.
36. Terman, D.S., Yamamota, Y., Mattioli, M. et al. (1980). J. Immunol. 124, 795.
37. Snyder, H.W., Jr., Jones, F.R., Day, N.K. et al. (1982). J. Immunol. 128, 2776.
38. Snyder, H.W., Jr., Singhal, M.C., Hardy, W.D., Jr. (1984). J. Immunol. 132, 1538.
39. Snyder, H.W., Jr., Singhal, M.C., Yoshida, L.H. et al. (1985). Molec. Immunol., in press.
40. Hellström, K.E., Hellström, I., Snyder, H.W., Jr. et al. (1985). Contemp. Top. Immunobiol. 15, in press.

41. Liu, W.T., Engelman, R.W., Trang, L.Q. et al. (1984). Proc. Natl. Acad. Sci. 81, 3516.
42. Day, N.K., O'Reilly-Felice, C., Hardy, W.D., Jr. et al. (1980). J. Immunol. 125, 2363.
43. Liu, W.T., Good, R.A., Trang, L.Q. et al. (1984). Proc. Natl. Acad. Sci. 81, 6471.
44. Harper, H.D., Sjöquist, J., Hardy, W.D., Jr. et al. (1985). Cancer 55, 1863.
45. Kiprov, D.D., Lippert, R., Jones, F.R. et al. (1984). J. Biol. Response Mod. 3, 341.
46. Kiprov, D.D., Lippert, R., Sandstrom, E. et al. (1985). J. Clin. Apheresis, in press.

BOVINE LEUKEMIA VIRUS VACCINE

Janice Miller

National Animal Disease Center
Ames, Iowa

Compared to the vaccination attempts described in other
animal species, not much attention has been given to such
research in the bovine. Part of the reason for this lack of
interest is that some countries had established relatively successful bovine leukosis control programs several years before
the bovine leukemia virus (BLV) was identified. In this volume,
Dr. Van Der Maaten has described the eradication effort in Den-
mark, which was based on elimination of herds that had cattle
with persistent lymphocytosis ("Pathogenesis of Bovine Retrovirus
Infection"). In other European countries the programs were less
stringent in that only the individual affected animals were eliminated. Despite the recognized insensitivity of hematologic
testing, the method was sufficiently effective to keep leukosis
prevalence quite low, and when serological tests for BLV infection became available, it was not difficult to incorporate them
into the test and slaughter protocols. In contrast, the United
States has never had any type of leukosis control and the prevalence of BLV infection is so high, especially in dairy cattle,
that an eradication program is not economically feasible. Therefore, we felt that an effort should be made to determine whether
a BLV vaccine would be biologically possible.

421

I am going to describe our experiments first because we were the first group to attempt BLV prophylaxis in 1978 (1). That study was very limited, as you will see, so we repeated and expanded the work in 1983 (2). In between our reports, Patrascu et al. (3) published results of an experiment in Romania that was almost identical to our 1978 report except they used a much larger number of animals.

The BLV antigen was prepared from cell culture fluid of a persistently infected fetal lamb kidney (FLK) cell line that was established several years ago by Dr. Van Der Maaten. We use a different culture procedure for making the feline leukemia virus vaccine, because if we grow FLK cells in serum-free medium they produce plenty of infectious virus but very little soluble glycoprotein. To get a reasonable antigen yield it is necessary to grow the cells in medium that is supplemented with at least 5% fetal calf serum. Because the cell culture produces infectious virus in addition to antigen, we use either acetylethylneimine or binary ethylenimine for inactivation. Selection of these chemicals was based on research with foot and mouth disease virus, which showed that viral nucleic acid was affected, whereas antigenicty of proteins was not.

As an adjuvant we have used only aluminum hydroxide gel, although others have used incomplete Freund's. The problem with oil adjuvants is that the intense tissue reaction may cause a problem in animals that are intended for slaughter. Each dose of vaccine contained 0.3 to 0.4 mg of viral glycoprotein. Virus challenge was accomplished by inoculation of infected lymphocytes, rather than cell-free virus, because that appears to be the way BLV is transmitted naturally. The number of lymphocytes used for challenge has varied from 2500 to 4,000,000.

In our experiments, three different systems were used for evaluating the results of vaccine challenge: syncytium induction assay (SIA) in cat cells; glycoprotein antigen production in

TABLE I. Immunization of Cattle with Antigens
in Culture Fluid from FLK Cells

| Treatment | Miller and Van Der Maaten | | Patrascu et al. |
	(1)	(2)	(3)
Vaccine and challenge	1/4[a]	10/12	2/20
Challenge only	2/2	8/8	8/8
Vaccine only	ND[b]	1/4	ND

[a]No. infected/no. tested.

[b]Not done.

lymphocyte culture, as detected with radioimmunoassay (RIA); bioassay in sheep. Although we believe bioassay is the most sensitive indicator of BLV infection, it is rather expensive so we did
not use it when both the SIA and RIA were positive.

The results of our 1978 and 1983 experiments are presented in
Table I. The first trial was limited to four animals but three of
them appeared to be protected by the vaccine. The second study
was less successful. One reason may have been that we used a
100-fold higher dose of infected lymphocytes for the challenge.
Another factor was that our virus inactivation treatment apparently was inadequate because one of four vaccinated cattle that
were not challenged became infected. Before starting the experiment we had inoculated a sheep with the vaccine and did not find
evidence of infectivitiy. Obviously, however, that was an insufficient testing procedure. Even though it was difficult to interpret the protective effect of our vaccine, because of the problem
with incomplete inactivation, we believe that immunization
altered the course of BLV infection in many animals. When we compared SIA results for the year following challenge, only 21.8% of

the tests were positive in vaccinated as compared to 87.5% in
controls. It appeared that even though vaccinated animals became
infected (whether through vaccination or challenge) the number of
infected lymphocytes in their blood was reduced.

The experiment conducted in Romania was much more successful than ours (Table I). They tested their antigen extensively
for virus inactivation before trying to vaccinate with it, and
they showed apparently complete protection in 18 of 20 animals
after challenge. In comparing their vaccination protocol to ours,
I noticed that seven of their animals received oil-adjuvanted
material, which may have improved the immune response. Another
difference in their experiment was that the challenge of infected
lymphocytes was given intramuscularly. We have never tried to
infect cattle by that route, and it may not be as effective as
the subcutaneous inoculation procedure we use. I think the evaluation of vaccinates for infection was very thorough, because
each test involved inoculation of blood into three sheep. Most
cattle were tested at 10 weeks post challenge but some were
tested twice, at 7 and 32 weeks post challenge. The results were
quite consistent in that blood from infected cattle caused seroconversion in each recipient sheep.

Regarding the immune response of vaccinated cattle, they produce antibody to the viral glycoprotein, with neutralizing titers
up to 1:128. This serological reaction is a disadvantage in terms
of the potential usefulness of such a vaccine because vaccinated
cattle could not be easily differentiated from infected cattle.
The carbohydrate component of the BLV glycoprotein is necessary
for a precipitating reaction to occur so we thought that if we
used just the protein as a vaccine we might protect cattle without causing them to seroconvert. However, as shown in Table II
antigen treated vith glycosidases did not prevent infection.

Recently Dr. Misao Onuma published a paper describing the
vaccination of sheep with several different BLV preparations (5;

TABLE II. Immunization of Cattle with Glycosidase-treated
BLV Glycoprotein[a]

Treatment	Result
Vaccine and challenge	6/8[b]
Challenge only	5/8

[a]See Ref. 4.

[b]No. infected/no. tested.

Table III). He started with culture fluid from FLK cells but concanavalin A Sepharose was used to separate the p24 and glyco-protein antigens. In addition to these soluble immunogens he used two cell preparations as vaccines. One cell line was the FLK and the other was SF28, an infected sheep cell line that is BLV transformed but does not produce virus. The soluble antigens were inactivated with acetylethylenimine and cells were fixed with 2.5% glutaraldehyde. Each sheep was given three injections, the first in an oil adjuvant. The concentration of soluble antigen was similar to that used in our experiments and the other vac-cines contained about 50,000,000 cells. For the challenge he used 10,000 infected lymphocytes, given subcutaneously. Results were fairly clear-cut, as shown in Table III. The sheep vac-cinated with p24 antigen or with SF28 cells did not make anti-body to glycoprotein antigen, and were not protected against the challenge. In contrast, sheep vaccinated with glycoprotein or with FLK cells made antibody to glycoprotein and were protected. I should point out that the SIA was used to check for infection and a more sensitive evaluation, such as bioassay, might have shown some of the sheep were not protected.

The only other work done on a BLV vaccine was done in Russia (Table IV). Parfanovich and her colleagues (6) purified virus on

TABLE III.   Immunization of Sheep with Soluble
and Cellular Antigens of BLV[a]

| Antigen | Result | |
	Antibody[b]	Infection[c]
p24	0/3[d]	3/3
Glycoprotein	3/3	0/3
FLK cells	3/3	0/3
SF28 cells	0/3	3/3

[a]See Ref. 5.

[b]To glycoprotein by AGID.

[c]SIA.

[d]No. positive/no. tested.

sucrose gradients and then tested several methylated amino acids as inactivating agents. They selected one that they felt gave sufficient inactivation with maximum antigen preservation. Aluminum hydroxide was used as an adjuvant and two injections were given. Protein content of the vaccine was similar to that used in our experiments but total viral protein was quantitated, not just glycoprotein. The challenge inoculum was either cell-free BLV or infected lymphocytes but in the results it is not clear which was used in various experiments so I have pooled them for analysis. The authors concluded that vaccinated cattle were completely protected against challenge, but this probably could be considered questionable because of the method used to test vaccinates for infection. Blood lymphocytes were cultured with phytohemagglutinin and then examined by electron microscopy for virus-like particles, and I think most people would agree that such an assay is relatively insensitive. Notice that infection was detected in only half of the nonvaccinated challenged controls, which is the sort of result one might expect with an inadequate test system. If that is the case, it is likely that at least some of the

TABLE IV. Immunization of Cattle and Sheep
with Inactivated BLV[a]

Treatment	Result
Cattle	
Vaccine and challenge	0/16[b]
Challenge only	12/24
Sheep	
Vaccine and challenge	0/27
Challenge only	32/36

[a]See Ref. 6.

[b]No. positive/no. tested (electron microscopy).

vaccinates were also infected. The Russian group also did some vaccine trials in sheep but they are difficult to interpret because the controls shown are from experiments done previously in other laboratories.

Before concluding, I should mention some experiments in which attempts were made to use noninfected lymphoid cells to protect animals. Dr. Gordon Theilen used a lymphoblastoid cell line that was derived from a case of calf form lymphosarcoma (non-BLV infected). He gave two or three injections of these cells, mixed with aluminum hydroxide, and then challenged with infected lymphocytes. Results of the first two experiments looked promising (Table V), especially since the vaccine did not cause seroconversion and therefore would not interfere with serological tests for diagnosis of BLV infection. The mechanism of protection, in the absence of viral-specific stimulation, was not apparent. Subsequently, however, in a third experiment a control group was added

TABLE V. Immunization of Cattle with Non-BLV
Lymphoid Cell Line[a]

Treatment	Expts. 1 and 2[a]	Expt. 3[b]
Vaccine and challenge	1/9[c]	2/12
Challenge only	7/9	9/12
Adjuvant and challenge	ND[d]	3/12

[a]See Refs. 7 and 8.

[b]Not published.

[c]No. infected/no. tested (antibody to BLV glycoprotein by AGID).

[d]Not done.

that received only aluminum hydroxide. As you can see (Table V),
the adjuvant was just as protective alone as when mixed with the
lymphoid cells. This experiment has not been reported but I think
it is important to know about it when considering results of the
published work.

A different lymphoid cell line, also from a calf lymphosarcoma, was used by Roberts et al. (9,10) to immunize sheep (Table
VI). Although a slight protective effect was observed in the
period shortly after vaccination, a subsequent study in cattle
showed no protection.

At our last international bovine leukosis meeting in 1982,
we had a rather spirited discussion regarding the requirements
a BLV vaccine would have to fulfill to be acceptable. It was
unanimously agreed that such a vaccine would have to be noninfectious, nononcogenic and prevent persistent infection. The debat-
able issue was whether it could be used if it interfered with the
serological tests commonly used to detect BLV-infected cattle. In

TABLE VI. Immunization of Sheep with Non-BLV Infected
Lymphoid Cell Line[a]

Treatment	Result
Vaccine and challenge	
4 weeks	1/4[b]
8 weeks	3/4
12 weeks	3/4
Challenge only	4/4

[a]See Ref. 9.

[b]No. positive/no. tested (antibody to BLV glycoprotein).

places like the United States, where there is a very high prevalence of BLV, it probably would be necessary to use a subunit
glycoprotein vaccine and then use the p24 antigen for serological
testing to detect infection. However, infected cattle do not have
high antibody titers to p24, so a very sensitive test such as
ELISA or RIA would be required, and there are only one or two
research laboratories in the country that could perform these
assays. Furthermore, our European colleagues have expressed doubt
that their animal health regulatory agencies would ever allow the
importation of vaccinated animals and currently that is the major
reason that United States cattle producers are even interested
in BLV. I think after considering these problems, you will understand why we are not too enthusiastic about the potential for
controlling this virus by vaccination.

REFERENCES

1. Miller, J.M. and Van Der Maaten, M.J. (1978). Ann. Rech. Vet.
   9, 871.
2. Miller, J.M., Van Der Maaten, M.J. and Schmerr, M.J.F.
   (1983). Am. J. Vet. Res. 44, 64.
3. Patrascu, I.V., Coman, S., Sandu, I. et al. (1980). Rev.
   Roum. Med-Virol. 31, 95.

4. Miller, J.M., Van Der Maaten, M.J. and Schmerr, M.J.F.
   (1984). In "Fifth International Symposium on Bovine Leukosis," p. 507. Commission of the European Communities,
   Luxembourg.
5. Onuma, M., Hodatsu, T., Yamamoto, S. et al. (1984). Am. J.
   Vet. Res. 45, 1212.
6. Parfanovich, M.I., Zhdanov, M., Lazarenko, A.A. et al.
   (1983). Br. Vet. J. 139, 137.
7. Theilen, G.H., Miller, J.M., Higgins, J. et al. (1982). In
   "Fourth International Symposium on Bovine Leukosis," p. 547.
   Martinus Nijhoff, Boston.
8. Theilen, G.H., Ruppanner, R.N., Miller, J.M. et al. (1984).
   In "Fifth International Symposium on Bovine Leukosis,"
   p. 493. Commission of the European Communities, Luxembourg.
9. Roberts, D.H., Lucas, M.H., Sands, J. et al. (1982). Vet.
   Immunol. Immunopathol. 3, 635.
10. Roberts, D.H., Lucas, M.H., Sands, J. et al. (1984). In
    "Fifth International Symposium on Bovine Leukosis," p. 481.
    Commission of the European Communities, Luxembourg.

SIMIAN VACCINE

Murray B. Gardner

Department of Pathology
School of Medicine
University of California
Davis, California

My role will be fourfold. I am going to play the historian, although I do not really consider myself an elder citizen. I have lived through a bit of retrovirus history and shall say something from that perspective. I shall say a few words about SAIDS and AIDS and their similarities and differences and something new about the comparison of AIDS viruses and, finally, I shall end up on the AIDS vaccine rationale, laying the groundwork for what is coming.

I have stood up at meetings since 1968 as an advocate for the study of retroviruses, defending why I, an M.D., would be working with wild mice, parakeets, cats, monkeys and what not, trying to figure out what is happening with their retroviruses. I always have had to explain why we could not find these viruses in man and promise that they were going to be there, even if they were lurking in the deep. I have had to explain to my mother, kids and friends why I was studying things that apparently did not have anything to do with humans.

Now it is the other way around. Retroviruses are indeed presenting themselves with vengence on the human scene and are drawing attention because of their causative role in AIDS. I read the local newspaper and see the headline "AIDS Toll Rises, Vaccine

Hopes Fade." My wife says, "I thought you were going to make a vaccine. Haven't you even tried yet?" My kid comes home from school and says, "I was going to give a report on the future of AIDS vaccination. Is it already over? You cannot do it?" Then I pick up the latest *Time* magazine and I read about the "AIDS Virus as a Rosetta Stone." It says all sorts of things that are timely and topical about AIDS, about how science will triumph over the dread disease. According to *Time*, we have an epidemic that has not yet struck the general population, 6500 cases so far, fatal in about half of those cases. The article talks about the Pasteur group, mentions Jean-Claude Chermann, Dr. Montagnier's colleague, and says that he considers HTLV-III (human T cell lymphotropic virus type III) and LAV (lymphadenopathy-associated virus) to be "like two brothers." You read a little farther. It talks about a spectrum of outcomes. Although nobody as yet apparently has recovered from AIDS, some with mild disease (AIDS-related complex [ARC]) do get better. We read that the vast majority of infected people have no symptoms and that about 50% of the gay men in San Francisco and New York now have HTLV-III antibodies but only about 10% or so of them are destined to get AIDS each year.

What should we tell the people who test positive for the antibodies? We must not lead such people to conclude wrongly that they are doomed. The reference to the rosetta stone means that individuals who have antibodies to the AIDS virus carry a badge of honor telling their employers, insurance companies and landlords that they are homosexuals or drug abusers. Then as if that were not enough, the same *Time* magazine tells me that non-A, non-B hepatitis may be caused by a retrovirus. My head is swimming.

During the 1970s the National Cancer Institute (NCI) made the biggest effort imaginable to find retroviruses in humans. It was coordinated to some fashion, and we pulled together, sharing our resources. Oh, there was competition, but still we tried together and made a noble effort under Robert Huebner, Wally Rowe and

John Moloney. This effort paid off with Gallo's isolation of
HTLV-I in 1979, but by then the Virus Cancer Program was dead.
Now is the time we really need that teamwork. The National Institute of Allergy and Infectious Diseases (NIAID) has taken the
ball and is running with it.

Let me review the four eras of tumor virology that Wally Rowe
outlined. It is very poetic. We seem to have gone almost back to
the beginning. The first era was when Peyton Rous showed that
avian sarcoma virus fulfilled Koch's postulates and thus proved
for the first time that a virus could cause cancer. However,
Koch's postulates could not be met so easily with other viruses.
This led to the second era, dominated by the rabbit Shope papil-
loma and the mouse mammary tumor viruses, during which investigators began to carve out those cofactors that had to be present in
order for the virus to produce disease. In other words, you never
had a one-to-one relationship of virus to disease. Other influ-
ences (e.g., hormones, cell genes) tipped the balance for the
host or the virus. That era continued until about 1950 and cul-
minated in Ludwig Gross's isolation and thorough study of the
murine leukemia virus. Then, following the lead of the Cal Tech
phage people, Dulbecco, Rubin and colleagues showed that the DNA
tumor viruses (polyoma, adenovirus) and then RNA tumor viruses
(avian and murine leukemia and sarcoma viruses) could be grown
in cell culture; they worked up the basis for viral interference,
quantitative focus formation assays and mixture of defective and
helper viruses. Huebner described the DNA tumor virus antigens
and antibodies. This was the third major era. The fourth era, the
one that most of us got in on, was based on the realization that
not only were RNA tumor viruses important in nature, but because
they encoded reverse transcriptase enzyme, these fascinating
things had the ability to be genes on the one hand and viruses on
the other. The genetic inheritance of these retrovirogenes was
the trigger for formation of the NCI Virus Cancer Program. Based

primarily on the finding that leukemia and mammary tumor virus
genes were inherited in AKR and in GR inbred mice, respectively,
it was suspected that the inheritance of analogous viral genes
and their later activation were going to be very important in the
generality of human cancers. When Huebner came to Los Angeles in
1968, he said to me, "You know, we have got to get people working
on RNA tumor viruses." I said, "Sure, we will do it. What are
they?" He said, "There has been all this work on DNA tumor
viruses, millions of dollars spent on polyoma and SV40 that don't
cause any disease in nature. Let's study something that causes
cancer in the real world. These RNA tumor viruses are out there
in nature causing cancer in chickens, mice, cats and cows. There
has to be unity in nature; we cannot have these things in so many
species and not have them in man." So we went after virtually
every animal and human in Los Angeles. From 1968 to 1978 we
checked out parakeets, dogs, cats, wild rats, wild mice and zoo
animals. We found the virus in some species (e.g., cats, wild
rodents); we did not find it in others (e.g., parakeets, dogs,
humans). We found that viruses of this type caused not only cancer, mostly lymphomas and sarcomas, but also a variety of other
diseases, including immunosuppression. We looked by every conceivable assay at all possible human tissues. We sent material
to everybody's ice box. After 12 years, we had not found a human
retrovirus. So we were out of business and the whole Virus Cancer
Program came tumbling down in 1980. Much to his credit, Gallo
hung in there and finally his lab at the NCI did isolate a human
virus in 1979. Shortly thereafter the Japanese identified the
first bonafide human RNA tumor virus, HTLV-I. The key event leading to this accomplishment was the discovery by Frank Ruscetti,
then in Gallo's lab, of the T cell growth factor which facili-
tated the tissue culture growth of T lymphocytes harboring HTLV-
I. Gallo's lab was thus in a position to isolate other T cell

tropic human retroviruses, such as HTLV-III. Those are the four
major chapters of the story leading up to 1981.

The fifth era now in full blast is that of molecular virology
using recombinant DNA technology. Think about it. We have studied
avian leukosis virus for 80 years and still do not have all the
answers. We have been studying the mouse mammary tumor for
50 years and we still do not understand many things about that
virus. With murine leukemia virus (MuLV), it has been 35 years
and it too remains an unfolding story; with feline leukemia virus
(FeLV), 20 years; and with HTLV-I, only 4 years. With the AIDS
viruses, a brand new biology is only 1 year old. It is an excit-
ing new chapter in retrovirology. No one knows where it is going
to lead. The simian model of AIDS (SAIDS) and its associated
type D retrovirus also make up a new, remarkable biology with
many parallels to human AIDS.

No apologies need be given for the potential importance of
the inherited RNA tumor virus genes, but all known retroviral
diseases still seem to be due to the horizontally transmitted
viruses as first found in the Peyton Rous era. These viruses are
fulfilling Koch's postulates and behaving like other infectious
viruses acquired by the animal from who knows where, getting in
and out of the target cells but not being inherited as genetic
elements. Cofactors may be all important in determining who gets
sick and who does not. It is therefore appropriate that research
on AIDS be supported, at least in part, by NIAID because it is
indeed an infectious disease.

Let me highlight probably the most dramatic thing that has
happened with the simian model of AIDS at the University of
California, Davis. Rhesus macaques in one cage (north corral #1)
had a 40% death rate in 1981 to 1982 from a wasting disease with
multiple infections (now called SAIDS). Similar focal disease
outbreaks had happened since the late 1960s, but in each
instance, the veterinarians thought that they were caused by an

environmental factor in the soil or water or by a dietary deficiency. The researchers did not investigate an underlying infectious etiology. They held on to the resistant animals and thus in
retrospect fueled the next epidemic when new animals were exposed
to these carriers. The reason that the disease was not thoroughly
investigated was that there was no recognized human disease such
as AIDS to call attention to it.

This AIDS-like disease in monkeys has many different manifestations, such as diarrhea, weight loss and failure to thrive. It
was called the wasting disease, the low protein syndrome, what
have you, but the whole picture was not put together until a few
Kaposi-like solid tumors occurred. How long would it have been
before human AIDS would have been discovered had it not been for
the cluster of homosexuals with Kaposi sarcoma that Gotlieb et
al. uncovered in 1981? Occurrence of these solid tumors was the
tip-off that something unusual was going on in the monkeys and
humans. With that in mind we began to look for an infectious
agent in the monkey. To prove an infectious etiology, we divided
the north corral #1 into two parts, making a cage inside a cage
separated by a 10-foot barrier of chain-linked fencing, and we
added new monkeys to each cage. A year later all 23 monkeys
exposed directly to the affected cage mates had died of SAIDS,
confirmed histologically, serologically and virologically. Ten
feet away, all 22 animals were alive and healthy 1 year later and
not a single animal seroconverted or became virus infected. A
distance of 10 feet was all that it took to protect against the
spread of this highly contagious disease. Spread of this disease
obviously required close physical contact. The monkeys rub, bite,
scratch and climb over each other and spill the virus out of
their saliva. Just as in FeLV in cats, we believe that saliva is
the major route by which the virus is spread among monkeys. We
now know that 20% of the animals in that cage are persistently
infected with the SAIDS virus, that 80% have antibody to this

virus and that 60% have antibody but no detectable virus. All
monkeys over 3 years of age are antibody positive. A few young
animals get the virus, fail to develop antibody and quickly die
off. All monkeys in this cage get infected in time; the majority
make antibodies, get rid of the virus and remain well. About 20%
of the animals remain persistently infected in the face of antiviral antibodies and these include ill animals as well as healthy
carriers. If you want to set up a vaccine experiment, you can add
immunized and control monkeys to this cage and certainly expect
to see a meaningful difference if the vaccine works. Rhesus
monkeys inoculated with the tissue culture purified type D virus
develop a spectrum of disease patterns just like those we see in
the naturally occurring SAIDS outbreak and what you might expect
from any infectious disease, including AIDS. Some animals die
within 2 to 3 months with severe immune depletion and opportunistic infections. Other animals remain chronically ill over many
months with weight loss, anemia, generalized lymphadenopathy,
splenomegaly, hypoproteinemia, diarrhea, gingivitis and depressed
lymphoid mitogenic responsiveness, but they hang on to life.
Occasionally, an animal snaps back, recovers lymphoid responsiveness and becomes reasonably healthy. Such recovered animals have
high titers of virus neutralizing antibody and are nonviremic in
contrast to the persistently infected monkeys in which neutralizing antibody is at low titer or absent. We isolate virus easily
from multiple tissues of the infected animals, most readily from
peripheral blood lymphocytes (PBL) and saliva. Whether the seem-
ingly immune and recovered animal has latent but potentially
activatable type D retrovirus in places such as bone marrow macrophages must yet be determined. The similarities of this simian
model to FeLV in infected multicat households is striking. However, the amount of virus in PBL and tissues other than salivary
gland is rather low, considerably less than in most FeLV-infected
cats or MuLV-infected mice. The early, intermediate and end

stages of SAIDS and AIDS are pathologically almost undistinguish-
able, as are many of the clinical, epidemiologic and virologic
features. There are differences, however. The simian type D virus
does not have the restricted T4 lymphotropism as seen with the
AIDS viruses. The monkey virus grows in both T4 and T8 and B
cells as well as in macrophages, fibroblasts and epithelial
cells. The infected monkeys do not show as marked a hyperimmune
polyclonal B cell immune response compared to that often seen in
infected humans. SAIDS has a lesser incidence of Pneumocystis
carinii and Kaposi's sarcoma than does AIDS.

You can use Southern blots and the molecularly cloned Mason-
Pfizer monkey virus (MPMV) or SAIDS type D virus probes to look
at SAIDS virus genes in the rhesus tissues, although there is a
background of inherited related sequences. The endogenous-related
sequences are mostly in the gag and pol regions, so env-specific
clones are cleaner. We can detect SAIDS proviral DNA in PBL,
spleens and salivary glands. We can distinguish different strains
of SAIDS type D virus from each other and from MPMV. Type D viral
polymorphism apparently occurs in SAIDS at several West Coast
centers and one strain of this virus (type 2) appears to be
linked to the retroperitoneal fibrosis seen in association with
SAIDS in monkeys at Oregon and Washington. HTLV-I may be latent
in some of these monkeys, as it surely is at the New England
Center, but we have not found any association between HTLV-I and
SAIDS in our animals. Nor do we have any evidence of an HTLV-III-
related virus in our SAIDS animals at Davis.

We obtained the frozen rhesus breast tumor that was the
initial source of the original MPMV isolate in 1970. We reisolated this virus from that tumor, put it in monkeys and produced
fatal SAIDS, thus confirming the initial transmission studies
with this virus in the early 1970s. By restriction mapping the
recovered virus was shown to be identical to the original MPMV.
Interestingly, the original MPMV is no longer recovered from

monkeys with spontaneous SAIDS. All the type D isolates are now
related to MPMV in the core antigens but are distinct in the
envelope antigens. We are confident that this family of type D
viruses possesses immunosuppressive properties and is the primary agent of SAIDS at our California Primate Center and probably at the Oregon and Washington centers as well.

Having found this remarkable type D virus causing SAIDS in
our monkeys, we were, of course, struck by the similar appearance of the human AIDS extracellular virus particles under the
electron microscope. We compared the three prototype human AIDS-
associated retroviruses, LAV, HTLV-III and ARV, one to another
and to the SAIDS virus. We wanted to compare the human isolates
for strain variability because of the implications for immuno-
diagnostics and vaccines. We looked at the three human viruses
by several techniques, including electron microscopy, immunofluorescence and Western blotting, using a battery of sera from
infected humans. A molecularly cloned probe of ARV was obtained
from the Chiron lab and used to compare the restriction maps of
these viruses. The three human isolates were indistinguishable
by electron microscopy, immunofluorescence and immunoblotting.
Any one of them could thus serve as a target for serologic surveys. Genetically, they were also very similar, with LAV and
HTLV-III being almost identical. Morphologically, they also
looked like visna and other lentiviruses with which they may yet
show some relatedness. However, the SAIDS type D viruses showed
no immunologic or genetic relatedness to the human viruses in
these same assays. Furthermore, the SAIDS virus maturates as an
intracytoplasmic A particle, a feature not seen in the AIDS
viruses. Thus, these immunosuppressive retroviruses were unique
to each species.

There exists an obvious rationale for preparing a vaccine
against AIDS. The disease is not going to go away on its own.
Its incidence is increasing steadily. We have identified the

causative virus, but much remains to be learned about the natural
history. Although infected humans do make antibodies which recognize the envelope as an immune target, virus production tends to
persist in most. It is not yet known whether neutralizing antibodies can be induced that will protect against this disease, but
precedence from natural retroviral infection in animals indicates
that vaccine protection against human AIDS is by no means impos-
sible. Furthermore, the recombinant DNA industry will be putting
its novel technologies to work on this problem. SAIDS and other
animal retroviral models will continue to serve as a vital link
between the test tube and the human. Therefore, a commitment to
take on this problem with optimism and teamwork is in order.

HUMAN AIDS
IN THE CHIMPANZEE

TRANSMISSION OF AIDS TO CHIMPANZEES:
INFECTION, DISEASE AND IMMUNE RESPONSE[1]

Jorg W. Eichberg, David A. Lawlor,
Ronald C. Kennedy, Gordon R. Dressman

Virology and Immunology Department,
Southwest Foundation for Biomedical Research,
San Antonio, Texas

Harvey J. Alter

Department of Transfusion Medicine
Clinical Center

W. Carl Saxinger

Laboratory of Tumor Cell Biology
National Cancer Institute
National Institutes of Health
Bethesda, Maryland

INTRODUCTION

Acquired immune deficiency syndrome (AIDS) is a recently
recognized human disease whose incidence in the United States is
rapidly increasing (1). The disease is characterized by diverse
immunological abnormalities, including lymphocyte dysfunction and
depletion of the T helper subpopulation of lymphocytes (2,3). A

---

[1]This work was supported by Contracts N01-HB-2-7004 and
N01-CL-1-2115 and Grant HL-32505 from the National Heart, Lung,
and Blood Institute, Bethesda, Maryland.

443

virus is now recognized as the etiologic agent of this disease
and is referred to by different research groups as human T cell
lymphotropic virus type III (HTLV-III) (4), lymphadenopathy-
associated virus (LAV) (5) or AIDS-related retrovirus (ARV) (6).
Although epidemiologic observations suggest that sexual transmission of HTLV-III is the primary mode of transmission of AIDS to
homosexuals and bisexuals, an increase in the number of cases
classified as transfusion-associated AIDS has been reported
(7-10). Thus, persons who receive blood transfusions or blood
components are increasingly at risk for developing AIDS.

Overall, it is apparent that AIDS is an escalating disease of
devastating proportions. An animal model for this disease would
have several major benefits, including: 1) safety and efficacy
testing of potential HTLV-III vaccines, 2) testing potential
methods of HTLV-III inactivation in contaminated blood products
and reagents, 3) elucidation of the role of the immune system in
protecting individuals against AIDS and 4) elucidation of the
mechanisms whereby HTLV-III infection is transformed into
clinical disease.

Our laboratories have recently transmitted AIDS to chimpanzees with plasma from human AIDS patients (11). In addition,
chimpanzees have also been experimentally infected with HTLV-III
and LAV (12,13). In our investigations involving the transmission
of transfusion-associated AIDS, two of three chimpanzees given
plasma from patients with AIDS or pre-AIDS demonstrated serum
antibodies to HTLV-III 10 to 12 weeks after inoculation. These
antibodies continue to persist 2 years following the initial
infection. One of these two animals also developed lymphadenopathy that persisted for 32 weeks. During this 32 week
period of active lymphadenopathy, his total number of T cells
(OKT3 or T3) and T helper cells (OKT4 or T4) as well as the ratio
of T4/T8 lymphocytes were depressed. No opportunistic infection
was noted during or after this immune depression. This study

demonstrated the risk involved in the use of cell plasma and
blood products in the transmission of transfusion-associated
AIDS, and demonstrated the susceptibility of the chimpanzee to
HTLV-III infection and the ability to simulate the human lymphadenopathy syndrome in this animal species.

MATERIALS AND METHODS

Inoculation of Animals

Three chimpanzees (X114, X132, X133) were inoculated with
plasma (3 ml/kg or 150 ml) from each of three patients with AIDS
or with the AIDS-related complex (ARC). A fourth animal served
as control, receiving plasma from normal human donors. Prior to
inoculation, all animals were seronegative for anti-HTLV-III
antibodies, had normal T3 and T4 levels and T4/T8 ratios and
were clinically normal.

As summarized in Table I chimpanzees X114 and X132 were each
inoculated three times with 150 ml individual aliquots of plasma
obtained from different patients with ARC or AIDS. The anti-HTLV-
III antibody titer of each inoculum is also given in Table I.
Chimpanzee X133 was used in a two-phase experiment. First,
repeated inoculations of cryoprecipitate were administered to
determine if the immunologic abnormalities frequently observed in
hemophiliacs could be induced in this manner in an animal model
and to determine if multiple exposures to foreign antigens might
enhance susceptibility to AIDS. The intermittent administration
of 39 units of cryoprecipitate did not result in the development
of anti-HTLV-III antibodies or immune abnormalities. At weeks 26,
31 and 32, this animal received a total of 150 ml of lymphocyte-
rich plasma from each of three human AIDS or ARC donors. Donor 1
was an ARC patient with lymphadenopathy whose plasma was also
administered to chimpanzee X114.

TABLE I. Description of Human Plasma Sources Used for Chimpanzee Inoculation

Chimpanzee number	Time of inoculation	Volume (3 ml/kg)	Donor plasma description	Anti-HTLV-III antibody titer
X132	Day 1	150 ml	ARC	>1:1,000,000
	2	150 ml	Kaposi's sarcoma	1:770,000
	3	150 ml	Opportunistic infection	1:73,000
X114	Day 1	150 ml	ARC	1:215,000
	2	150 ml	Kaposi's sarcoma	1:48,000
	3	150 ml	Opportunistic infection	1:930,000
X133	Weeks 1–24	39 units	Cryoprecipitate in 11 sequential injections	
	Week 26 (1)[a]	150 ml	Lymphocyte-rich ARC	1:215,000
	31 (7)	150 ml	Lymphocyte-rich Kaposi's sarcoma	1:24,000
	32 (8)	150 ml	Lymphocyte-rich opportunistic infection	>1:1,000,000
X140	Day 1	50 ml	Normal plasma	Negative
	2	50 ml	Normal plasma	Negative
	3	50 ml	Normal plasma	Negative

[a]Parentheses indicate weeks after inoculation shown in Figure 1.

Chimpanzee X140 served as control, receiving 50 ml of plasma on three consecutive days from each of three normal (150 ml total volume) anti-HTLV-III antibody-negative donors.

Antibody Determination

Antibodies to HTLV-III were determined in a solid-phase enzyme-linked immunosorbent assay (ELISA) with the H9 HTLV-III clone as described in detail (11,14). Assays were performed in duplicate, and the end point titers of positive samples were determined using two-fold dilutions. Selected samples were tested for the presence of IgM antibodies to HTLV-III with the substitution of a μ-chain specific antihuman IgM reagent. Antibodies to cytomegalovirus and Epstein-Barr virus were performed as previously described (11).

Lymphocyte Subpopulation Assay

Ficoll-Hypaque banded peripheral blood mononuclear cells were pelleted and treated with 2 ml of Tris-ammonium chloride for 2 minutes at room temperature to lyse residual erythrocytes. The cells were repelleted and suspended in 2 ml of RPMI-FCS. The cells were washed once with phosphate-buffered saline (PBS) and sodium azide (PBS-NaN$_3$) and 10^7 cells were evenly distributed into each of five 12 × 75 mm tubes. The cells were centrifuged and the pellets resuspended with 0.1 ml of the appropriately diluted fluorescein isothiocyanate (FITC) conjugated antibody. B lymphocyte (sIg marker) enumeration was done by a direct fluorescence procedure using an FITC goat antihuman immunoglobulin (Meloy, Springfield, Virginia). Cells were incubated in the dark for 30 minutes on ice and washed three times with PBS-NaN$_3$ prior to mounting on glass microscope slides. T lymphocyte subpopulation enumeration was a two-step antibody staining procedure utilizing OKT3, OKT4 or OKT8 (Ortho Diagnostics, Raritan, New Jersey) reagents as the primary antibody and an FITC conjugate

of an IgG fraction of sheep antimouse IgG fraction (Cappel Laboratories, West Chester, Pennsylvania) in the second step. Both
incubations were performed in the dark for 30 minutes on ice. The
cells were subsequently washed three times with PBS-NaN$_3$ prior to
being mounted under coverslips. The slides were refrigerated in
the dark until fluorescent microscopic examination was performed.
The 40X fluorite objective of a Nikon fluorescent microscope was
used to score 100 to 200 cells for fluorescence. Control fluorescence (cells incubated with PBS-NaN$_3$ in the first step and FITC-
conjugated sheep antimouse IgG in the second step) was routinely
less than 3%. Data are expressed as the percentage of lymphocytes
positive for fluorescence minus percentage of lymphocytes nonspecifically stained with the second staining antiglobulin
reagent.

Statistical Methods

The normal percentages for T3, T4, T8 and surface immunoglobulin (sIg) levels along with the ratio of T4/T8 were determined from 17 chimpanzees in our colony that had not undergone
AIDS experimentation. No anti-HTLV-III activity was found in
these sera and the percentage of each cell surface marker along
with the standard deviation (SD) was determined. Significantly
depressed levels of the individual cell surface markers were considered to be values greater than 2 SD below the mean. Because
2 SD in the T4/T8 ratio approaches the mean, a nonparametric
statistical test was used to determine significant differences.
A single-factor analysis of variance by ranks (Kruskal-Wallis
test) was performed (15). Significant levels of depression were
determined when p was <0.05.

RESULTS

All four chimpanzees were seronegative for antibodies to
HTLV-III, had normal percentages of T cell subpopulations and
normal mitogen responses prior to inoculation. The antibody
response observed in these animals is depicted in Figure 1. The
early appearance of anti-HTLV-III IgG antibodies in chimpanzee
X132 was followed by a continuous decline to baseline values by
week 28 post inoculation. An IgM antibody response was not
observed in this animal. This immune response pattern was consistent with passive transfer of antibodies to this animal from
the inoculum. No disease was observed in chimpanzee X132.

The humoral immune patterns of chimpanzee X114 (Fig. 1) also
was consistent with a passive transfer of IgG antibodies present
in the donor's plasma. However, development of anti-HTLV-III IgM
antibodies was noted during week 12. This was followed by an
anti-HTLV-III of the IgG class by week 18. The IgG activity
plateaued by week 36 and has remained at this level for at least
2 years post inoculation. The specificity of this antibody for
HTLV-III was confirmed by Western blot and by blocking the ELISA
reactivity with an HTLV-III-specific sheep antiserum (11,16).

Bilateral inguinal lymphadenopathy and a lesser degree of
cervical adenopathy was observed in chimpanzee X114, 24 weeks
after inoculation (14 weeks after active antibody development).
The size of the lymph nodes progressed to 6 × 4 cm which persisted for 22 weeks before gradually diminishing. The total duration of the lymphadenopathy was 32 weeks. An inguinal lymph node
biopsy, performed at week 33 post inoculation, showed severe
lymphoid hyperplasia as characteristically seen in human ARC (1).

A control lymph node biopsy was done prior to inoculation
on each chimpanzee revealing normal histology. Special stains,
including giemsa, periodic acid-Schiff, methenamine silver and
Fite, were performed to study sections for the presence of

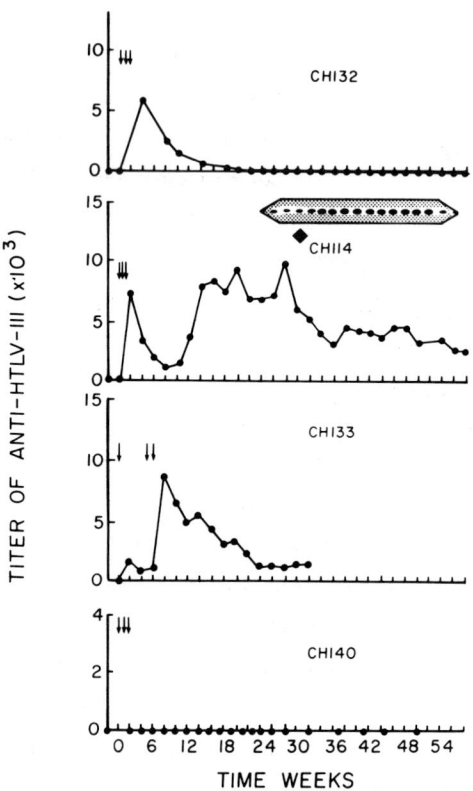

Fig. 1. Clinical and serologic results in chimpanzees X132, X114, X133 and control animal X140. Antibody to HTLV-III was measured in an ELISA and is expressed as the reciprocal titer. Lymphadenopathy is indicated by shaded bar and a significant (<0.05) decrease in T4/T8 ratios (♦) as determined by the Kruskal-Wallis test (15). The arrows indicate time of inoculation with plasma sources described in Table I.

mycobacteria, fungi, Pneumocystis carinii or other micro-organisms. No microorganisms, typically found in opportunistic infections, were found in these specially stained sections. Also no antibody seroconversion for cytomegalovirus or Epstein-Barr virus were demonstrated.

The third chimpanzee (X133) underwent the two-phase experiment described above (Table I). The intermittent administration
of 39 units of single-donor cryoprecipitate did not result in the
development of antibodies to HTLV-III. In the second phase of
this experiment, animal X133 was inoculated with 150 ml aliquots
of lymphocyte-enriched plasma obtained from three human donors.
An anti-HTLV-III response similar to that observed in chimpanzee
X114 developed. This animal developed an active HTLV-III antibody
response on the basis of: 1) the initial appearance of IgM antibodies to HTLV-III at week 4, which persisted through week 16,
and 2) the plateau of IgG antibody activity beginning at week 26
which has persisted 1½ years post infection.

The control animal, chimpanzee X140, did not develop any
specific anti-HTLV-III antibody response (Fig. 1). Fifteen
uninoculated chimpanzees from the Southwest Foundation for Biomedical Research (SFBR) colony were analyzed as background controls. All were found to be negative for antibody to HTLV-III.
In a previous survey of T and B cell subsets of normal chimpanzees at SFBR (17), we established the mean and SD for T3, T4, T8
and sIg markers as 68.9 ± 6.4%, 43.5 ± 7.5%, 47.0 ± 5.8% and
10.1 ± 2.1%, respectively. The mean and SD for the T4/T8 ratio
was 0.96 ± 0.27. It is important to note that chimpanzees have
about the same percentages of T3 and T4 cells as seen in man, but
have higher percentages of T8 cells, resulting in a calculated
ratio of T4/T8 for normal animals of approximately 1.0.

The relative percentage of lymphocytes positive for each of
the above markers (T3, T4, T8 and sIg) were determined at 2 week
intervals for the four animals in this study. The time periods
for each animal at which these values deviated from the mean by
more than 2 SD is summarized in Table II.

Total T lymphocyte numbers are predicted by the reactivity
with reagent OKT3. In chimpanzee 114, the relative number of T
cells was decreased at four time points during the study period

TABLE II. Summary of Lymphocyte sIg Status in Chimpanzees
Inoculated with Plasma Obtained from Individuals
with AIDS or Pre-AIDS or from Normal Donors

| Chimpanzee number | sIg | Time periods (weeks) with significant changes (>2 SD) | | |
| | | Cell surface markers | | |
		T3	T4	T8
X114	--[a]	2, 6, 24, 52	24, 30, 32, 34	--
X132	--	--	--	--
X133	--	--	--	--
X140	--	--	2	--

[a]No significant changes were noted.

of 64 weeks: first at weeks 2 and 6, and then again at weeks 24
and 52. Whether the active infection resulted in a loss of T cell
numbers or rather reflects a laboratory artifact in this animal
remains to be determined. However, the values did not correlate
with other markers such as anti-HTLV-III responses or the development of lymphadenopathy.

In this regard the time periods at which significant
decreases of the T4 population were noted is interesting. These
included two periods: one at week 24 and a second which lasted
from week 30 to 34. The first significant loss of T4 helper
lymphocytes correlated with the descending portion of the first
active antibody response and preceded development of the first
signs of lymphadenopathy. The second decrease (weeks 30 to 34)
again followed a peak of antibody activity and correlated with
the development of massive lymphadenopathy (Fig. 1). It is of
note that a significant decrease of the T4/T8 ratio was also
noted at weeks 30 to 32 (Fig. 1).

DISCUSSION

Since our first report on the transmission of HTLV-III infection with human plasma to chimpanzees (11), several other laboratories have successfully infected chimpanzees with purified HTLV-III, LAV or ARV (12,13,18). It is clear that the chimpanzee is easily infected with the agent of AIDS. Our study is unique in that it demonstrates HTLV-III infection can be transmitted by cell-poor blood products. In addition, to our knowledge, chimpanzee X114 is the only animal that demonstrated significant lymphadenopathy with immunologic abnormalities. It is noteworthy that the lymphadenopathy in this chimpanzee was transient, yet anti-HTLV-III titers remained constant for a period of 60 weeks post inoculation. In this regard, Laurence et al. (19) reported on a single ARC patient with generalized lymphadenopathy who remained seropositive against LAV despite gradual resolution of the lymphadenopathy and related disease symptoms.

Because the actual time of exposure to HTLV-III is generally not known, longitudinal T cell subset studies in human AIDS patients usually have been started only after the appearance of clinical symptoms (e.g., weight loss, fever, lymphadenopathy, Kaposi's sarcoma and opportunistic infections). The ability to infect the chimpanzees with HTLV-III should allow for a more precise delineation of the temporal relationship between T cell abnormalities and the onset of HTLV-III infection and disease. HTLV-III has a tropism for helper T cells (T4), and destruction of this cell population results in the immune abnormalities seen in AIDS--namely, decreased T4 cells, a low T helper/T suppressor ratio (T4/T8) and low proliferative responses to mitogens and antigens. However, other virus infections and diseases (e.g., hepatitis and cytomegalovirus) may cause low T4/T8 ratios, at least temporarily (20,21). Therefore, T cell enumeration serves only as corroborative evidence of AIDS.

Chimpanzee X114 developed clinical disease simulating the human lymphadenopathy syndrome as evidenced by: 1) massive lymphadenopathy with severe lymphoid hyperplasia on biopsy, 2) depression of T3 and T4 cells and a concomitant decrease in the T4/T8 ratio and 3) a temporal relationship between the onset of disease and the most severe T cell abnormalities. At the peak of lymphadenopathy the relative numbers of T4 cells decreased significantly for a period of 6 weeks. These data are not presented herein, but the abnormalities in T cells were associated with marked impairment of responses to the mitogens phytohemagglutinin, pokeweed and concanavalin A, and occasional reduction of natural killer cell activity (11).

As seen in human AIDS, T cells subset enumeration in our experimently infected animals correlated with infection and disease status. The temporal sequence of the development of anti-HTLV-III activity and the concomitant decrease of the T4 lymphocyte numbers suggest an interesting correlation. Peaks of antibody activity were noted at week 20 and again at week 30 (Fig. 1). On the other hand a significant decreased level of T4 cells were noted at weeks 24 and 30 to 34 (Table II). Active viral replication may well stimulate antibody production which then could result in the destruction of the infected target cell, e.g., T4 lymphocytes.

These results show that the chimpanzee is susceptible to HTLV-III infection and disease and that the ranges of immunologic abnormalities seen in these animals resemble, to a degree, those seen in various stags of pre-AIDS in humans. The data also imply that some AIDS patients positive for antibodies to HTLV-III are not infectious or that susceptibility to AIDS may be determined by other host or environmental factors. The spontaneous recovery in chimpanzee 114 also suggests that AIDS may not be a relentlessly progressive disease. Most important, this animal model will allow for evaluation of interventive measures, particularly

inactivation methods for blood products, antiviral therapy and
vaccine efficacy.

ACKNOWLEDGMENT

Our appreciation to Dr. Abe Macher of the National Cancer
Institute for performing special histopathologic studies on the
lymph node biopsy.

REFERENCES

1. Update: Acquired immunodeficiency syndrome (AIDS)--United
   States. (1984). MMWR 32, 688.
2. Gottlieb, M.S., Schroff, R., Schanker, H.M. et al. (1981).
   N. Engl. J. Med. 305, 1425.
3. Lane, H.C., Masur, H., Edgar, L.C. et al. (1983). N. Engl.
   J. Med. 309, 453.
4. Popovic, M., Sarngadharan, M.G., Read, E. et al. (1984).
   Science 224, 497.
5. Barré-Sinoussi, F., Chermann, J.C., Rey, F. et al. (1983).
   Science 220, 868.
6. Levy, J.A., Hoffman, A.D., Kramer, S.M. et al. (1984).
   Science 225, 840.
7. Ammann, A.J., Wara, D.W., Dritz, S. et al. (1983). Lancet 1,
   956.
8. Feorino, P.M., Kalyanaraman, V.S., Haverkos, H.W. et al.
   (1984). Science, 225, 69.
9. Jaffe, H.W., Francis, D.P., McLane, M.F. et al. (1984).
   Science 223, 1309.
10. Curran, J.W., Lawrence, D.N., Jaffe, H. et al. (1984).
    N. Engl. J. Med. 310, 69.
11. Alter, H.J., Eichberg, J.W., Masur, H. et al. (1984). Science
    226, 549.
12. Francis, D.P., Feorino, P.M., Broderson, J.R. et al. (1984).
    Lancet 2, 1276.
13. Gajdusek, D.C., Amyx, H.L., Gibbs, C.J., Jr. et al. (1985).
    Lancet 1, 55.
14. Saxinger, C. and Gallo, R.C. (1983). Lab. Invest. 49, 371.
15. Zar, J.H. (1974). "Biostatistical Analysis." Prentice-Hall,
    Englewood Cliffs, New Jersey.
16. Towbin, H., Staehelin, T. and Gordon, J. (1979). Proc. Natl.
    Acad. Sci. 76, 4350.
17. Eichberg, J.W., Lawlor, D.A. and Alter, H.J. (1984). Fed.
    Proc. 43, 1914.

18. Eichberg, J.W., Alter, H.J., Levy, J.A. (1985). In "Proceed-
    ings of the International Conference on Acquired Immuno-
    deficiency Syndrome (AIDS)." Atlanta, Georgia, in press.
19. Laurence, J., Brun-Vezinet, F., Schutzer, S.E. et al. (1984).
    N. Engl. J. Med. 311, 1269.
20. Lemm, G., Salzer, K. and Warnatz, H. (1983). Clin. Exp.
    Immunol. 52, 250.
21. Mildvan, D., Mathur, U., Enlow, R.W. et al. (1982). Ann.
    Intern. Med. 96, 700.

ANIMAL MODELS OF HUMAN DISEASE
INDUCTION OF PERSISTENT HUMAN T LYMPHOTROPIC RETROVIRUS INFECTIONS IN NONHUMAN PRIMATES AND EQUINES INOCULATED WITH TISSUES FROM AIDS PATIENTS OR PURIFIED VIRUS GROWN IN VITRO

Clarence J. Gibbs, Jr.
D. Carleton Gajdusek
Leon G. Epstein
David M. Asher
Jaap Goudsmit

Laboratory of Central Nervous System Studies
Intramural Research Program
National Institute of Neurological
and Communicative Disorders and Stroke
National Institutes of Health
Bethesda, Maryland

Acquired immune deficiency syndrome (AIDS) is a slow infection caused by a human T lymphocyte retrovirus (HTLV-III/LAV). In the main adults at risk are homosexual males, intravenous drug abusers and heterosexual contacts of HTLV-III/LAV seropositive individuals. The majority of juvenile cases of AIDS have occurred in children born to mothers that are intravenous drug abusers that have AIDS, AIDS-related complex or the asymptomatic HTLV-III/LAV seropositive carriers of the virus. A number of AIDS cases have occurred in patients of all age groups that are hemophiliacs or who have been the recipients of blood transfusions with HTLV-III/LAV contaminated blood.

Characteristic signs of clinical AIDS include lymphadenopathy, weight loss, severe diarrhea, muscle weakness, neoplasms and a number of varied opportunistic infections which have

in the past complicated the identification of the etiological
agent of the disease. Most importantly has been the recognition
that greater than 40% of all adults and children with AIDS
develop an associated undifferentiated global progressive
encephalopathy. In newborns and young children with clinical AIDS
this newly recognized neurological disease is characterized by a
marked loss of developmental milestones, impaired growth, weakness and the development of pyramidal tract signs, ataxia and
seizures. In adults the disease is characterized by cerebral
atrophy, progressive dementia and the frequent development of
paresis, spasticity and seizures. Histopathological examination
of brain tissue taken at autopsy revealed microglial nodules,
macrophage infiltration and multinucleated giant cells which on
electron microscopic examination were shown to contain virus
particles morphologically indistinguishable from HTLV-III/LAV
virus. The presence of HTLV-III virus in brain tissue of patients
with AIDS encephalopathy was further confirmed by in situ
hybridization using an HTLV-III probe and by transmission of the
virus to chimpanzees given a single injection of human brain
homogenate. Since the finding of HTLV-III/LAV virus in the brains
of AIDS encephalopathy has profound implications on the development of putative chemotherapy and vaccines, the need to establish
a suitable animal model for studying the pathogenesis of AIDS and
its associated encephalopathy is obvious.

In an attempt to develop a suitable animal model a total of
36 chimpanzees and 57 Old World and New World monkeys of nine
different species (M. mulatta, M. arctoides, M. radiata,
M. fascicularis, C. sabacus, E. patas, C. albrifrons, S. sciureus
and A. geoffroyi) and six horses have been inoculated with HTLV-
III/LAV/IDAV-2-infected cell cultures or with tissues from
patients that have been diagnosed as having AIDS. To date only
chimpanzees have been found to be uniformly susceptible to infection with the virus.

Eleven chimpanzees were inoculated on primary passage with HTLV-III/LAV/IDAV-2-infected cell cultures. Each of the 11 chimpanzees developed specific antibodies to the virus, regardless of the strain used. Strains of HTLV-III virus were reisolated from the leukocytes of seven of the 11 chimpanzees when cocultivated with H9 cells. Second and third serial passages of the virus utilizing heparinized whole blood or tissues from seropositive chimpanzees were successful in five of five and four of five chimpanzees, respectively.

Multiple isolations of HTLV-III virus were obtained from eight chimpanzees over a period of 90 to 180 days following their inoculation. Serial passage of the virus was successfully accomplished from three chimpanzees using whole blood collected 60 to 90 days after inoculation indicating persistent infection and prolonged viremia in the presence of high titers of specific antibody much like that which occurs in sheep infected with visna virus.

Fifteen of the 36 chimpanzees were inoculated with homogenates of tissues from AIDS patients including brain, lymph nodes, spleen, other viscera and plasma. Seven of these 15 chimpanzees became persistently infected and developed antibodies to HTLV-III/LAV virus. Of particular importance has been the isolation of the virus from packed leukocytes of two chimpanzees inoculated intracerebrally and intravenously with brain homogenates from two AIDS patients, respectively. Virus was first recovered on days 7 and 14 after inoculation and the animals remained persistently infected over the next several months of observation.

Six chimpanzees inoculated on primary passage with HTLV-III virus infected cell culture material developed specific antibodies and a persistent viremia as early as 8 days following inoculation which has persisted for more than 1 year. Serial passage has been easily accomplished by intravenous inoculation of whole blood from chimpanzees as soon as antibodies were

detected in their blood. Moreover, the long-term persistent
viremia permits isolation and serial passage of the virus for
well over 1 year from the time of inoculation of the donor animal. Our experience to date indicates that viremic animals probably remain infected for several years without developing overt
signs of clinical disease supporting the observation that humans
can be asymptomatic carriers of the virus.

Immunoglobulin-G (IgG) response to HTLV-III/LAV virus was
determined on serial serum specimens collected over several
months from chimpanzees inoculated with purified virus and tissues from patients dying with AIDS using an enzyme-linked immunosorbent assay (ELISA). In chimpanzees inoculated with virus grown
in vitro a fairly constant pattern of antibody development was
noted, i.e., there was an initial rise in titer which occurred
over a period of 4 to 6 weeks following inoculation and titers
continued to rise until all gag and env gene products were recognized. In contrast, chimpanzees inoculated with tissues from AIDS
patients initially developed a transient peak antibody titer
10 to 12 weeks after inoculation, which lysed to lower levels
over the next 8 to 10 weeks. This was followed by a second
gradual sustained rise, which has been maintained with fluctuating titers for more than 1.5 years. Overall the titers in animals
inoculated with human tissues were lower (1:75-1:150) than those
in chimpanzees inoculated with virus grown in vitro (1:500-
1:1000). This suggested to us that antibody titers were a function of the quantity of viable virus in the inoculum.

All animals have been under clinical observation for more
than 2 years. None of the seropositive chimpanzees has developed
significant weight loss, lymphadenopathy, tumors, severe opportunistic infections, subacute encephalopathy or sustained immunodeficiency. One infant chimpanzee died 5 months after inoculation
with LAV following an illness characterized by 6 days of bouts of
bloody diarrhea with Strongyloides stercoralis and Balantidium

coli in the feces. This was followed by clinical acute encephalitis with high lymphocytosis. Extensive neuropathological
studies failed to elicit any unusual findings. It is of interest
to note that this animal's lymphocytes were positive for HTLV-III
virus and whole blood from this animal induced HTLV-III infection
in a previously uninfected chimpanzee.

Although a sustained immune deficiency syndrome has not been
observed in any of the chimpanzees, a transient depression of in
vitro lymphocyte function was noted in two animals, and a transient lymphocytosis in five of the animals.

It is of significance to note that we have not detected antibodies to HTLV-III/LAV virus in the sera from any of the more
than 50 nonhuman primates of nine different species inoculated
with the same inoculum that went into the chimpanzees. We have,
however, successfully isolated HTLV-III virus from the leukocytes
of three seronegative rhesus monkeys on repeated occasions. Further, two seronegative squirrel monkeys and one seronegative
patas monkey inoculated with HTLV-III have died unexpectedly
without signs of immune deficiency or opportunistic infection.
The squirrel monkeys on necropsy were observed to have significantly enlarged mesenteric lymph nodes and attempts to isolate
virus in vivo and in vitro are underway.

In summary, we have successfully infected chimpanzees with
HTLV-III/LAV virus, the etiological retrovirus of AIDS, by the
inoculation of tissues of patients dying with the disease or with
purified virus grown in vitro. Animals appear to remain persistently infected for more than 2 years and possibly for life. It
is clear that the virus also serves as the primary cause of a
newly recognized neurological disease--AIDS encephalopathy. This
finding has profound influence on the development of chemotherapeutic and immunophylactic regimens for use in humans. The identification of asymptomatic seropositive animals that are persistently viremic suggests that similar carrier states exist in the

human population and the detection of viremia in asymptomatic
seronegative rhesus monkeys further strengthens this observation.

Since it is clear that AIDS is a virus-induced slow infection, continued surveillance of all inoculated animals for 3 to
5 years will be necessary to determine if clinical disease with
immune deficiency will become manifest.

In an effort to broaden the experimental host range for HTLV-
III/LAV retrovirus we have taken advantage of the obvious similarities of the viruses to the virus of visna and the virus of
equine infectious anemia (EIA) which induce persistent viremias
in the presence of high levels of antibodies in sheep and horses,
respectively. We have recently inoculated six EIA-negative horses
with purified HTLV-III virus and homogenates of tissues taken at
autopsy from patients that have died with confirmed cases of
AIDS. Four of the six horses have developed specific antibodies
to HTLV-III virus and have remained negative for antibodies to
EIA. Tests for detection of viremia are underway. The animals
have remained asymptomatic during the 8 months they have been
under observation.

SELECTED REFERENCES

1. Gajdusek, D.C., Amyx, H.L. and Gibbs, C.J., Jr. (1984).
   Lancet 1, 1415.
2. Gajdusek, D.C., Gibbs, C.J., Jr., Amyx, H.L. et al. (1985).
   Lancet 1, 55.
3. McClure, H., Swenson, B., King, F. et al. (1984). MMWR 33,
   442.
4. Alter, H.J., Eichberg, J.W., Masur, H. et al. (1984). Science
   226, 549.

Index